ORDER FORM

FOOD-MEDICATION INTERACTIONS SEVENTEETH EDITION

NAME:_____

INSTITUTION:_____

ADDRESS:_____

CITY: _____ STATE:____ email:____

ZIP:_____

PHONE: (   )_____ QUANTITY: FMI____ @____ _____

PLEASE NOTIFY ME OF NEW EDITIONS - CHECK HERE ☐

D1800824

Food-Medication Interactions 17th EDITION

PRICES:

1-4 @ $33.95 EACH
5-10 @ $32.95 EACH
11+ @ $32.50 EACH

SHIPPING & HANDLING:
$9.00 FOR THE FIRST BOOK
$2.00 EACH ADDITIONAL BOOK - UP TO SIXTEEN
$41.00 FOR ORDERS OF 17+ BOOKS
CANADA- ADD $5.OO PER BOOK

☐ AMEX ☐ MasterCcard ☐ VISA ☐ Discover

CREDIT CARD NUMBER _____

EXPIRATION DATE_____

SIGNATURE_____

SHIPPING & HANDLING

PENNSYLVANIA RESIDENTS
ADD 6% SALES TAX $ _____

TOTAL ENCLOSED $ _____

PREPAYMENT REQUIRED.

CHECKS MUST BE IN US FUNDS DRAWN ON A US BANK.
ENCLOSE THIS ORDER FORM WITH YOUR CHECK, MONEY ORDER
OR CREDIT CARD INFORMATION TO:

FOOD-MEDICATION INTERACTIONS
PO BOX 204
BIRCHRUNVILLE, PA 19421-0204
PHONE: 800-746-2324 FAX 610-827-7669
email: foodmedint@aol.com website: foodmedinteractions.com

CREDIT CARD BILLING ADDRESS _____

CITY _____ , **STATE** _____ **ZIP** _____

SEE OTHER SIDE FOR SOFTWARE ORDER FORM

PDA (BLACKBERRY, iPhone, iPad or Windows Smartphone, Droid & WINDOWS SOFTWARE ORDER FORM

SEND SOFTWARE TO:

NAME: _____

INSTITUTION: _____

ADDRESS: _____

CITY: _____ STATE: _____ ZIP: _____

PHONE: ( ) _____ PC SOFTWARE: _____ @ _____ $ _____

BLACKBERRY ☐ iPhone ☐ PALM ☐ POCKET

PC ☐ ____ @ _____ $ _____

SHIPPING & HANDLING	$ _____
PENNSYLVANIA RESIDENTS ADD 6% SALES TAX	$ _____
TOTAL ENCLOSED	$ _____

PC SOFTWARE REQUIREMENTS: **PDA or SMARTPHONE**

REQUIREMENTS:

WINDOWS NT/2000/XP/VISTA
16 MB RAM   **1 MB FREE RAM**
33 MB FREE HARD DISK
PENTIUM CPU OR HIGHER
PRICE: **PRICE:**
$129.95 $89.95

NETWORK COMPATIBLE
CALL FOR MULTI-USER PRICING

SHIPPING AND HANDLING:
$11.00 PER PROGRAM
$25.00 PER PROGRAM ORDER-CANADA
INTERNATIONAL - EMAIL US

☐ AMEX   ☐ MasterCard   ☐ VISA   ☐ DISCOVER

CREDIT CARD NUMBER _____

EXP DATE _____

SIGNATURE_____

CREDIT CARD NUMBER _____

EXPIRATION DATE_____

PREPAYMENT REQUIRED.

CHECKS MUST BE IN US FUNDS DRAWN ON A US BANK.
ENCLOSE THIS ORDER FORM WITH YOUR CHECK, MONEY ORDER
OR CREDIT CARD INFORMATION TO:
FOOD-MEDICATION INTERACTIONS
PO BOX 204
BIRCHRUNVILLE, PA 19421-0204
PHONE: 800-746-2324 FAX 610-827-7669
email: foodmedint@aol.com website: foodmedinteractions.com

SEE OTHER SIDE FOR BOOK ORDER FORM

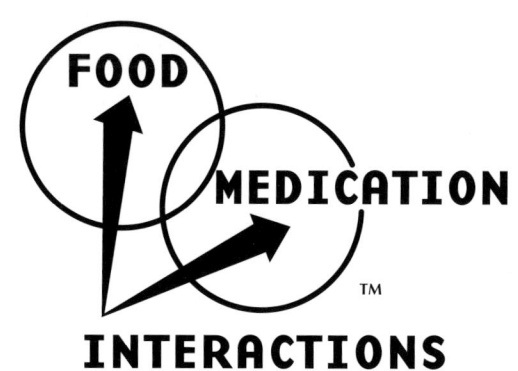

FOOD MEDICATION INTERACTIONS

17th Edition
by
ZANETA M. PRONSKY, MS, RD, LDN, FADA
&
SR JEANNE P. CROWE, PHARM D, RPH

2

Published and distributed by: FOOD-MEDICATION INTERACTIONS
                                PO Box 204
                                Birchrunville, PA 19421-0204 Phone: 800-746-2324

Library of Congress Control Number: 202932772
ISBN: 0-9710896-5-5 (978-0-9710896-5-5)   Printed in USA

First Edition, 1978   Third Edition, 1981   Fifth Edition, 1986
Second Edition, 1979   Fourth Edition, 1983   Sixth Edition, 1988
Authors: Dorothy Powers, RD & Ann O. Moore, MS, RD

Seventh Edition, 1991
Author: Ann Moore Allen, MS, RD

Eighth Edition Copyright © 1993   Eleventh Edition Copyright © 2000 Fourteenth Edition Copyright © 2006
Ninth Edition Copyright © 1995   Twelfth Edition Copyright © 2002   Fifteenth Edition Copyright © 2008
Tenth Edition Copyright © 1998   Thirteenth Edition Copyright © 2004
Author: Zaneta M. Pronsky, MS, RD, LDN, FADA

Sixteenth Edition Copyright © 2010
Seventeeth Edition Copyright © 2012 2nd Printing
Authors: Zaneta M. Pronsky, MS, RD, LDN, FADA & Sr Jeanne P. Crowe, PharmD, RPh

Contact the author/publishers for orders,
 information about **Computerized Food-Medication Interactions** software PC or PDA, reference information at:
FOOD MEDICATION INTERACTIONS
PO Box 204
Birchrunville, PA 19421-0204
or (610) 827-7800 or (800) 746-2324.
e-mail: foodmedint@aol.com, website: www.foodmedinteractions.com

AUTHORS: Zaneta M. Pronsky, MS, RD, LDN, FADA, Consultant Dietitian; Former Chief Research Dietitian, Clinical Research Center, Indiana University Medical Center, Indianapolis, IN

Sr. Jeanne P. Crowe, PharmD, RPh, Clinical pharmacist, pharmacist immunizer, author, lecturer. Pharmacist advisor for the Greater Philadelphia Area Celiac/Sprue Support Group, Former Director of Pharmacy, Camilla Hall Nursing home, Immaculata, PA

EDITORS:
Dean Elbe, BSc (Pharm), BCPP, PharmD, Clinical Pharmacist, Child & Adolescent Psychiatry, Children's & Women's Hospital of British Columbia, Vancouver, BC, Canada; Clinical Instructor UBC Faculty of Pharmaceutical Sciences, University of British Columbia, Vancouver, BC, Canada
and also the author of the Grapefruit Interaction Table.

Sol Epstein, MD, FRCP, FACP, Professor of Medicine and Geriatrics, Mt. Sinai School of Medicine, NYC, NY and Osteoporosis Specialist Abington Endocrine Associates, Willow Grove, PA

Laboratory Table Author: William Roberts, MD, PhD, Medical Dir Automated Core Laboratory, ARUP Laboratories; Professor of Pathology, University of Utah, Salt Lake City, UT

Tables Editor: Keith Ayoob, EdD, RD, FADA, Assoc. Professor, Dept Pediatrics, Albert Einstein College of Medicine, Bronx, NY

Advisors: Veronica S.L. Young, PharmD, MPH, Asst. Director, Drug Information Service, The University of Texas Health Science Center at San Antonio, San Antonio, TX; Clinical Assistant Professor, University of Texas, College of Pharmacy, Austin, TX

PREFACE

Any procedure or practice described in this book should be applied by the healthcare practitioner under appropriate supervision in accordance with professional standards of care used with regard to the unique circumstances that apply in each practice situation. Due to space limitations, it is impossible to include all contraindications, warnings or precautions, particularly those pertaining to pediatric or geriatric use. Pregnancy and lactation information are directly from manufacturer's information and should be confirmed with the physician before any drug is used or avoided by a pregnant or lactating woman. Care has been taken to confirm the accuracy of information presented and to describe generally accepted practices. However, the authors, editors and publishers cannot accept responsibility for errors or omissions or for any consequences from applications of the information in this book and make no warranty, expressed or implied, with respect to the contents of the book.

Every effort has been made to ensure that the information herein is in accordance with current recommendations and practices. Because of ongoing research, changes in government regulations and the constant flow of information on drug interactions, reactions and therapy, the reader is cautioned to check the package insert of each drug for indications, dosages, warnings and precautions, particularly if the drug is new or infrequently used.

Contact the author/publisher for orders or information about
Computerized **Food-Medication** **Interactions** software for **PC** or
PDA Software Program (Blackberry, iPhone, Droid or Windows Mobile Smartphones),
requests about specific references
or suggestions for improvements at:

> **Food-Medication Interactions**
> PO Box 204, Birchrunville, PA 19421-0204
> Phone (610) 827-7800 or (800) 746-2324.
> Fax: (610) 827-7669
> e-mail: foodmedint@aol.com
> Web Site: www.foodmedinteractions.com

TABLE OF CONTENTS

1. Guide to the Use of This Book .... Inside Front Cover
2. Micronutrient Food Sources .... Inside Back Cover
3. **Abbreviations and Symbols** **402**
4. Introduction 6
5. Mechanisms of Interactions 7
6. Guidelines for Counseling Medicated Patients 13
7. Medical Nutritional Therapy to Aid in the Relief of Medication Side Effects 15
8. FDA Pregnancy Categories 18
9. **Food-Medication Interactions** **19**
10. Tables: Laboratory Values 354
        Comparison of Height-Weight Tables 370
        Segmental Weights for Limbs, Calculation of Desirable Body Weight, BMI 371
        Nutritional Assessment Standards for Adults 372
        Potential Interactive Ingredients 374
        Drug-Alcohol (Ethanol) Interactions 376
        Caffeine Content of Foods and Beverages 379
        Potential Gluten Containing Ingredients of Medication 380
        High Oxalate Food Sources 381
        High Phytate Food Sources 382
        Pressor Agents 383
        Osmolalities of Selected Beverages and Foods 384
        pH and Acid Content of Beverages 385
        Magnesium (Mg) Sources 386
        Potassium (K) Sources, Vitamin K Sources 387
        Grapefruit-Drug Interactions 390
        Drugs Not Compatible with Tube Feeding 393
11. **References** **394**

INTRODUCTION TO <u>FOOD</u> <u>MEDICATION</u> <u>INTERACTIONS</u>

Medications can affect and be affected by food. Recognition of the interaction of drugs and nutrition plays a vital role in the expanding medical services available for patients. The Joint Commission on Accreditation of Health Care Organizations and other agencies are currently focusing more attention on this topic by mandating that health care professionals document and advise patients about food-medication interactions.

Patients must be assessed individually for the effect of food on medication action and the effect of medication on nutritional status. These two aspects of medication use can be complicated by: special diets, nutritional supplements, non-nutrients in food, excipients in medications, alcohol intake, tube feeding, underlying illness, polypharmacy, general physical condition and other factors.

Please note that food and medication interactions are only possibilities. Inclusion of an effect does <u>not</u> imply that this effect will occur in each patient. An effect is included if the reported incidence is $\geq 1\%$ more than that reported with a placebo. If the % incidence is available, the effect is <u>underlined</u> if the incidence is $\geq 5\%$. The effect is <u>CAPITALIZED</u> and <u>UNDERLINED</u> if the incidence is $\geq 20\%$.

Medications in the same pharmaceutical class generally exhibit similar effects. Therefore, master drug monographs have been created. **Differences among drugs within the same class are emphasized in the master monographs**. For example, **diazepam (Valium)** is referred to **Benzodiazepines; benazepril (Lotensin)** to **Angiotensin Converting Enzyme Inhibitors**; and **oxybutynin (Ditropan)** to **Bladder Control Agents**.

The following sections provide a review of various aspects of food-medication interactions to enable the health professional to optimize dietary and drug regimens. Included are "Guidelines for Counseling Medicated Patients" and "Medical Nutritional Therapy to Treat Medication Side Effects". Laboratory Values and reference tables are added to provide instant access to supplemental information which augments the text.

Before using the **<u>Food-Medication Interactions</u>** book, please review the following sections: the **<u>Guide to the Use of the Book,</u> inside the front cover**, and the <u>Table of Contents</u> (page 5). Drugs are listed alphabetically by generic and Trade names (capitalized). Every effort has been made to include the most commonly used medications with the most recent information available.

MECHANISMS OF FOOD MEDICATION INTERACTIONS

The study of the **absorption, distribution, metabolism** and **excretion** of drugs is referred to as **pharmacokinetics**.
The study of the **absorption, distribution, metabolism** and **excretion** of nutrients is **nutrient kinetics**.

Absorption: Process by which a drug/nutrient proceeds from the site of administration to the systemic circulation.
Distribution: Movement of the drug/nutrient from one location to another in the body.
Metabolism: Process by which the drug/nutrient is chemically changed by the action of enzymes most commonly in the intestinal tract and the liver. The metabolite may become more active, less active or as active as the parent compound.
Excretion: Process by which the drug/nutrient or metabolites are removed from the body, primarily by the kidneys.

EFFECT OF FOOD/NUTRIENTS ON MEDICATION KINETICS

Effect of Food/Nutients on Medication Absorption

The presence of food in the stomach may decrease the rate and/or extent of drug absorption. Examples:
- The absorption of the antiosteoporosis drug **alendronate** (**Fosamax**) is decreased 60% with coffee or juice.
  It is NOT absorbed at all when ingested with or up to 2 hours after a meal.
  It should be taken with plain water at least 30 minutes before first food or beverage of the day.
  Absorption is optimal if taken 2 hours before the first food or beverage of the day.
- A high fiber diet may decrease the absorption of tricyclic antidepressants such as **amitriptyline** (**Elavil**).
  The drug appears to be adsorbed by the fiber, preventing the drug from moving out of the intestinal tract.

Chelation between certain drugs and divalent/trivalent cations Ca, Mg, Al, Fe, Zn decreases drug absorption. Example:
- **Ciprofloxacin** (**Cipro**) forms an insoluble complex with Ca in some dairy products; Ca, Fe, Mg or Zn in supplements; or Ca, Al and/or Mg antacids, decreasing drug absorption.

The presence of food in the stomach may enhance the absorption of some drugs. Examples:
- The absorption of **cefuroxime axetil** (**Ceftin**) is significantly higher when given with food than in a fasting state. The prescence of food appears to enhance dissolution and absorption of the drug.
- A high fat meal results in an 82% greater C_{max} for **cinacalcet** (**Sensipar**) used for hyperparathyroidism in dialysis patients.

Effect of Food/Nutrients on Medication Distribution

Low serum albumin concentrations result in clinically significant decrease of drug binding sites. This may increase the free fraction of highly protein bound drugs. Examples:
- Hypoalbuminemia (< 3g/dL) provides fewer binding sites for highly protein bound drugs such as **phenytoin** (**Dilantin**)- 90% bound and **warfarin** (**Coumadin**)- 99% bound. A higher unbound or "free" fraction of drug is available as compared to an individual with normal serum albumin. Only the unbound drug can cause a pharmacologic effect, the higher unbound fraction will have a greater drug effect.
  For **warfarin** this can induce bleeding, while higher unbound **phenytoin** levels can cause CNS toxicity.

Effect of Food/Nutrients on Medication Metabolism

Food may alter the metabolism of some drugs. Examples:
- Concurrent ingestion of food and **propranolol** (**Inderal**) reduces first pass metabolism of the drug. This interaction results in higher serum drug levels.
- Grapefruit inhibits metabolism of some drugs such as **amiodarone** (**Cordarone**) by inhibiting activity of cytochrome P450 3A4 isoenzymes in the intestinal wall. Serum drug levels increase, may become toxic.
- The natural product **St John's wort**, used as an antidepressant, is believed to induce cytochrome P450 3A4. Blood levels of drugs metabolized by this enzyme will be lower if **St John's wort** is also taken on a routine basis, thus causing therapeutic failure. Affected drugs include the antiretroviral **indinavir** (**Crixivan**), oral contraceptives, and the immunosuppressants **cyclosporine** (**Neoral**) and **tacrolimus** (**Prograf**).

Effect of Food/Nutrients on Medication Excretion

Foods and nutrients may alter the renal excretion of some drugs and affect blood levels of some drugs. Example:
- **Lithium** (**Eskalith**) and sodium are reabsorbed at the same sites in the kidney. High sodium intake increases sodium excretion and thereby **lithium** excretion. Low sodium intake causes sodium retention and **lithium** retention.

Pharmacogenomics: Individual Differences In Drug Disposition

- **Pharmacogenomics** studies how an individual's genetic inheritance affects drug metabolism and the pharmacologic effect of the drug on the body. Pharmacogenomics seeks to determine genetic variations in individuals to increase drug efficacy and safety while decreasing drug toxicity.
- Rates of metabolism, drug-receptor sensitivity, and efficacy of drug transporters will determine in part how an individual responds to a specific drug as compared to other individuals.
- Genetic variation(s) in drug metabolizing enzymes will affect rates of metabolism and drug concentrations.
EXAMPLES:
  Fluoxetine (**Prozac**) is metabolized by CYP2D6. CYP2D6 poor metabolizers may have an exaggerated response to and adverse effects due to high levels of unmetabolized drug. Ultra-rapid CYP2D6 metabolizers may have poor

therapeutic response due to a low level of the drug.

Codeine is metabolized to **morphine** by CYP2D6 resulting in analgesia.
CYP2D6 ultra rapid metabolizers may have an exaggerated response to **codeine** with a greater incidence of adverse effects. CYP2D6 poor and ultra poor metabolizers may experience therapeutics failure.

Warfarin is metabolized by CYP2C9. CYP2C9 poor metabolizers and ultra-poor metabolizers may experience bleeding and other toxic effects from usual doses of warfarin.

Proton pump inhibitors such as **omeprazole (Prilosec)** are metabolized by CYP2C19.
Poor metabolizers have higher drug concentrations and increased ulcer healing rates.
CYP2C19 rapid metabolizers have decreased ulcer healing rates.

Phenytoin (Dilantin) is metabolized by CYP2C9. CYP2C9 poor and ultra-poor metabolizers will experience high drug concentrations and toxic effects from usual doses of **phenytoin**.

- Genetic variation(s) in drug-receptors may determine efficacy or toxicity of a drug. An individual may have an exaggerated response, an expected response or no response to a drug based on the genetic changes expressed in drug-receptor(s) of the individual.
  EXAMPLE: Genetic variations in Beta-2 receptors contribute to the response to Beta-2 agonists such as **albuterol (Proventil HFA)**.
- Genetic variation(s) in drug transporters may determine if the drug molecule reaches the intended target in the body in adequate concentrations.
  EXAMPLE: The drug-transporter P-glycoprotein contributes to drug excretion into urine, bile, and intestinal lumen. Genetic variation of P-glycoprotein is responsible for greater bioavailability of **digoxin (Lanoxin)**.

EFFECTS OF MEDICATIONS ON FOOD/NUTRIENT KINETICS
Effect of Medication on Nutrient Absorption

Drug complexes with nutrients preventing the absorption of drug, nutrient or both. Examples:
- Antibiotics **tetracycline** and **ciprofloxacin (Cipro)** chelate with divalent or trivalent cations, Ca, Mg, Fe, Zn.
- Antihyperlipidemic, bile acid sequestrant **cholestyramine (Questran)** adsorbs fat soluble vitamins A, D, E, K.

Drug alters gastric acidity. Examples:
- Prolonged use of antiulcer/antiGERD drugs such as a proton pump inhibitor eg: **pantoprazole (Protonix)** or a histamine H_2 receptor antagonist eg: **ranitidine (Zantac)** may decrease absorption of vitamin B_{12}, thiamin and Fe which are optimally absorbed in an acid environment

Drug damages mucosal surface.
- Medication induced gastro-intestinal mucosal damage by antineoplastic drugs may cause decreased nutrient absorption.

Effect of Medication on Nutrient Metabolism

Drug increases the metabolism of nutrients resulting in higher requirements and danger of deficiency. Example:
- Anticonvulsants **phenobarbital** and **phenytoin** (**Dilantin**) increase the rate of metabolism of folic acid, vitamins D and K. Long term use may thus lead to deficiencies and bone disorders such as osteoporosis.

Drug causes vitamin antagonism. Examples:
- Antituberculosis drug **isoniazid** (**INH**) inhibits the conversion of **pyridoxine** (**vitamin B$_6$**) to the active form. Unless a **pyridoxine** supplement is prescribed, pyridoxine deficiency and peripheral neuropathy may occur.

Effect of Medication on Nutrient Excretion

Drug increases the urinary loss of nutrients. Example:
- Loop diuretics, such as **furosemide** (**Lasix**), increase excretion of Na, K, Cl, Mg, Ca.

Drug decreases the urinary excretion of nutrients. Example:
- Thiazide diuretics increase excretion of most electrolytes, but enhance renal reabsorption of Ca causing decreased excretion of Ca.

MODIFICATION OF MEDICATION ACTION

Enhancement of Medication Action

Foods or additives have effects similar to those of a drug, enhancing the effects or toxicity of the drug. Examples:
- High caffeine intake may increase the adverse effects of **theophylline**, **methylphenidate** (**Ritalin**) ie nervousness, tremor, insomnia.
- Tyramine, dopamine or other vasoconstrictors (pressor agents) in food enhance the toxic effects of MAO inhibitors, such as **tranylcypromine** (**Parnate**). This effect may cause a hypertensive crisis, which can be fatal.

Antagonism of Medication Action

Nutrient or food component may oppose the desired action of the drug. Examples:
- Vitamin K aids the production of clotting factors in direct opposition to the action of **warfarin** (**Coumadin**).
- The immunosuppressant effects of drugs like **cyclosporine** (**Neoral**) and **azathioprine** (**Imuran**) may be blunted by the immunostimulatory properties of natural products such as echinacea and saw palmetto.
- Caffeine is a stimulant which counteracts the antianxiety effects of benzodiazepines.

Diet counteracts the effect of the drug. Examples:
- High fat diet counteracts the effect of antihyperlipidemic drugs such as **pravastatin** (**Pravachol**), **atorvastatin** (**Lipitor**), and **fenofibrate** (**Tricor**).

Authors: Zaneta M. Pronsky, RD, MS, LDN, FADA and Sr. Jeanne Patricia Crowe, PharmD, RPh

Gastrointestinal Effects

Drug may impair salivary flow causing dry mouth and increased caries, stomatitis, glossitis. Example:
- Tricyclic antidepressants such as **amitriptyline** (**Elavil**) cause dry mouth and sour or metallic taste.

Drug may be secreted into the saliva. Example:
- The antibiotic **clarithromycin** (**Biaxin**) enters the saliva causing a bitter taste.

Drug may suppress natural oral bacteria resulting in oral candidiasis. Examples:
- Antibiotics, such as **tetracycline**, **cephalexin** (**Keflex**) and other cephalosporins may result in oral yeast overgrowth i.e. candidiasis, especially with long term use.

Drug may cause dysgeusia (abnormal or impaired sense of taste). Examples:
- Antibiotic **metronidazole** (**Flagyl**) and the hypnotic/sleep aid **eszopicolone** (**Lunesta**) can cause an unpleasant metallic taste in the mouth.

Drug may damage rapidly proliferating cells. Example:
- The cytotoxic effects of antineoplastics such as **cisplatin** or **methotrexate** cause stomatitis, glossitis, gingivitis, ulcers of the oral mucosa and esophagitis.

Drug may cause dysphagia.
- Drug induced dry mouth/throat and/or mucositis lead to swallowing problems.

Drug may irritate the stomach mucosa causing distress, nausea, vomiting, bleeding, ulceration. Example:
- Nonsteroidal anti-inflammatory drugs (NSAID) such as **acetylsalicylic acid** (**aspirin**) or **ibuprofen** (**Advil**, **Motrin**) may cause stomach irritation, sometimes leading to sudden, serious gastric bleeding.

Drug may affect intestinal peristalsis. Example:
- Anticholinergic drugs (antipsychotics, antihistamines) slow peristalsis causing constipation.

Drug may destroy intestinal bacteria.
- Antibiotics such as **clindamycin** (**Cleocin**) may cause C. difficile overgrowth, leading to pseudomembranous colitis.

Appetite Changes

Drug may suppress appetite. Example:
- Stimulants, such as amphetamines (**Dexadrine**, **Adderall**) used to treat ADHD, suppress appetite and may delay children's growth.

Drug may increase appetite. Examples:
- Tricyclic antidepressants such as **amitriptyline** (**Elavil**), and most antipsychotic drugs, such as **olanzapine** (**Zyprexa**) or **clozapine** (**Clozaril**) stimulate appetite and weight gain.

Metabolic Effects

Drug may cause or exacerbate glucose intolerance and lead to or aggravate diabetes. Examples:
- Antipsychotic **olanzapine** (**Zyprexa**) or corticosteroids affect glucose regulation leading to new onset diabetes, insulin/glucose intolerance/type 2 diabetes (now a <u>class</u> <u>warning</u> for all second generation antipsychotics). Diabetes may occur independently of weight gain.

Drug may lead to lipid abnormalities such as elevated cholesterol and/or triglycerides. Examples:
- Antipsychotics **chlorpromazine** (**Thorazine**) and **olanzapine** (**Zyprexa**) may cause elevated lipids. Antipsychotic **risperidone** (**Risperdal**) may cause elevated triglycerides.

Renal/ Urinary Effects

Drug can cause urinary retention/hesitation.
- Antidepressant **duloxetine** (**Cymbalta**) label was recently updated due to 78 unique postmarketing cases of urinary retention/hesitancy. Twenty six of the 78 cases reported serious outcomes: catheterization and/or hospitalization.
- Bladder control agents such as **oxybutynin** (**Ditropan**) or **tolterodine** (**Detrol**) are designed to decrease urgency and frequency of urination, but can result in retention.
- Anticholinergic drugs (antipsychotics, antidepressants, antihistamines) can cause retention/hesitancy due to their anticholinergic effect.

Drug can cause increased frequency.
- Osteoporosis treatment **calcitonin** (**Miacalcin**) or antirejection drug **tacrolimus** (**Prograf**) can ↑ urinary frequency.

Drug can cause renal failure, often acute.
- Acute renal failure has been reported with all NSAIDS eg: **ibuprofen** (**Advil Motrin**)

<u>Authors:</u> Zaneta M. Pronsky, RD, MS, LDN, FADA and Sr. Jeanne Patricia Crowe, PharmD, RPh
   Edited by Keith-Thomas Ayoob, EdD, RD, FADA

GUIDELINES FOR COUNSELING MEDICATED PATIENTS

The following guidelines provide information about potential food-medication interactions.
Examples illustrate possible diet adjustments. Patient counseling for any medication should include:

1. Pertinent medication **information**: The **name of the drug, drug indications**, and **duration** of therapy.
   eg **Ciprofloxacin (Cipro)**, Antibiotic, 10 day therapy.

2. **When** and **how** to take the drug:
   eg Take the drug in the AM; PM; 6 hours before bedtime; on an empty stomach; 1 hour before or 2 hours after meals; or with food, meals or specific beverages.
   eg Food decreases absorption of bisphosphonate **alendronate (Fosamax)**.

   MNT: Take at least 30 minutes before any food or beverage except water.

3. Expected **side effects** and dietary suggestions to relieve symptoms of side effects:
   See next section, <u>Medical Nutrition Therapy</u>, pages 15-17.

4. **Nutritional problems** that may arise from medication use, especially if dietary intake is inadequate:
   eg Potassium-depleting diuretics, eg **furosemide (Lasix)** may cause hypokalemia, hypomagnesemia &/or hyponatremia.

   MNT: Increase intake of high potassium and high magnesium foods, see tables pages 387 & 386.
   Avoid low Na diet if hyponatremia occurs

5. **Dietary changes** that may alter **drug action** (particularly after drug has reached steady-state):
   eg Inconsistent intake of **vitamin K**-containing foods may affect the anticoagulant action of **warfarin (Coumadin)**.

   MNT: Maintain consistent intake of foods high in **vitamin K**, see table p 388.

6. **Foods and beverages to avoid or limit** while taking the drug:
   eg To prevent a hypertensive crisis, avoid foods high in tyramine or other pressor amines with an MAOI such as **phenelzine sulfate (Nardil)**.

   MNT: Provide information on specific foods to avoid or limit, see table p 383.

7. **Advice on alcohol ingestion:** Concurrent intake of some medications with beer, wine, other alcoholic beverages or alcohol used in cooking may modify the effects of both or may produce undesirable side effects.
   eg A **disulfiram**-like reaction results from concurrent alcohol and **metronidazole (Flagyl)** use.

   MNT: Provide patient with information on alcohol interactions and possible sources of alcohol, see table p 376.

8. Possible **interactions** between medications and **vitamin, mineral** and other **food supplements:**
   eg Concurrent administration of a calcium supplement or other divalent/trivalent cation and an antibiotic such as **tetracycline** or **ciprofloxacin** may impair the absorption of both the calcium and the antibiotic.
   MNT: Take antibiotic 2 hours before or 6 hours after ingestion of divalent/trivalent cations, eg: Ca, Mg or Fe.
   eg **St. John's wort** induces CYP3A4, lowering **cyclosporine (Neoral)**, **simvastatin (Zocor)** blood levels/effectiveness.
   MNT: Do not take **St. John's wort (SJW)** while taking affected drugs.
9. The importance of following a **special diet prescription** for treatment of a medical condition:
   eg Antihyperlipidemic drug, eg **atorvastatin (Lipitor)**, therapy is an adjunct to a low cholesterol, low fat diet.
   eg A prescribed diabetic diet is an adjunct to antidiabetic medication such as **insulin** or **metformin (Glucophage)**.
   Drug therapy is <u>not</u> a substitute for dietary regulation.
10. A **personal dietary prescription** pertains to that person only.
    Do not follow dietary suggestions prescribed for others:
    eg Dietary restrictions with potassium-depleting diuretics differ from those with potassium-sparing diuretics. Serious adverse effects occur if diet prescriptions are interchanged.
11. Before modifying a drug or diet prescription, the prescribing physician must be consulted.
12. For in-depth nutritional information, consult a **Registered Dietitian**.
13. For questions regarding drug action or possible side effects, consult a **Registered Pharmacist**.

Revised 2007: Zaneta M. Pronsky, MS, RD, LDN, FADA and Christine Hamilton Smith, PhD, RD.

MEDICAL NUTRITION THERAPY TO TREAT MEDICATION SIDE EFFECTS

Prior to implementing MNT, consult the physician or pharmacist for evaluation of a possible adverse drug effect. These suggestions are intended to reinforce rather than replace information provided by the health professional.

Loss of Appetite

1. Question patient regarding factors contributing to appetite loss, such as depression.
2. Educate the patient about the importance of an adequate, well-balanced diet.
3. Create a pleasant environment for eating. If possible, eliminate distractions and time pressure.
4. If early satiety occurs or meals are not well-tolerated, offer small, frequent, attractive meals or snacks.
5. Provide variety in color, texture, taste and temperature.
6. Enhance flavors by using seasonings. Marinate meats in sauces or fruit juices.
7. Encourage weakened patients to select foods that require minimal eating effort.
8. Use nutritional supplement products (liquid, pudding, bars, cereal, baked products) between meals.

Taste/Smell Dysfunction

1. If permissible, mask the taste of a drug with food, pulpy fruits (applesauce, crushed pineapple), fruit juices or milk. Water, lemon juice, water ice, sugarless gum or candy can be used as mouth rinses.
2. To enhance food flavors and aroma, use highly flavored foods, seasonings, sauces.
   Acidic foods/beverages may awaken ability to taste foods.

Dry or Sore Mouth (may lead to decreased salivation, tooth decay, gum disease, fungal infection)

1. Stress good oral hygiene. Do dental care cautiously to minimize mucosal damage. Severe or long-term problem causes ill-fitting dentures and changes in chewing ability and eating habits.
2. Decrease dry or salty foods/snacks. Moisten (dunk) dry foods in beverages or swallow with liquid.
3. Offer moist, bland, soft foods: mashed potatoes, custards, puddings, fruit whips or smoothies. Add milk-based sauces, gravies or syrups to food. Avoid spicy, rough textured or highly acidic foods.
4. Lick or suck ice chips. Incorporate cold foods or beverages into meals or snacks: sherbets, ice cream, ice milk, frozen yogurt, water ices, sorbets, popsicles. Add cold melons, applesauce or other cold fruit.
5. Suggest sugarless gum/candy. Warm water rinses or saliva substitutes may help.

Appetite Stimulation or Weight Gain

1. Assess weight gain as a possible reversal of depression-induced weight loss.
2. Educate the patient that certain drugs may increase appetite and the desire for sweets.
3. Encourage a slow rate of eating (at least 20 minutes to finish first portions of a meal).

4. Encourage low calorie foods, lettuce salads, fresh fruit and vegetables, diet beverages, low calorie snacks.
5. Incorporate high fiber foods or snacks which may contribute to early satiety.
6. Instruct patient or food provider to control access to specific high calorie foods, snacks or beverages.
7. Emphasize low fat/fat free condiments such as fat free salad dressing or Lite mayonnaise.
8. Encourage additional water in place of high calorie drinks to total at least 6-8 cups fluid per day.

Epigastric Distress (stomach discomfort, heartburn or indigestion)

1. Remain upright for 30 minutes after taking drug (particularly if drug causes GI irritation).
2. Limit or eliminate foods or beverages that may contribute to epigastric distress such as alcohol, liqueurs, caffeinated beverages, decaffeinated coffee, colas, onions, peppermint, chocolate, pepper, garlic, chili powder, acidic or spicy food. Use of soft or bland food may be helpful.
3. Offer small quantities of food at frequent intervals in a relaxed environment. Avoid overeating.
4. Avoid extremely hot or extremely cold foods or liquids (may stimulate acid secretion).
5. Avoid greasy, fried or fatty foods (may delay gastric emptying).
6. Evaluate the intake of milk or cream (may stimulate acid secretion).
7. Avoid eating for at least one hour before bedtime.
8. If patient is overweight, suggest a low-calorie diet and exercise program to promote weight loss.

Nausea/Vomiting (dehydration, weight loss, inadequate nutrient intake, electrolyte imbalance)

1. Honor food preferences. Disliked foods may aggravate nausea.
2. Offer small quantities of easily digestible foods at frequent intervals. Eat slowly.
3. Reduce food volume at meals. Serve liquids after meals and limit liquid intake with meals.
4. Suggest intake of toasted or dry enriched white bread, crackers or graham crackers, cooked or dry ready-to-eat cereals. To reduce nausea, eat one of these foods early in the morning or before rising.
5. Offer cold, clear or carbonated liquids (ginger ale) or non-acidic juices. Avoid lukewarm beverages.
6. Cold foods may be better tolerated than hot foods, and bland foods better than spicy foods.
7. Avoid any fried, greasy or fatty foods (may delay gastric emptying).
8. If nausea occurs at consistent times each day, reschedule meal and snack times.

Diarrhea

1. Focus on fluid and electrolyte replacement with products such as Gatorade or Pedialyte.
2. During the acute phase of diarrhea, solid food may be withheld for 24 hours or longer. Fluids may be limited to clear liquids.
3. Intake of frequent, small amounts of bland foods (crackers, plain toast) may be allowed as tolerated.
4. Initially restrict or avoid caffeine, alcohol, spicy foods, fatty foods, concentrated sweets, raw fruits or vegetables, fried foods, bran & whole grain cereals, nuts, beans, relishes.
5. Evaluate tolerance to dairy products. Return to normal diet gradually.

Gastrointestinal Gas (flatulence and/or belching)

1. Discourage swallowing large amounts of air such as eating fast, chewing gum, or talking while chewing.
2. Encourage patient to avoid flatulogenic foods such as beans, bran, cabbage, cauliflower, broccoli, onions, peppers, radishes, apples, celery, eggplant.
3. Encourage use of alpha-D-galactosidase enzyme (Beano) when consuming potentially flatulogenic foods.
4. Limit consumption of carbonated beverages.

Constipation

1. Avoid prolonged use or overuse of cathartics, laxatives or enemas which can cause laxative dependence.
2. Gradually increase fiber (vegetables, fruits, whole grain cereals) in the diet. May use bran in moderation.
3. Maintain adequate fluid intake, especially water.
4. Stress the importance of daily exercise, regular meals, defecation reflex recognition and regularity.

Glucose Intolerance/Diabetes

1. Carbohydrate controlled diet to balance starch/sugar intake with medication action.
2. Reduce fat to (< 30% of calories) and saturated fat (< 10% of calories). Increase fiber in the diet.
3. Educate about eating during special events, sick days, menu substitutions or hypoglycemia.
4. Emphasize adequate fluid intake and beverages appropriate for diabetic diet.
5. Use alcohol only with caution and under advice from physician.
6. If patient is overweight, suggest a low-calorie, high fiber diet for weight loss.
7. Stress the importance of a treatment regimen of medication use, daily exercise, regular meal/snack times.

Hyperlipidemia (elevated cholesterol and/or triglycerides)

1. Provide patient information about fat/cholesterol content of food.
2. Limit fat to 30% of calories, 10% from saturated fats.
3. Limit cholesterol to less than 300 mg/day, preferably less than 200 mg.
4. Greatly reduce or avoid concentrated sweets (sucrose), especially if triglycerides are elevated.
5. Increase soluble fiber (eg oat bran) in the diet.
6. Increase intake of food high in omega-3 fatty acids (eg: walnuts, salmon, flax seed).
7. Avoid alcohol or use only under advice from physician
8. Stress the importance of exercise, start with realistic short increments with eventual goal of one hour total per day.
9. If patient is overweight, suggest a low-calorie, high fiber diet for weight loss.

Revised and updated 2007 by Authors and Editors.

FDA pregnancy categories

Category	Level of risk with drug exposure	Examples
A	Controlled studies in women fail to demonstrate risk in the first trimester (and there is no evidence of risk in later trimesters) and possibility of fetal harm appears remote.	thyroid hormones folic acid pyridoxine
B	Animal reproduction studies have not demonstrated fetal risk, but there are no controlled studies in pregnant women. Animal reproduction studies have shown adverse effect that was not confirmed in controlled studies on women in first trimester. There is no evidence of risk in later trimesters.	metronidazole famciclovir clindamycin didanosine, acyclovir
C	Studies in animals have revealed adverse effects on fetus and there are no controlled studies in women. In some cases, studies in women and animals are not available. Drugs in this category should be given only if potential benefit justifies risk to fetus.	ciprofloxacin corticosteroids foscarnet, indinavir dronabinol, filgrastim
D	There is positive evidence of human fetal risk, but the benefits for pregnant women may be acceptable despite the risk, as in life-threatening diseases for which safer drugs cannot be used or are ineffective. An appropriate statement must appear in the "warnings" section of the labeling of the drugs in this category.	cytarabine daunorubicin etoposide bleomycin
X	Studies in animals or humans have demonstrated fetal abnormalities or adverse reaction reports indicate evidence of fetal risk. The risk of using the drug in pregnant women clearly out-weighs any possible benefit. The drug is contraindicated in women who may become pregnant.	cyclophosphamide megestrol thalidomide ribavirin

Patients/clients who are pregnant or who are attempting to become pregnant should always consult with their physician(s) and possibly their pharmacist before taking any medication including OTC (over the counter) products and/or "herbal/natural products."

FOOD MEDICATION INTERACTIONS

MEDICATION INDICATION(S), Classification & Pharmacologic Action

abacavir (ABC)
Ziagen
Tab- Na starch glycolate
Soln- saccharin,
  sorbitol, propylene
  glycol = 50 mg/mL,
  citric acid

ANTIRETROVIRAL (HIV/AIDS), NRTI
Drug: Take s̄ regard to food.
Nutr: Anorexia.
Oral/GI: <u>N/V</u>, abdominal pain, diarrhea.
S/Cond: Caution c̄ alcohol- ↑ drug levels due to ↓ elimination.
Not c̄ lactation. Caution c̄ ↓ mild hepatic func. Not c̄ moderate or severe
↓ hepatic func. Not c̄ HLA-B*5701 genetic variant- testing recommended
before drug use.[1]
Pregnancy: Category C.
Other: <u>Allergic</u> <u>reaction</u> (can be fatal), <u>fever</u>, <u>rash</u>,
pharyngitis, dyspnea, cough, hypotension, headache, weakness,
insomnia, pancreatitis, ENT infections, depression,
hepatomegaly c̄ steatosis & lactic acidosis (can be fatal),
(↑ in women, obesity). Rare- SJS, TEN, renal failure, hepatic failure.
Blood/Serum: ↑ <u>TG</u>, ↑ AST, ↑ ALT, ↑ alk phos, ↑ GGT, ↑ CPK,
↑ amylase, anemia, ↓ neutrophils. Rare- lactic acidosis.

abatacept
Orencia
Vial- maltose 500 mg

ANTIARTHRITIC, Rheumatoid Arthritis (Adult or Juvenile) Parenteral (IV)
T-lymphocyte activation inhibitor
Drug: Dosage based on body weight.
Oral/GI: Dyspepsia, <u>nausea</u>.
S/Cond: Not c̄ lactation. Caution c̄ geriatric. Caution c̄ COPD or TB.
Pregnancy: Category C.
Other: <u>Headache</u>, <u>URTI</u>, nasopharyngitis, other infections, dizziness,
cough, back pain, HTN, rash, extremity pain, flushing, dyspnea.
Urinary: UTI.
Monitor: For acute infusion reaction, infection.

Abelcet	ANTIFUNGAL	See **amphotericin B p 34**
Abilify	ANTIPSYCHOTIC (Second Generation)	See **aripiprazole p 41**
Abraxane	ANTINEOPLASTIC, Antimitotic Agent	See **paclitaxel p 242**
Abstral	ANALGESIC, Narcotic, Opioid	See **fentanyl p 139**

acamprosate
Campral (DR)
Tab- Na starch glycolate

ALCOHOL ABUSE DETERENT
    Drug: Take s̄ regard to food. Take TID c̄ meals to ↑ compliance.
    Nutr: Anorexia, ↑ appetite, ↑ wt.
    Oral/GI: Taste changes, N/V, dyspepsia, abdominal pain, flatulence, diarrhea.
    S/Cond: Avoid alcohol. Not c̄ lactation. Caution c̄ moderate ↓ renal func, not c̄ CrCl < 30 mL/minute. **Pregnancy:** Category C.
    Other: Headache, weakness, edema, chills, back pain, impotence, HTN, suicidal thinking or behavior.

acarbose
Precose
Tab- starch

ANTIDIABETIC AGENT- TYPE 2 Diabetes, Alpha-glucosidase Inhibitor
    Drug: Take c̄ first bite of each main meal. Titrate dose to ↓ GI side effects. Do not take c̄ digestive enzymes, eg amylase or pancreatin.[1]
    Diet: Prescribed diabetic diet.
    Nutr: Delays abs of dietary disaccharides & complex CHO.
    Oral/GI: Abdominal pain, DIARRHEA, FLATULENCE, borborygmus.
    S/Cond: Limit alcohol. Not c̄ lactation. Caution c̄ moderate ↓ renal func. Not c̄ severe ↓ renal func or hepatic cirrhosis.
    Not c̄ diabetic ketoacidosis.
    Not c̄ IBS, malabsorption syndrome or intestinal obstruction.
    Does not cause hypoglycemia when used as single agent.
    In combination c̄ other agents, use only glucose to treat hypoglycemia.
    Pregnancy: Category B. **Other:** Hepatotoxicity.
    Blood/Serum: ↓ *FASTING GLUCOSE*, ↓ *POSTPRANDIAL GLUCOSE*, ↓ *Hb A1$_C$*, slightly ↓ HCT. ↑ AST, ↑ ALT at higher doses. **Monitor:** Glucose, HbA1$_C$. AST & ALT q 3 months for first year, then periodically.

| **Accupril** | ANTIHYPERTENSIVE | See **Angiotensin Converting** |
| quinapril | | **Enzyme Inhibitors p 36** |

Accuretic	ANTIHYPERTENSIVE, DIURETIC	See **Angiotensin Converting**
quinapril & hydrochlorothiazide Combination drug		**Enzyme Inhibitors p 36**
		See **hydrochlothiazide p 166**

| **Accutane** | ANTIACNE | See **isotretinoin p 181** |
| previous brand name | | |

acebutolol
Sectral
Cap- starch

ANTIHYPERTENSIVE, ANTIARRHYTHMIC, Cardioselective Beta-Blocker c̄ ISA
Drug: Take s̄ regard to food. **Diet:** ↓ Na, ↓ cal may be recommended.
Avoid natural licorice, see p 374.
Oral/GI: Pharyngitis, dyspepsia, N/V, constipation, diarrhea, flatulence.
S/Cond: Not c̄ lactation.
Caution c̄ diabetes- may mask signs of hypoglycemia.
May reduce insulin release in response to hyperglycemia.[6]
Caution c̄ ↓ renal or ↓ hepatic func. Caution c̄ geriatric- ↓ dose.
Caution c̄ asthma/bronchospasm. **Pregnancy:** Category B.
Other: ↓ _BP_ c̄ possible hypotension. Fatigue, headache, dizziness,
drowsiness, bradycardia, depression, chest pain, edema, insomnia,
abnormal dreams, rash, cough, anxiety. < 1%- joint/muscle pain.
Blood/Serum: + ANA. ↓ chol, ↓ LDL. Rare- ↑ AST, ↑ ALT, ↑ bil,
↑ alk phos, ↑ LDH.
Urinary: ↑ frequency.
Monitor: BP, cardiac func, glucose c̄ diabetes. Possibly renal or hepatic func.

| **Aceon** | ANTIHYPERTENSIVE | See **Angiotensin Converting** |
| perindopril | | **Enzyme Inhibitors p 36** |

acetaminophen (APAP)   ANALGESIC, ANTIPYRETIC   Oral and Parenteral (IV only)
  Aspirin Free Anacin   **Drug:** May take $\bar{s}$ regard to food. Food slightly delays abs of SR form.[6]
  Tab- starch,   May open cap & mix $\bar{c}$ small amount drink or soft food.
  cornstarch,   Do not mix $\bar{c}$ hot drink, causes bitter taste.[2]
  propylene glycol   **Diet:** In one study, Vit C $\geq$ 3 g/day $\downarrow$ excretion 75%- $\uparrow$ risk of toxicity.[93]
  Aspirin Free Excedrin   Caffeine $\uparrow$ rate of abs & effect of drug.[108]
  Cap- 65 mg caffeine   **Oral/GI:** No GI bleeding.
  Tylenol   **S/Cond:** Avoid alcohol[13] or limit to < 3 drinks/day.
    Caution $\bar{c}$ $\downarrow$ hepatic func.
  Ofirmev   Chronic alcoholics - do not exceed 2 g/day[7] due to $\uparrow$ risk of hepatotoxicity.
  IV soln- mannitol,   **Pregnancy:** Category B.
  cysteine   **Other:** Rare- pancreatitis.[1] Rare- hepatotoxicity - can be fatal
($\uparrow$ risk in adults $\bar{c}$ dose > 4 g/day).[2]
Blood/Serum: Hemolytic anemia, $\downarrow$ WBC, $\uparrow$ bil, $\uparrow$ LDH, $\underline{AST}$,
$\uparrow$ <u>ALT</u>, $\uparrow$ PT/INR. False $\downarrow$ or $\uparrow$ glucose $\bar{c}$ some glucometers.
Urinary: <u>False</u> $\downarrow$ <u>glucose</u> $\bar{c}$ <u>chemstrips</u>.

Check brand for alcohol, aspartame, saccharin, sorbitol, starch, sucrose, sulfites or tartrazine.

---

acetylsalicylic acid   ANALGESIC, NSAID   See **aspirin p 44**

Aciphex   ANTIULCER, ANTIGERD, ANTISECRETORY See **Proton Pump Inhibitors p 268**
  rabeprazole

Actemra   ANTIARTHRITIC, Rheumatoid Arthritis (Adult or Juvenile) Parenteral only (IV)
    Interleukin-6 (IL-6) inhibitor   See **tocilizumab p 317**

actinomycin-D   ANTINEOPLASTIC, Antibiotic   See **dactinomycin p 100**

Actiq   ANALGESIC, Narcotic, Opioid, Transmucosal system See **fentanyl p 139**

Activella   HORMONE, Estrogen + Progestin   See **Hormone Therapy p 165**
  estradiol & norethindrone acetate

| **Actonel** | OSTEOPOROSIS TREATMENT, PAGET'S DISEASE TREATMENT | |
| risedronate | | See **Bisphosphonates, Oral p 59** |

Actonel with Calcium	OSTEOPOROSIS TREATMENT	
risedronate		See **Bisphosphonates, Oral p 59**
calcium carbonate	**Actonel** Tab- lactose. **Ca** Tab- starch	See **calcium carbonate p 70**

One week treatment pack = 1**Actonel** (35 mg) & 6 **ca carbonate** 500 mg each

| **Actos** | ANTIDIABETIC AGENT | See **thiazolidinediones p 312** |
| pioglitazone | | |

ACTOplus Met	ANTIDIABETIC AGENT, ANTIHYPERGLYCEMIC AGENT	
pioglitazone	Combination drug	See **thiazolidinediones p 312**
metformin	Tab	See **metformin p 210**

acyclovir
Zovirax
Cap- lactose,
cornstarch
Tab- Na starch glycolate
Susp- sorbitol

Generic brand
Tab- starch free
Parenteral-
500 mg vial-
 50 mg (2.18 mEq) Na
1000 mg vial-
 98 mg (4.26 mEq) Na

ANTIVIRAL (Herpes, Chickenpox, Shingles) Oral, Ointment or Parenteral (IV)
Drug: May take c̄ food. Take c̄ full glass water.
Diet: Insure adequate fluid intake/hydration, 2-3 L/day,[26] unless
otherwise directed. **Nutr:** Anorexia.
Oral/GI: N/V, abdominal pain, constipation, diarrhea.
S/Cond: Caution c̄ lactation. Caution c̄ ↓ renal func.
Pregnancy: Oral & IV- Category B. Ointment- Category C.
Other: Headache, dizziness, fatigue, edema, rash, confusion (↑ in geriatrics),
agitation, hallucinations, paresthesia, tremors.
IV only- ↓ BP, acute renal failure (more common c̄ bolus infusion).
Blood/Serum: Transient c̄ IV– ↑ BUN, ↑ crea, ↑ AST, ↑ ALT.
Rare- dyscrasias.
Urinary: Rare- crystalluria, hematuria.
Monitor: Renal func c̄ IV.

| **Adalat/Adalat CC** | ANTIANGINA, ANTIHYPERTENSIVE (CC form) | |
| | Ca Channel Blocker | See **nifedipine p 229** |

adalimumab
Humira
mannitol 9.6 mg/syringe

ANTIARTHRITIC (Rheumatoid or Psoriatric Arthritis), TNF Inhibitor Parenteral only (SC)
Oral/GI: Nausea, abdominal pain.
S/Cond: Not c̄ lactation. Caution c̄ CHF, immune or demyelinating disorder.
Pregnancy: Category B.
Other: <u>Rash</u>, rhinitis, sinusitis, flu syndrome, weakness, headache, back pain, URTI, HTN, allergic reaction.
Rare- lupus-like syndrome, TB, malignancies (eg lymphoma), serious infection (can be fatal).
Blood/Serum: ↑ chol, ↑ alk phos. Rare- dyscrasias.
Urinary: UTI, hematuria. **Monitor:** For active TB prior to & during treatment.

Adcirca
tadalafil

PULMONARY ARTERIAL HYPERTENSION TREATMENT
Tab- lactose   See listing for **sildenafil p 292**

Adderall/Adderall XR

ANTI-ADHD, Stimulant   See **amphetamines p 33**

---

adefovir
Hepsera
Tab- lactose, starch

CHRONIC HEPATITIS B TREATMENT, NRTI
Drug: Take s̄ regard to food.
Oral/GI: Dyspepsia.
S/Cond: Not c̄ lactation. Caution c̄ ↓ renal func.
Pregnancy: Category C.
Other: <u>Acute exacerbation of hepatitis after discontinuation of drug.</u>
Rare- nephrotoxicity, lactic acidosis, hepatomegaly c̄ steatosis.
Blood/Serum: ↑ crea. Rare- dyscrasias.
Urinary: Hematuria.
Monitor: Baseline & periodic renal func, hepatic func.

Adipex-P

APPETITE SUPPRESSANT, ANTIOBESITY   See **phentermine p 255**

Adriamycin

ANTINEOPLASTIC, Antibiotic   See **doxorubicin p 117**

Advair Diskus
Diskus- lactose

ANTIASTHMA, COPD TREATMENT   See **fluticasone p 144**
Combination drug   See **salmeterol p 286**

Advicor	ANTIHYPERLIPIDEMIC Combination of SR **niacin** & **lovastatin**	See **niacin** p 228 See **HMG-CoA Reductase** **Inhibitors** p 164
Advil	ANTIARTHRITIC, ANALGESIC, NSAID	See **ibuprofen** p 170
Aggrenox Cap- cornstarch, lactose, sucrose, 25 mg Tab **aspirin**	PLATELET AGGREGATION INHIBITOR	See **dipyridamole** p 113 See **aspirin** p 44
Agrylin	THROMBOCYTHEMIA TREATMENT	See **anagrelide** p 36
Alavert	ANTIHISTAMINE	See **loratadine** p 199

albuterol
  Accuneb
  Inhalation Soln
  Generics-
  Syrup- propylene glycol
  Oral soln- saccharin
  Tab- cornstarch, lactose,
  potato starch
  Proventil HFA Aerosol
  alcohol
  Ventolin HFA Aerosol
  VoSpire ER (SR)
  Tab- Ca Sulfate, lactose,
  propylene glycol

ANTIASTHMA, BRONCHODILATOR, Sympathomimetic, Beta-2 agonist
Oral (Tab, Syrup, Soln), Inhalant (Aerosol, Soln)
Drug: If GI distress occurs, take c̄ food. Swallow SR tabs whole c̄ liquid- do not crush, chew or break.
Diet: Limit caffeine/xanthine, see p 379. **Nutr:** ↑ appetite, anorexia.
Oral/GI: Inhalant- Peculiar taste, sore/dry throat.
Oral- N/V, dyspepsia, diarrhea.
S/Cond: Not c̄ lactation. Caution c̄ HTN or CV disorders.
Caution c̄ diabetes. Caution c̄ ↓ renal func, hyperthyroidism or seizures.
Pregnancy: Category C.
Other: TREMOR, NERVOUSNESS, palpitations, tachycardia, headache, dizziness, angina, muscle cramps, nosebleed, insomnia, hyperactivity especially in children, paradoxical bronchospasm.
Inhalant- ear infection, URTI, chest pain.
Blood/Serum: ↓ K, ↑ glucose, ↓ chol, ↓ LDL, ↑ HDL.[100] SR tab- ↓ HgB, ↓ HCT, ↓ WBC, ↑ AST.

Aldactazide	ANTIHYPERTENSIVE, DIURETIC Combination drug	See **spironolactone** p 297 See **hydrochlorothiazide** p 166
Aldactone	ANTIHYPERTENSIVE, DIURETIC	See **spironolactone** p 297

Aldoril
  only generic available

ANTIHYPERTENSIVE, DIURETIC
  Combination drug

See **methyldopa p 213**
See **hydrochlorothiazide p 166**

alefacept
  Amevive
  preservative free pwd
  sucrose 12.5 mg

PSORIASIS TREATMENT, Immunosuppressive Agent   Parenteral (IM, IV)
  Oral/GI: Nausea.
  S/Cond: Not c̄ lactation. Not c̄ HIV, systemic malignancy or infection.
  Not c̄ low CD4+ T-lymphocyte count. **Pregnancy:** Category B.
  Other: Chills (↑ c̄ IV use), pharyngitis, allergic reaction, dizziness, ↑ cough,
  itching, muscle pain, CV events, MI, infection, malignancy.
  Injection site reaction (↑ c̄ IM).
  Blood/Serum: ↓ CD4+ T-lymphocyte, ↑ AST, ↑ ALT.
  Monitor: CD4+ T-lymphocyte a wk before use & q 2 wk during 12 wk
  treatment. Hepatic func.

alendronate
  Fosamax

OSTEOPOROSIS TREATMENT, PAGET'S DISEASE TREATMENT
                    See **Bisphosphonates, Oral p 59**

Aleve

ANTIARTHRITIC, ANALGESIC, NSAID   See **naproxen sodium p 224**

alfuzosin
  Uroxatral

BPH TREATMENT   See **Alpha₁-Adrenergic Blockers
                    p 28**

Alimta

ANTINEOPLASTIC, Antifolate   See **pemetrexed p 248**

aliskiren
  Tekturna
  Tab

ANTIHYPERTENSIVE, Direct Renin Inhibitor
  Drug: Take once a day consistently c̄ or s̄ food.[1] High fat meals ↓ abs by 71%.
  Oral/GI: Dyspepsia, GERD, abdominal pain, diarrhea.
  S/Cond: Not c̄ lactation. Caution c̄ severe ↓ renal func.
  Pregnancy: Category C- 1ˢᵗ trimester. Category D- 2ⁿᵈ & 3ʳᵈ trimesters.
  Blood/Serum: ↑ K in diabetics. < 1%- ↓ Hgb, ↑ K, ↑ CPK, ↑ uric acid.
  Monitor: Electrolytes & renal func in diabetics.

Alkeran

ANTINEOPLASTIC, Alkylating Agent, Nitrogen Mustard See **melphalan p 207**

Allegra

ANTIHISTAMINE   See **fexofenadine p 141**

Allegra-D (SR)　　　　ANTIHISTAMINE, DECONGESTANT　　　See **fexofenadine p 141**
  Tab 12 hr- starch　　　　　Combination drug　　　　　　　　See **pseudoephedrine p 269**
  Tab 24 hr- starch free　　**Drug:** Swallow whole on empty stomach.
　　　　　　　　　　　　Nutr: Food ↓ rate & extent of abs of SR form.[6]

Alli (OTC)　　　　　WEIGHT CONTROL AGENT, Lipase Inhibitor　　See **orlistat p 238**

allopurinol　　　　　ANTIGOUT, Xanthine Oxidase Inhibitor　　Oral or Parenteral (IV)
  Zyloprim　　　　　IV form used to control ↑ uric acid caused by chemotherapy.
  Tab- lactose,　　　　**Drug:** If GI distress occurs, take c̄ food or milk, preferably after meals.
   cornstarch　　　　**Diet:** Drink 2.5 - 3 L fluids/day to produce 2 L urine per 24 hr.[13]
  Aloprim (IV)　　　Avoid large doses Vit C to ↓ potential for renal calculi.[13]
  preservative free　　**Nutr:** To ↓ risk of xanthine calculi, maintain neutral or slightly alkaline urine.
　　　　　　　　　　Oral/GI: Taste loss/changes, N/V, gastritis, abdominal pain, diarrhea.
　　　　　　　　　　S/Cond: Limit alcohol. Caution c̄ lactation. Caution c̄ ↓ renal or ↓ hepatic func.
　　　　　　　　　　Pregnancy: Category C. **Other:** Drowsiness, headache, rash, fever.[7]
　　　　　　　　　　Rare- renal failure /insufficiency, peripheral neuropathy, neuritis,
　　　　　　　　　　paresthesia, myopathy, SJS, jaundice, hepatitis, severe dermatitis/necrolysis.
　　　　　　　　　　Blood/Serum: ↓ _URIC ACID_. < 1%- dyscrasias, ↑ alk phos, ↑ AST,
　　　　　　　　　　↑ ALT, ↑ bil, ↑ BUN, ↑ crea.
　　　　　　　　　　Urinary: ↓ _URIC ACID_. Rare- xanthine crystalluria, renal calculi.[26]
　　　　　　　　　　Monitor: CBC, uric acid. Renal & hepatic func, especially in the first
　　　　　　　　　　months of use.

almotriptan　　　　ANTIMIGRAINE, Serotonin 5-HT$_1$ Receptor Agonist　See **Antimigraine p 39**
  Axert

Aloprim　　　　　ANTIGOUT, Xanthine Oxidase Inhibitor　　See **allopurinol above**

Alora　　　　　　HORMONE　　　　　　　　　　　　　　See **Hormone Therapy p 165**

Aloxi　　　　　　ANTIEMETIC, ANTINAUSEANT　　　　　See **palonosetron p 243**

Alpha₁ Adrenergic Blockers ANTIHYPERTENSIVE[a], BPH TREATMENT[b]

Drug: prazosin or **terazosin-** Take first dose HS in bed to prevent first dose syncope.
Take XL brand c̄ breakfast to ↑ blood levels. Take s̄ regard to food.
alfuzosin- Take c̄ same meal each day. Do not crush or chew.
silodosin- take c̄ a meal.
tamsulosin- Take 1/2 hr after same meal each day. Swallow cap whole- do not open, crush or chew.
Diet: For antihypertensive- ↓ Na, ↓ cal diet may be recommended. Avoid natural licorice, see p 374.
alfuzosin, silodosin & **tamsulosin** only- Theoretical interaction c̄ grapefruit/related citrus, see p 390.
Nutr: Slightly ↑ wt c̄ **doxazosin** or **terazosin.**
Oral/GI: Dry mouth, dyspepsia, nausea, abdominal pain, diarrhea, constipation.
S/Cond: Avoid alcohol.[7] Caution c̄ lactation. 90-99 % serum pro bound.
alfuzosin- Not c̄ moderate or severe ↓ hepatic func. Caution c̄ severe ↓ renal func.
doxazosin- Caution c̄ ↓ hepatic func. **prazosin-** Caution c̄ ↓ renal func.
silodosin- Not c̄ severe ↓ hepatic func. Caution c̄ moderate ↓ renal func. Not c̄ severe ↓ renal func.
terazosin- Caution c̄ ↓ hepatic or ↓ renal func.[13]
Pregnancy: alfuzosin, tamsulosin, sildosin- Category B. **doxazosin, prazosin, terazosin-** Category C.
Other: ↓ _BP_ c̄ possible hypotension (rare c̄ **alfuzosin** or **terazosin**), <u>dizziness</u>, <u>weakness</u>,
fatigue, headache, URTI, rhinitis, pharyngitis. Rare- syncope, ↑ c̄ first dose.
alfuzosin- ↑ <u>QT</u> <u>INTERVAL</u>.
doxazosin- <u>DROWSINESS</u>, edema, arrhythmias, ataxia.
prazosin- <u>Palpitations</u>, <u>drowsiness</u>, edema, blurred vision, depression, nervousness, paresthesia, rash, nosebleed.
sildosin- <u>RETROGRADE EJACULATION</u>.
tamsulosin- ↑ cough, back pain, insomnia, ↓ vision.
terazosin- Blurred vision, drowsiness, edema, palpitations, paresthesia, back or joint pain.
Blood/Serum: doxazosin- Slightly ↓ chol, ↓ LDL, ↓ TG, ↑ HDL, ↓ WBC.
       prazosin- + ANA. Transient ↓ WBC, ↑ uric acid, ↑ BUN.[6]
       terazosin- Slightly ↓ Hb, ↓ HCT, ↓ WBC, ↓ alb, ↓ TP, ↓ chol, ↓ LDL, ↓ VLDL. <1%- ↓ platelets.
Urinary: BPH patients- ↑ _FLOW_, ↓ _RESIDUAL URINE_, ↓ _FREQUENCY_, ↓ _NOCTURIA_, ↑ _EASE OF STARTING MICTURITION_.
prazosin- ↑ <u>VMA</u>. **Monitor:** BP.

alfuzosin[b]	**Uroxatral** (ER) Tab- mannitol, castor oil
doxazosin[a, b]	**Cardura** Tab- lactose, Na starch glycolate **Cardura XL** Tab
prazosin[a]	**Minipress**/Cap- starch, sucrose

sildosin[b]	**Rapaflo** Cap- starch	
tamsulosin[b]	**Flomax** Cap- trace alcohol	
terazosin[a, b]	**Hytrin** Cap-mineral oil	**Terazosin** Tab- some brands contain lactose

alprazolam
   Xanax/Xanax XR
   Niravam

ANTIANXIETY, ANTIPANIC   See **Benzodiazepines p 54**

Altace
   ramipril

ANTIHYPERTENSIVE   See **Angiotensin Converting Enzyme Inhibitors p 36**

Altoprev
   lovastatin

ANTIHYPERLIPIDEMIC   See **HMG-CoA Reductase Inhibitors p 164**

aluminum hydroxide & magnesium hydroxide   ANTACID, ANTIFLATULENT if c̄ simethicone
Drug: Take 1 hr after meals & HS. Chew tab well. **Diet:** Take Fe or Fol suppl separately by 2 hr.[13]
Take separately from citrus fruit/juice or Ca citrate by 3 hr- juice ↑ Al abs.[9a] **Nutr:** ↓ abs of Fol, P & Fe.
Oral/GI: Chalky taste, rare- constipation, diarrhea. **S/Cond: Mylanta Maximum Strength** thickens some TF.[8]
Not c̄ ESRD- ↑ Mg & ↑ Al. LT use in dialysis may cause encephalopathy, neurotoxicity, osteomalacia.
Pregnancy: Avoid chronic high dose.[13] Aluminum hydroxide- Category C.[2]
Blood/Serum: ↓ P, ↓ K, ↑ gastrin,[13] ↑ Mg, ↓ Ca c̄ LT use, ↑ Al c̄ LT use in ESRD.

   Di-Gel- (simethicone) Susp- saccharin, sorbitol. Tab-mannitol, saccharin.
   Gelusil- (simethicone) Chew Tab- mannitol, sorbitol, sugar.
   Maalox Regular/Maalox Max- (simethicone) Reg Susp- saccharin Ca, sorbitol.
                    Max Susp- saccharin Na or Ca, sorbitol.
   Mylanta/ Mylanta Maximum Strength- (simethicone) Susp- sorbitol, saccharin Na.
                     Extra strength susp- saccharin Na, sorbitol.

See "Guide to the Use of This Book" inside front cover.

amantadine
Symmetrel
Tab- Na starch glycolate
Syrup- 3.2 g
 sorbitol/5 mL

ANTIPARKINSON, ANTIVIRAL (influenza A), ANTI EPS
    Drug: Take at least 4 hr before bedtime to prevent insomnia.
    Nutr: Anorexia.
    Oral/GI: Dry mouth, dry nose, <u>nausea</u>, constipation.
    S/Cond: Avoid alcohol. Not c̄ lactation. ↑ risk of dental problems, see p 15.
    Caution c̄ ↓ renal or ↓ hepatic func, CHF, edema, seizures or psychosis.
    Pregnancy: Category C.
    Other: <u>Dizziness</u>, <u>insomnia</u>, blurred vision, depression, ataxia,
    orthostatic hypotension, agitation, confusion, fatigue, headache,
    peripheral edema, livedo reticularis, hallucinations, anxiety.
    Rare- CHF, psychosis, NMS.
    Blood/Serum: Rare- ↑ alk phos, ↑ AST, ↑ ALT, ↑ bil, ↑ GGT, ↑ CPK,
    ↑ LDH[7], ↑ BUN, ↑ crea.
    Urinary: ↑ frequency, retention.
    Monitor: BP.

Amaryl
 glimepiride

ORAL HYPOGLYCEMIC   See **sulfonylureas p 299**

Ambien/Ambien CR

SLEEP AID, Hypnotic   See **zolpidem p 351**

AmBisome

ANTIFUNGAL, ANTIPROTOZOAL   See **amphotericin B p 34**

Amerge
 naratriptan

ANTIMIGRAINE, Serotonin 5-HT$_1$ Receptor Agonist   See **Antimigraine p 39**

Amevive

PSORIASIS TREATMENT, Parenteral (IM, IV)   See **alefacept p 26**

amikacin
 Amikin (brand name
 discontinued)
 Vial-
 0.66% Na bisulfite

ANTIBIOTIC, Aminoglycoside   Parenteral only (IM or IV)
    Diet: Insure adequate fluid intake/hydration to ↓ renal damage.
    Oral/GI: N/V. **S/Cond:** Dose based on IBW.
    In obesity, dose based on IBW + 0.4 (TBW-IBW).[12]
    Not c̄ lactation. Caution c̄ ↓ renal func, dehydration or hypocalcemia.[6]
    Pregnancy: Category D.
    Other: <u>OTOTOXICITY</u>, neurotoxicity, muscle weakness, nephrotoxicity, ataxia.

Rare- hypotension.
Blood/Serum: ↑ crea. Rare- anemia, eosinophilia.[7]
Urinary: Pro, ↓ specific gravity, RBC, WBC, cast, ↓ output.
Monitor: Renal & auditory func. Drug serum levels.

amiloride & hydrochlorothiazide

ANTIHYPERTENSIVE, DIURETIC (**amiloride** K-sparing; **HCTZ** K-depleting)
Tab- lactose, starch
See listing for **triamterene p 322**
See **hydrochlorothiazide p 166**

aminophylline

ANTIASTHMA, BRONCHODILATOR, Methylxanthine
See listing for **theophylline p 311**

amiodarone
Cordarone
Tab- lactose, starch
Generic brands-
IV- benzyl alcohol =
   20.2 mg/mL
Pacerone
400 mg Tab-
   lactose, cornstarch
100 & 200 mg Tab-
   lactose, cornstarch,
   Na starch gycolate

ANTIARRHYTHMIC   Oral or Parenteral (IV)
Drug: Take Tab consistently c̄ or s̄ meals. High fat food ↑ rate of abs & C_{max} of drug.
Diet: Avoid grapefruit/related citrus,[3a] see p 390. Avoid SJW,[4] see p 286.
Nutr: Anorexia. **Oral/GI:** Abnormal taste, smell & salivation, NAUSEA/VOMITING, abdominal pain, constipation.
S/Cond: Not c̄ lactation. Not c̄ hypokalemia or hypomagnesemia.
96% serum pro bound. Caution c̄ geriatric.[84] Caution c̄ ↓ hepatic func.[6]
TF ↓ drug level by 70%.[113] **Pregnancy:** Category D.
Other: ATAXIA, pulmonary toxicity (fatal in 10% of cases), cough, hepatotoxicity, dizziness, tremor, fatigue, blurred vision, paresthesias, photosensitivity, bradycardia, ↑ QT interval, CHF, insomnia, proarrhythmia (can be fatal), headache, flushing, edema, optic neuropathy, hypo or hyperthyroidism, blue-gray skin tone c̄ LT use.
Hypotension, SJS c̄ IV (< 1% c̄ oral).
Blood/Serum: ↑ Alk Phos, ↑ AST, ↑ ALT, ↑ T_4, ↑ T_3, ↑ TSH, ↑ crea, dyscrasias, coagulation abnormalities.
Monitor: Hepatic, pulmonary & thyroid func. Ophthalmic exams. BP c̄ IV.

Amitiza

CHLORIDE CHANNEL ACTIVATOR   See **lubiprostone p 201**
   for chronic idiopathic constipation

amitriptyline
Elavil (generics only)

ANTIDEPRESSANT   See **Tricyclic Antidepressants p 323**

amlodipine
  Norvasc
  Tab- Na starch glycolate

ANTIHYPERTENSIVE, ANTIANGINA, Ca Channel Blocker,
                                        dihydropyridine derivative
  Drug: Take s̄ regard to food. May take c̄ food to ↓ GI distress.
  Diet: ↓ Na, ↓ cal may be recommended. Avoid natural licorice, see p 374.
  No significant interaction c̄ grapefruit/related citrus, see p 390.
  Oral/GI: Dysphagia, nausea, cramps.
  S/Cond: Not c̄ lactation. 93% serum pro bound. Caution c̄ ↓ hepatic func.
  Pregnancy: Category C.
  Other: ↓ _BP_ c̄ possible hypotension. <u>Edema</u>, dizziness, flushing,
  drowsiness, palpitations, muscle pain, rash.
  Monitor: BP.

amoxicillin
  Generic brands
  Susp- 1.67 g sucrose/5 mL
  Teva brand Chew Tabs-
   lactose, mannitol, sugar
  Cap
  Dispermox
   Dispersible Tab-
   aspartame. Gluten free
  Trimox
   Susp- sucrose

ANTIBIOTIC, Penicillin
  Drug: Food does not affect abs. May take c̄ food to ↓ GI distress.
  Chew tab- crush or chew. Dissolve dispersible tab in 10 mL water, milk,
  formula or juice, do not chew or swallow whole.
  Nutr: Prebiotics may ↓ GI side effects.[29]
  Oral/GI: N/V, <u>diarrhea</u>.
  Rare- stomatitis, glossitis, oral candidiasis or pseudomembranous colitis.
  S/Cond: Caution c̄ lactation. Caution c̄ ↓ renal func.[13]
  Pregnancy: Category B.
  Other: <u>Rash</u>, rare- allergic reaction (can be fatal).
  Blood/Serum: Anemias, dyscrasias, ↑ AST, ↑ ALT.
  Monitor: LT use- renal & hepatic func. CBC c̄ diff.[6]

**amoxicillin and
clavulanate potassium**

  Generic brands only

ANTIBIOTIC, Penicillin   See **amoxicillin above**
  Drug: Take at the start of a standard meal to ↓ GI upset, but not c̄
  high fat meal. High fat ↓ abs of clavulanate.
  (Standard meal = 612 cal, 89 g CHO, 25 g fat, 14 g pro).
  Chew tab- crush or chew. Swallow XR Tab whole.
  Tab 250, 500 & 875 mg contain 25 mg (0.63 mEq) K, starch
  Pwd for Susp & Chew-Tab 125 mg contain 6 mg (0.16 mEq) K/5 mL susp or Tab
  Pwd for Susp & Chew-Tab 200 mg contain 5 mg (0.14 mEq) K/5mL susp or Tab

Pwd for Susp & Chew-Tab 250 mg contain 13 mg (0.32 mEq) K/5mL susp or Tab
Pwd for Susp & Chew-Tab 400 mg contain 12 mg (0.29 mEq) K/5 mL susp or Tab
All Pwd for Susp & Chew-Tabs- saccharin Na & mannitol
200 & 400 mg Pwd for Susp- also contain aspartame
200 & 400 mg Chew-Tabs- also contain aspartame

Amphetamines
Adderall/Adderall XR
dextroamphetamine &
amphetamine
Adderall Tab- sucrose,
lactose, cornstarch
Adderall XR Cap-
sugar spheres
(sucrose & starch),
Kosher gelatin

Dexedrine
dextroamphetamine
Spansule (SR)-
cetyl alcohol,
sugar spheres
(sucrose & starch),
propylene glycol

Didrex
(appetite suppressant/anorectic)
benzphetamine Tab- lactose, sorbitol

ANTI-ADHD, ANTINARCOLEPSY, APPETITE SUPPRESSANT, CNS Stimulant
Drug: Swallow SR form whole early in the day. As anorectic, take 1/2-1 hr before meals. For other uses (eg ADHD) take c̄ or after meal.
Diet: Limit caffeine,[17] see p 379. Avoid high dose Vit C.
Acidifying agents (eg cranberry) ↓ abs, ↑ excretion & ↓ half life of the drug.
Alkalinizing agents (eg Na bicarbonate, $CaCO_3$, antacids) ↑ abs, ↓ excretion & ↑ half life.
As anorectic, low cal diet essential.
Nutr: <u>Anorexia</u>, ↓ wt. ↓ <u>growth in children</u>.[17]
Oral/GI: <u>Dry mouth</u>, metallic taste, stomach pain/cramps, nausea, diarrhea, constipation.
S/Cond: Avoid alcohol.[17] Not c̄ lactation. Caution c̄ HTN.
May be habit forming. Caution c̄ seizures or diabetes.
Caution c̄ geriatric.[84] Benzphetamine - not for ≤ 12 y.o.
Pregnancy: Category C. Benzphetamine- Category X.
Other: <u>Palpitations</u>, <u>restlessness</u>, <u>tremor</u>, ↑ <u>BP</u>, <u>nervousness</u>, <u>chills</u>,[17] dizziness, insomnia, blurred vision, tachycardia, headache, ↑ sweating, motor or verbal tics, euphoria, dyskinesia, over stimulation.
Blood/Serum: ↑ corticosteroids, ↑ T_4 c̄ heavy use.
Urinary: Acidification ↑ drug excretion. Alkalinization ↓ excretion.
False steroid results.
Monitor: BP. Children's growth.

A

amphotericin B
  Abelcet- lipid-based
  (lipid complex form)
  AmBisome- lipid-based
  (liposomal complex form)
  52 mg chol,
  900 mg sucrose/vial

  Amphotec- lipid-based
  (cholesteryl form)
  Fungizone-
  (deoxycholate form)

ANTIFUNGAL, ANTIPROTOZOAL   Parenteral (IV)
CRYPTOCOCCAL MENINGITIS TREATMENT in HIV (**AmBisome** only)
Lipid based forms- less nutrient depletion & less nephrotoxicity than deoxcholate form.
  Diet: Insure adequate fluid intake/hydration.
  ↑ K, ↑ Mg, ↑ Ca diet or K, Mg &/or Ca suppl.
  Nutr: <u>ANOREXIA</u>, ↓ <u>WEIGHT</u>.
  Oral/GI: <u>NAUSEA/VOMITING</u>, <u>stomach pain</u>, <u>dyspepsia</u>, <u>GI hemorrhage</u>, <u>DIARRHEA</u>.
  S/Cond: Not c̄ lactation. > 90% serum pro bound. Caution c̄ ↓ renal func.
  Do dental care cautiously- ↑ risk of bleeding.
  Pregnancy: Category B.
  Other: <u>FEVER</u>, <u>NEPHROTOXICITY</u> (↑ c̄ DEOXYCHOLATE FORM), <u>CHILLS</u>, <u>RASH</u>,
  <u>DYSPNEA</u>, <u>headache</u>, <u>blurred vision</u>, <u>muscle pain</u>, <u>HTN</u> or <u>hypotension</u>,
  <u>tachycardia</u>, <u>chest pain</u>, <u>weakness</u>, <u>back pain</u>, <u>edema</u>, <u>cough</u>,
  <u>sweating</u>, <u>lung disorder</u>, <u>anxiety</u>, <u>confusion</u>, <u>insomnia</u>,
  peripheral neuropathy, arrhythmias.
  Blood/Serum: <u>Anemia</u>, ↑ <u>BUN</u>, ↑ <u>CREA</u>, ↑ <u>GLUCOSE</u>, ↓ <u>K</u>, ↓ <u>Mg</u>, ↑ Na,
  ↓ <u>Ca</u>, ↑ alk phos, ↑ bil, ↑ AST, ↑ ALT, ↑ GGT.
  Urinary: ↑ <u>K</u>, ↑ uric acid, pro, hematuria.
  Monitor: Electrolytes, Mg, renal & hepatic func, CBC & platelets.

ampicillin
  Parenteral- 64 mg
  (2.78 mEq) Na/g to
  78 mg (3.39 mEq) Na/g
  Some caps- lactose
  Pwd for susp-
   sucrose

ANTIBIOTIC, Penicillin   Oral or Parenteral (IM or IV)
  Drug: Take c̄ 8 oz water on empty stomach 1 hr before or 2 hr after meal.
  Food ↓ rate & extent of abs. Acid stable.
  Oral/GI: Taste changes, glossitis, stomatitis, oral candidiasis c̄ LT use,
  N/V, pseudomembranous colitis, <u>diarrhea</u>.
  S/Cond: Not c̄ lactation. Caution c̄ ↓ renal func.[13]
  Pregnancy: Category B.
  Other: <u>Rash</u>, rare- allergic reaction (can be fatal).
  Blood/Serum: Anemia, dyscrasias, ↑ AST, ↑ ALT, ↑ LDH, ↑ alk phos.
  Urinary: False + glucose ($CuSO_4$).
  Monitor: LT use- CBC c̄ diff, hepatic & renal func.

ampicillin &	ANTIBIOTIC, Penicillin	Parenteral only (IM or IV)
sulbactam	**Oral/GI:** Glossitis, stomatitis, oral candidiasis c̄ LT use, N/V,	
Unasyn	pseudomembranous colitis, diarrhea.	
115 mg (5.0 mEq)	**S/Cond:** Caution c̄ lactation.[10] Caution c̄ ↓ renal func.[13]	
Na/ 1.5 g	**Pregnancy:** Category B.	

ampicillin & sulbactam
Unasyn
115 mg (5.0 mEq)
Na/ 1.5 g

ANTIBIOTIC, Penicillin   Parenteral only (IM or IV)
  Oral/GI: Glossitis, stomatitis, oral candidiasis c̄ LT use, N/V,
  pseudomembranous colitis, diarrhea.
  S/Cond: Caution c̄ lactation.[10] Caution c̄ ↓ renal func.[13]
  Pregnancy: Category B.
  Other: Rash, rare- allergic reaction (can be fatal).
  Blood/Serum: Dyscrasias, anemia, ↑ AST, ↑ ALT, ↑ alk phos, ↑ LDH,
  ↓ alb, ↓ TP, ↑ BUN, ↑ crea.
  Urinary: False + glucose (CuSO$_4$).
  Monitor: LT use- CBC c̄ diff, hepatic & renal func.

amprenavir
Agenerase

ANTIRETROVIRAL (HIV/AIDS), Protease Inhibitor, Sulfonamide
  withdrawn from market 10/07 due to low usage   See **fosamprenavir p 144**

Ampyra

MULTIPLE SCLEROSIS TREATMENT, Broad spectrum potassium blocker
  to improve walking in MS pts   See **dalfampridine p 100**

Amrix

  SKELETAL MUSCLE RELAXANT   See **cyclobenazprine p 95**
  ER once daily formula

Amturnide
Tab polyethylene glycol

ANTIHYPERTENSIVE AGENT, Combination drug
              Pregnancy: Category D   See **aliskiern p 26**
                                                         See **amlodipine p 32**
                                                         See **hydrochlorothiazide p 166**

Anacin

ANALGESIC, ANTIPYRETIC, NSAID   See **aspirin p 44**
  Tab- 400 mg **aspirin**, 32 mg **caffeine**, starch See **caffeine p 67**
  Extra Strength Tab- 500 mg aspirin, 32 mg caffeine, starch, cornstarch
  Caplet- same + propylene glycol, simethicone

Anafranil
clomipramine

ANTIDEPRESSANT   See **Tricyclic Antidepressants p 323**

anagrelide
Agrylin
Cap- lactose

THROMBOCYTHEMIA (↑ Platelets) TREATMENT
    Drug: Take s̄ regard to food. **Nutr:** <u>Anorexia</u>.
    Oral/GI: Canker sore, <u>dyspepsia</u>, belching, gastritis, <u>abdominal pain</u>,
    N/V, <u>flatulence</u>, DIARRHEA, constipation, GI hemorrhage, black stool.
    S/Cond: Not c̄ lactation. Caution c̄ ↓ renal func or ↓ hepatic func.
    Caution c̄ cardiac disease. **Pregnancy:** Category C.
    Other: PALPITATIONS, HEADACHE, WEAKNESS, EDEMA, <u>chest pain</u>, tachycardia,
    dizziness, <u>dyspnea</u>, <u>paresthesia</u>, <u>pain</u>, <u>rash</u>, <u>back pain</u>, <u>fever</u>, pharyngitis,
    <u>cough</u>, <u>pulmonary infiltrates/fibrosis</u>, hypotension c̄ ↑ dose, HTN,
    cardiac changes, syncope, migraine, skin disease, bruising, hair loss,
    depression, drowsiness, insomnia, confusion, nervousness, amnesia,
    flu-like symptoms, vision changes, photosensitivity, tinnitus,
    respiratory changes.
    Blood/Serum: ↓ PLATELETS. Anemia, thrombocytopenia. Rare- ↑ AST, ↑ ALT.
    Urinary: Hematuria, dysuria.
    Monitor: Platelets q 2 days for 1st wk, then q wk until < 600,00/uL.
    CBC, renal & hepatic func especially during 1st two weeks.

Anaprox	ANTIARTHRITIC, ANALGESIC, NSAID	See **naproxen p 224**
anastrozole **Arimidex**	ANTINEOPLASTIC	See **Aromatase Inhibitors p 42**
Ancef	ANTIBIOTIC, **cefazolin sodium**	See **cephalosporins p 80**
Androderm (transdermal)	MALE HORMONE REPLACEMENT, PRIMARY HYPOGONADISM, HYPOGONADOTROPIC HYPOGONADISM, Androgen See **testosterone p 308**	
AndroGel (transdermal)	MALE HORMONE REPLACEMENT, PRIMARY HYPOGONADISM, HYPOGONADOTROPIC HYPOGONADISM, Androgen See **testosterone p 308**	
Angeliq	HORMONE	See **Hormone Therapy p 165**

    Combination drug **estradiol & drospirenone**

Angiotensin Converting Enzyme (Ace) Inhibitors
ANTIHYPERTENSIVE (a), CHF TREATMENT (adjunct) (b), To treat Left Ventricular Dysfunction/CHF POST MI (adjunct) (c), Acute MI adjunct (d), To treat diabetic nephropathy (e)
Drug: Take **captopril** or **moexipril** on empty stomach 1 hr before meals (food ↓ abs by 30-50%).

High fat meals ↓ the rate & extent of abs of **quinapril** 25-30%. Take other ACE Inhibitors s̄ regard to food.
Diet: Insure adequate fluid intake/hydration. ↓ Na, ↓ cal may be recommended. Avoid salt subs.
Caution c̄ K suppl. Caution c̄ Mg suppl c̄ **quinapril**. Caution c̄ IV iron- severe systemic reactions
reported.[3] Fe, Mg or Al ↓ **captopril** abs- take oral Fe or Mg suppl & **captopril** separately by at least 2 hr.[3]
Al-Mg antacids/suppl ↓ **captopril**, **fosinopril** abs- take separately.[9b] Avoid natural licorice, see p 374.
Nutr: Anorexia, ↓ wt reported c̄ **captopril**, **enalapril**, **lisinopril**, **ramipril**. Quinapril has high Mg content.
Oral/GI: Rare- dysgeusia (↑ c̄ **captopril**) (metallic or salty taste c̄ **captopril**), dry mouth, N/V,
abdominal pain, constipation, diarrhea. **S/Cond:** Limit alcohol. Caution c̄ lactation for **benazepril**,
moexipril, **quinapril**. Not c̄ lactation for other ACE Inhibitors. Caution c̄ ↓ renal or ↓ hepatic func.
Caution c̄ diabetics on insulin- ↓ glucose. Caution c̄ geriatric. **Benazepril**, **fosinopril**, & **quinapril** are
> 96% serum pro bound. Drug efficacy may ↓ & side effects may ↑ in Black patients.[105]
Drugs c̄ HCT- not c̄ anuria or sulfonamide allergy.
Pregnancy: Category C- 1st trimester. Category D- 2nd & 3rd trimesters.
Other: ↓ _BP_ c̄ possible hypotension, <u>COUGH</u>, dyspnea, syncope, rash, <u>dizziness</u>, <u>headache</u>, fatigue,
muscle pain, insomnia. < 1%, but can be fatal- angioedema (↑ incidence in Black patients),[105]
pancreatitis, hepatotoxicity/jaundice, acute renal failure, SJS.
Blood/Serum: ↑ <u>K</u>, ↓ Na, ↑ AST, ↑ ALT, ↑ alk phos, ↑ bil, anemia, ↓ WBC, rare- dyscrasias, + ANA,
↑ uric acid, ↓ glucose in diabetics on insulin. Transient ↑ BUN, ↑ crea.
Urinary: < 1% transient ↑ pro. **Captopril**- false + acetone. ↑ Zn.[11]
Monitor: BP, electrolytes, renal func, CBC c̄ diff, diabetics for ↓ glucose.

benazepril	**Lotensin** [a]	Tab- lactose, starch. 5, 10, 20 mg Tab- castor oil **Lotensin HCT** [a]* Tab- lactose, castor oil
captopril	**Capoten** [a b c e]	Tab-lactose
enalapril	**Vasotec** [a b]	Tab- lactose, starch. **Vaseretic** [a]* Tab- lactose, starch
enalaprilat	**Vasotec I.V.** [a]	benzyl alcohol = 9 mg/ml
fosinopril	**Monopril** [a b]	Tab- lactose
lisinopril	**Prinivil** [a b d]/**Prinzide** [a]*Tab- mannitol, starch **Zestril** [a b d]/**Zestoretic** [a]*Tab- mannitol, starch	
moexipril	**Univasc** [a]	Tab- lactose **Uniretic** [a]*
perindopril	**Aceon** [a]	Tab- lactose
quinapril	**Accupril** [a b]	Tab- lactose, gelatin, Mg stearate, $MgCO_3$. 5 mg Tab = 18 mg Mg, 10 mg Tab = 37 mg Mg, 20 mg Tab = 50 mg Mg, 40 mg Tab = 100 mg Mg
	Accuretic [a]*	Tab- lactose, Mg stearate, MgCO3
ramipril	**Altace** [a b]	Cap & Tab- starch
trandolapril	**Mavik** [a c]	Tab- lactose, cornstarch

* Also contain **hydrochlorothiazide**, see **p 166**

Angiotensin II Receptor Antagonists (ARB)   ANTIHYPERTENSIVE [a], CHF Treatment [b]
TYPE 2 DIABETIC NEPHROPATHY TREATMENT [c], LEFT VENTRICULAR DYSFUNCTION TREATMENT[d]
Drug: Take s̄ regard to food.
Diet: Caution c̄ K suppl or salt sub. ↓ Na, ↓ cal may be recommended. Avoid natural licorice, see p 374.
losartan only- caution c̄ grapefruit/related citrus,[3] see p 390. **Oral/GI:** Dyspepsia, abdominal pain, diarrhea.
S/Cond: Not c̄ lactation. 90-99% serum pro bound. Caution c̄ ↓ hepatic func or severe ↓ renal func, but
dosage change is not usually required.
(**losartan, telmisartan** or **candesartan** only- ↓ starting dose c̄ ↓ hepatic func).
Drugs c̄ HCT- not c̄ anuria or sulfonamide allergy.
Pregnancy: azilsartan, eprosartan, Diovan, Avalide- Category D. All others- Category C- first trimester.
Category D- 2nd & 3rd trimesters.
Other: ↓ _BP_ c̄ possible hypotension, dizziness, muscle/bone pain, URTI, rhinitis, pharyngitis.
Rare- angioedema, cough, rhabdomyolysis.
Blood/Serum: ↑ K (↑ incidence in CHF patients). Slightly ↓ Hb, ↓ HCT.
eprosartan only - ↑ TG. < 1%- slightly ↑ BUN, ↑ crea,↑ AST, ↑ ALT, ↑ bil, ↑ uric acid, ↓ neutrophils.
Monitor: BP, K, renal func.

azilsartan	**Edarbi**[a]/**Edarbyclor**[a] **	Tab- mannitol
candesartan	**Atacand**[a b]/**Atacand HCT**[a] *	Tab- lactose, cornstarch
eprosartan	**Teveten**[a]/**Teveten HCT**[a] *	Tab- lactose, starch
irbesartan	**Avapro**[a c]/**Avalide**[a] *	Tab- lactose, starch
losartan	**Cozaar**[a c]/**Hyzaar**[a] *	Tab- lactose, starch, 2-8 mg (0.05-0.2 mEq) K/Tab
olmesartan	**Benicar**[a]/**Benicar HCT**[a] *	Tab- lactose
telmisartan	**Micardis**[a b]	Tab- sorbitol
	Micardis HCT[a] *	Tab- sorbitol, lactose, maize starch, starch
valsartan	**Diovan**[a b d]/**Diovan HCT**[a] *	Tab

*Also contain **hydrochlorothiazide**, see p 166   **Also contains **chlorthalidone**, see p 82

anidulafungin Eraxis	ANTIFUNGAL	See **echinocandins** p 120
Antabuse	ALCOHOL DETERRENT	See **disulfiram** p 113
Antara	ANTIHYPERLIPIDEMIC, Fibrate	See **fenofibrate** p 138

ANTIMIGRAINE, Serotonin 5-HT$_1$ Receptor Agonist for <u>acute</u> migraine attack or cluster headache
  (**sumatriptan** is the only one indicated for cluster headache)
Drug: Take s̄ regard to food. Dissolve ODT on tongue c̄ or s̄ liquid, swallow saliva. Swallow regular tab whole.
Diet: Avoid SJW,[93] see p 286.
almotriptan & **eletriptan**- caution c̄ grapefruit/related citrus, see p 390.
Oral/GI: Dry mouth, nasal, jaw, mouth & throat discomfort, dysphagia, dyspepsia, N/V, abdominal
pain, diarrhea. Nasal spray: <u>BAD/UNUSUAL TASTE</u>.
S/Cond: Avoid alcohol. Caution c̄ lactation. Caution c̄ ↓ hepatic func or ↓ renal func.
Contraindicated c̄ most vascular disease, ischemic heart disease, CAD, uncontrolled HTN.
Pregnancy: Category C.
Other: Paresthesia/atypical sensations (↑ c̄ parenteral **sumatriptan**), headache, drowsiness, dizziness,
weakness, chest pain, jaw/neck tightness, back pain, chills, sweating, mildly ↑ BP, palpitation, tremor,
euphoria, vision changes, photophobia.

almotriptan	**Axert**	Tab- Na starch glycolate, mannitol, propylene glycol
eletriptan	**Relpax**	Tab- lactose
frovatriptan	**Frova**	Tab- lactose, Na starch glycolate
naratriptan	**Amerge**	Tab- lactose
rizatriptan	**Maxalt**	Tab- lactose, starch
	Maxalt MLT	Orally Disintegrating Tab (ODT)- gelatin, mannitol, aspartame (1.05 mg phenylalanine/5 mg)
sumatriptan	**Imitrex**	Tab Nasal Spray Parenteral (SC)
	Sumavel DosePro	Parenteral (needle free SC)
zolmitriptan	**Zomig**	Tab- lactose, Na starch glycolate
	Zomig-ZMT	Tab- aspartame (2.81 mg phenylalanine/2.5 mg), mannitol
	Zomig Nasal Spray	

Antivert	ANTINAUSEANT, ANTIVERTIGO Canadian brand also contains **niacin**	See **meclizine** p 205 See **niacin** p 228
Apidra **insulin glulisine**	ANTIDIABETIC, HYPOGLYCEMIC Short acting, rapid onset **insulin**	See **insulin** p 175

apomorphine **Apokyn** 1 mg Na metabisulfite/mL 5 mg benzyl alcohol/mL	ANTIPARKINSON for Hypomobility Episode Parenteral (SC) nonergoline dopamine agonist **Nutr:** <u>Dehydration</u> **Oral/GI:** <u>SEVERE NAUSEA/VOMITING</u>, <u>constipation</u>, <u>diarrhea</u>. **S/Cond:** Avoid alcohol. Not c̄ lactation. Caution c̄ ↓ heptic or ↓ renal func. Caution c̄ geriatric. Not c̄ sulfite allergy. **Pregnancy:** Category C. **Other:** <u>YAWNING</u>, <u>DYSKINESIA</u>, <u>DROWSINESS</u>, <u>DIZZINESS</u>, <u>RHINORRHEA</u>, <u>chest pain</u>, <u>CHF</u>, <u>edema</u>, <u>hallucination/confusion</u>, <u>depression</u>, <u>anxiety</u>, <u>insomnia</u>, <u>fatigue</u>, <u>headache</u>, <u>joint pain</u>, <u>limb/back pain</u>, <u>pneumonia</u>, ↑ <u>sweating</u>, <u>ecchymosis</u>, <u>weakness</u>, <u>dyspnea</u>, orthostatic hypotension, syncope. **Urinary:** <u>UTI</u>.	
aprepitant **Emend** (Oral) Cap- sucrose **fosaprepitant** (Prodrug of **aprepitant**) **Emend** for injection Pwd- lactose	ANTIEMETIC, ANTINAUSEANT, Substance P/Neurokinin-1 Receptor Antagonist Oral and Parenteral (IV) **Drug:** Take oral cap s̄ regard to food. **Diet:** Oral- caution c̄ grapefruit/related citrus, see p 390. **Nutr:** Anorexia. **Oral/GI:** Gastritis, <u>hiccups</u>, abdominal pain, diarrhea, constipation. **S/Cond:** Not c̄ lactation. > 95% plasma pro bound. **Pregnancy:** Category B. **Other:** <u>Weakness</u>, <u>fatigue</u>, dizziness, dehydration. Hypersensitivity infusion reactions (IV): erythema, dyspnea, flushing, rash, itching. **Blood/Serum:** ↑ ALT, ↑ AST, ↑ BUN, ↓ neutrophils. **Urinary:** Proteinuria.	
Aptivus	ANTIRETROVIRAL (HIV/AIDS), Protease Inhibitor	See **tipranavir p 316**
AquaMEPHYTON	VITAMIN	See **vitamin K p 342**
Aquasol A	VITAMIN	See **vitamin A p 336**
ara-C	ANTINEOPLASTIC, Antimetabolite	See **cytarabine p 98**
Aranesp **darbepoetin**	ANTIANEMIC long acting **erythropoetin**	See **epoetin alfa p 126**
Arcapta Neohaler **indacaterol**- lactose	COPD TREATMENT, Beta2 Agonist, (Not for rapidly deteriorating COPD or asthma) Pwd for inhalation, long acting See listing for **salmeterol p 286**	

Aredia pamidronate	HYPERCALCEMIA TREATMENT	See **Bisphosphonates, Parenteral p 60**

arformoterol
  Brovana
	COPD TREATMENT, Beta-2 Agonist
	  Inhalation Soln, long acting
		See listing for **salmeterol p 286**

Aricept/Aricept ODT	ANTIALZHEIMER'S, Acetylcholinesterase Inhibitor	See **donepezil p 116**
Arimidex anastrozole	ANTINEOPLASTIC	See **Aromatase Inhibitors p 42**

aripiprazole
  Abilify
  Tab- lactose,
   cornstarch
  Soln-
   200 mg fructose/mL,
   400 mg sucrose/mL,
   propylene glycol
  Discmelt (ODT)-
   acesulfame K,
   aspartame, xylitol

  Vial for IM

ANTIPSYCHOTIC (Second Generation), ANTIMANIC (To treat Bipolar Disorder),
    ANTIDEPRESSANT (added to other antidepressant), TREATMENT OF
    IRRITABILITY IN AUTISM, (pt 6-17 yr old)   Oral or Parenteral (IM)
  Drug: Take s̄ regard to food.
  Dissolve ODT on tongue c̄ or s̄ liquid, swallow saliva.
  Diet: Oral forms- theoretical interaction c̄ grapefruit/related citrus, see p 390.
  Insure adequate fluid intake/hydration.
  Nutr: ↑ <u>WEIGHT</u>, primarily c̄ baseline BMI < 23. Anorexia, ↓ wt.
  Oral/GI: ↑ salivation, N/V, constipation, dry mouth, dyspepsia.
  S/Cond: Avoid alcohol. Not c̄ lactation. 99% serum pro bound.
  Not c̄ dehydration. Caution c̄ dysphagia. Caution c̄ seizures.
  Caution c̄ geriatric. ↑ risk of mortality in geriatrics c̄ dementia.
  Pregnancy: Category C.
  Other: <u>Headache</u>, <u>insomnia</u>, <u>sedation</u>, <u>drowsiness</u> (↑ in <u>CHILDREN</u>),
  <u>akathisia</u>, <u>blurred vision</u>, fatigue, pain, ↑ or ↓ BP, rhinitis, cough,
  flu syndrome, headache, restlessness, dyskinesia, dystonia, fever, anxiety,
  tremor, slightly ↑ QT interval, tachycardia, dizziness, rash,
  muscle cramps, depression, nervousness, confusion, abnormal gait, edema,
  chest/neck pain. Rare- NMS.
  Blood/Serum: < 1%- ↑ glucose, ↑ bil, ↑ crea, ↑ CPK, ↑ BUN,
  ↑ prolactin, ↑ ALT, ↑ AST.
  Monitor: Baseline wt then monthly.
  Baseline BP, FBS, lipids then at 12 wk, then at least annually.[1]

A

Aromasin ANTINEOPLASTIC See **Aromatase Inhibitors below**
  exemestane

Aromatase Inhibitors ANTINEOPLASTIC (Estrogen or Progesterone Receptor Positive Breast Cancer
                              in postmenopausal women)
Drug: Take **anastrozole** or **letrozole** s̄ regard to food.
Take **exemestane** once daily after a meal (test meal was 40% fat).
Nutr: <u>Anorexia</u>, ↓ wt, ↑ <u>appetite</u>, ↑ wt.
Oral/GI: <u>Dry mouth</u>, <u>N/V</u>, <u>pain</u>, <u>diarrhea</u>, <u>constipation</u>.
S/Cond: Caution c̄ lactation. **exemestane** is 90% serum pro bound.
Pregnancy: Category D.
Other: <u>HOT FLASHES</u>, <u>bone,</u> <u>joint</u> or <u>muscle pain</u>, <u>stiffness</u>, ↓ <u>BMD</u>, <u>osteopenia</u>, <u>weakness</u>,
<u>dizziness</u>, <u>headache</u>, <u>chest pain</u>, <u>dyspnea</u>, <u>cough</u>, <u>rash</u>, <u>edema</u>, <u>depression</u>, <u>paresthesia</u>, HTN, drowsiness,
insomnia, anxiety, deep vein thrombosis.
Blood/Serum: ↓ <u>ESTRADIOL</u>, anemia, ↓ WBC, ↑ GGT, ↑ AST, ↑ ALT, ↑ alk phos, ↑ bil, ↑ chol, ↑ LDL, ↑ Ca.
Monitor: Hepatic func, lipids. Baseline BMD, then yearly.[6]

anastrozole	**Arimidex**	Tab- lactose, Na starch gycolate
exemestane	**Aromasin**	Tab- mannitol, Na starch glycolate, sucrose
letrozole	**Femara**	Tab- lactose, maize starch, Na starch glycolate

Artane (generic equivalents) ANTIPARKINSON See **trihexyphenidyl p 324**

ASA ANALGESIC, ANTIPYRETIC, ANTIARTHRITIC, NSAID See **aspirin p 44**

Asacol ANTI-INFLAMMATORY (in ulcerative colitis) See **mesalamine p 209**

ascorbic acid VITAMIN See **vitamin C p 339**

Ascriptin NSAID, ANALGESIC, ANTIPYRETIC (buffered) See **aspirin p 44**

asenapine
 Saphris
 Sublingual tab-
 mannitol, gelatin

ANTIPSYCHOTIC (second generation), ANTIMANIC (bipolar 1 treatment)

Drug: Place tab under tongue & allow to dissolve completely.
Do not take food or drink for $\geq$ 10 min after administration.

Nutr: <u>Weight gain</u>, ↑ appetite.

Oral/GI: <u>Oral</u> <u>hypoesthesia</u>, dry mouth, ↑ salivation, glossodynia, swollen tongue, oral parasthesia, <u>vomiting</u>, stomach discomfort, <u>constipation</u>. Rare- dysphagia.

S/Cond: Avoid alcohol. Not c̄ lactation. 95% serum pro bound. Hypoalbuminemia (< 3g/dL) may ↑ drug effects.
Not c̄ severe ↓ hepatic func. Caution c̄ diabetes- possible ↑ glucose.
Caution c̄ geriatric. ↑ risk of mortality in geriatrics c̄ dementia.
Caution c̄ seizure disorders. Not c̄ hypokalemia, hypomagnesmia or cardiac arrhythmias- may prolong QT interval.

Pregnancy: Category C.

Other: <u>Dizziness</u>, <u>insomnia</u>, <u>EPS</u>, <u>akathisia</u>, <u>somnolence</u>, anxiety, depression, headache, fatigue, orthostatic hypotension, HTN, toothache, tachycardia.
Rare- NMS.

Blood/Serum: ↑ glucose, ↑ chol, ↑ TG, ↑ ALT, ↑ prolactin, ↓ Na.

Monitor: CBC, BP, wt, Hb A1$_C$, FBS, lipids at baseline and periodically.

Asmanex Twisthaler
 Pwd-anhydrous lactose (contains milk pro)

ANTI-ALLERGIC RHINITIS, Corticosteroid

See listing for **beclomethasone p 51**

aspirin — ANALGESIC, ANTIPYRETIC, ANTIARTHRITIC, NSAID, TO PREVENT CVA OR MI

ASA, acetylsalicylic acid
Aspirin
Ascriptin (buffered)
Regular Strength Tab-
 325 mg aspirin,
 24 mg each Mg & AlOH,
 171 mg $CaCO_3$
Ascriptin Maximun Strength
 500 mg aspirin
 237 mg $CaCO_3$
 33 mg each Mg & AlOH
 Both Tabs- cornstarch,
 sugar, mannitol, starch,
 propylene glycol,
 saccharin Na, sorbitol
Bayer Children's Aspirin
 Chew Tab-
 81 mg aspirin, saccharin
Bayer Low Dose
Adult Strength
 Tab (delayed release)
 81 mg aspirin, lactose
Bufferin (buffered)
 Tab- cornstarch, propylene
 glycol, simethicone
Ecotrin- enteric-coated
 325 mg Tab- starch, simethicone,
 Na starch glycolate
 81 mg Tab-
 propylene glycol, starch

Platelet Aggregation Inhibitor

Drug: Take c̄ 8 oz water or milk, after meals or c̄ food to ↓ GI irritation. Food ↓ rate of abs.[4] Swallow enteric-coated tab whole.

Diet: Insure adequate fluid intake/hydration. ↑ foods high in Vit C[13] & Fol[11] c̄ LT high dose. Avoid or limit natural products which affect coagulation (eg garlic, ginger, gingko, ginseng or horse chestnut). Limit caffeine to ↓ GI effects. **Nutr:** Anorexia.

Oral/GI: May cause sudden, serious gastric bleeding. N/V, DYSPEPSIA, black tarry stools.

S/Cond: Avoid alcohol. Caution c̄ lactation. Caution c̄ diabetes. Not for patient prone to Vit K def, bleeding disorder or gastritis/ulcer. ≥ 90% serum pro bound at low serum conc. Caution c̄ G6PD def- risk of hemolytic anemia. Do dental care cautiously- ↑ risk of bleeding. Not recommended for children, except in Kawasaki disease. Not c̄ tartrazine allergy, severe anemia, severe ↓ renal or ↓ hepatic func. New recommendations-low dose- 81 mg aspirin for men age 45-79 & women age 55-79 & those over 80 c̄ no other GI risk factors. GI risk usually offset by prevention of initial MI or CVA.[1]

Pregnancy: Category D.[7] Contraindicated in last trimester.[2]

Other: Rare- allergic reaction (↑ risk c̄ urticaria, asthma, nasal polyps)[2], angioedema, Reyes syndrome (especially in children), tinnitus, hepatotoxicity. May contribute to Fe def anemia. LT use may cause occult fecal blood loss.[14]

Blood/ Serum: ↓ PLATELET AGGREGATION, ↑ bleeding time, ↓ T_4, ↓ or ↑ uric acid (dose-related), ↓ K, ↑ AST, ↑ ALT, ↑ alk phos, ↓ Fe,[7] ↑ BUN, ↑ crea. Rare- ↓ WBC, ↓ platelets, anemia. High dose- ↑ or ↓ glucose, ↑ PT/INR, ↓ Fol,[11] possible ↓ Vit C. ↓ C-REACTIVE PRO (if ↑ prior to aspirin use).[6]

Urinary: ↑ Vit C, ↑ K, false ↑ or ↓ glucose (method related) c̄ high dose aspirin. + Pro. **Monitor:** HCT & renal func c̄ LT use or high dose.[6]

Aspirin Free Anacin — ANALGESIC — See **acetaminophen p 22**

Atacand/Atacand HCT candesartan	ANTIHYPERTENSIVE See **Angiotensin II Receptor Antagonists p 38** **Atacand HCT** also contains **hydrochlorothiazide** see **p 166**

Atarax (previous brand name)   ANTIHISTAMINE, ANTIANXIETY   See **hydroxyzine p 169**

atazanavir
Reyataz
Cap- lactose

ANTIRETROVIRAL (HIV/AIDS), Protease Inhibitor
Drug: Must take $\bar{c}$ food to ↑ bioavailability.
(research meal = 357-721 cal & 8-38 g fat)
Take 2 hr before or 1 hr after Ca, Mg suppl or antacids.
Diet: Avoid SJW, see p 286. **Oral/GI:** Nausea.
Nutr: ↓ stomach acidity greatly ↓ bioavailability of drug.
S/Cond: Not $\bar{c}$ lactation. Caution $\bar{c}$ mild-moderate ↓ hepatic func.
Not $\bar{c}$ severe ↓ hepatic func, achlorhydria. **Pregnancy:** Category B.
Other: Jaundice/scleral icterus, fever, muscle pain, lipodystrophy,
ECG PR prolongation.
Rare- photosensitivity, lactic acidosis syndrome (↑ in female, obesity).[7]
Blood/Serum: ↑ <u>BILIRUBIN</u>, ↑ AST, ↑ ALT, ↑ glucose, ↑ amylase, ↑ TG,
↑ HDL, slightly ↑ or ↓ LDL, ↑ or ↓ chol.
Monitor: Hepatic func, if history of hepatitis B or C.

atenolol
Tenormin
Tab- starch

ANTIHYPERTENSIVE, ANTIANGINAL, To Treat ACUTE MI
Cardioselective Beta-Blocker   Oral or Parenteral (IV) IV generic only
Drug: Take $\bar{s}$ regard to food. Take separately from orange juice.[111]
Diet: ↓ Na, ↓ cal may be recommended. Avoid natural licorice, see p 374.
Take 2 hr before or 6 hr after Ca suppl[3] or antacids.[9b]
Nutr: Ca salts or orange juice[111] may ↓ abs.[3] **Oral/GI:** Nausea, diarrhea.
S/Cond: Caution $\bar{c}$ lactation. Caution $\bar{c}$ diabetes- may mask signs of
hypoglycemia.[13] May reduce insulin release in response to hyperglycemia.[6]
Caution $\bar{c}$ severe ↓ renal func. Caution $\bar{c}$ asthma/bronchospasm.
Pregnancy: Category D.
Other: ↓ <u>*BP*</u> $\bar{c}$ possible hypotension.
<u>Dizziness</u>, drowsiness, fatigue, bradycardia, depression.
Blood/Serum: ↑ TG, ↓ HDL, ↑ lipoproteins, ↑ K, ↑ uric acid, ↑ BUN.
Monitor: BP, cardiac func, glucose $\bar{c}$ diabetes. Possibly renal func, CBC.[13]

Ativan
  lorazepam

ANTIANXIETY

See **Benzodiazepines p 54**

atomoxetine
  Strattera
  Cap- starch

ANTI-ADHD, Non-Stimulant, Selective Norepinephrine Reuptake Inhibitor
  Drug: Take s̄ regard to meals. High fat meal ↓ rate, but not extent of abs.
  Diet: Insure adequate cal intake.
  Nutr: ↓ appetite, ↓ wt, DELAYED GROWTH IN CHILDREN.
  Oral/GI: Dry mouth, N/V, dyspepsia, abdominal pain, constipation,
  diarrhea, flatulence.
  S/Cond: Caution c̄ lactation. 98% serum pro bound.
  Caution c̄ HTN, cardiovascular disease or ↓ hepatic func.
  CYP2D6 poor metabolizers may need ↓ dose.
  Pregnancy: Category C.
  Other: Fatigue, insomnia, erectile dysfunction, hot flushes, drowsiness,
  headache, sinusitis, irritability, dizziness, hypotension, mood swings,
  tearfulness, paresthesia, tremor, palpitations, ↑ HR, ↑ sweating, chills,
  dermatitis, menstrual disorders, rigors, cough, ↑ BP.
  Very rare- jaundice, hepatic injury, CVA, hypotension, syncope,
  suicidal thinking & behavior.
  Urinary: Retention/hesitancy.
  Monitor: Children's growth. S/S of suicidal thoughts.
  Possibly genetic testing for CYP2D6 status prior to use or if ↑ side effects.

atorvastatin
  Lipitor

ANTIHYPERLIPIDEMIC

See **HMG-CoA Reductase Inhibitors p 164**

Atripla
  Tab

ANTIRETROVIRAL (HIV/AIDS)
  Combination drug

See **efavirenz p 121**
emtricitabine p 123
tenofovir p 306

Atrovent/Atrovent HFA

BRONCHODILATOR

See **ipratropium p 178**

Augmentin
  (brand name discontinued)

ANTIBIOTIC

See **amoxicillin & clavulanate potassium p 32**

Avandamet **rosiglitazone** & **metformin** Combination drug Tab- lactose, Na starch glycolate	ANTIDIABETIC AGENT	See **thiazolidinediones p 312** See **metformin p 210**
Avandaryl **rosiglitazone** & **glimepiride** Combination drug Tab- lactose, Na starch glycolate	ANTIDIABETIC AGENT	See **thiazolidinediones p 312** See **sulfonylureas p 299**
Avandia rosiglitazone	ANTIDIABETIC AGENT	See **thiazolidinediones p 312**

Avapro/Avalide
  irbesartan
	ANTIHYPERTENSIVE See **Angiotensin II Receptor Antagonists p 38**
	  Avalide also contains **hydrochlorothiazide,** see p 166	

Avastin	ANTINEOPLASTIC, Angiogenesis Inhibitor See **bevacizumab p 56**	
Avelox	ANTIBIOTIC, Fluoroquinolone	See **moxifloxacin p 222**
Aviane	ORAL CONTRACEPTIVE	See **Oral Contraceptives p 237**
Avinza	ANALGESIC, Narcotic, Opioid See **morphine p 221** Controlled-release oral **morphine** for once daily administration	

Avodart
  dutasteride
  Cap
	BPH TREATMENT, Androgen Hormone Inhibitor See listing for **finasteride p 142**
	  5 alpha-reductase inhibitor for treatment of prostate hyperplasia
	    Drug: Swallow whole s̄ regard to food.	

Avonex	MULTIPLE SCLEROSIS TREATMENT	See **interferon beta-1a p 178**

Axert
  almotriptan
	ANTIMIGRAINE
	  Serotonin 5-HT$_1$ Receptor Agonist
		See **Antimigraine p 39**

Axid/Axid AR nizatadine	ANTIULCER, ANTIGERD, ANTISECRETORY	See **Histamine H$_2$ Receptor Antagonists p 162**

Axiron
(transdermal)

MALE HORMONE REPLACEMENT, PRIMARY HYPOGONADISM, HYPOGONADOTROPIC HYPOGONADISM, Androgen See **testosterone p 308**

azacitidine
Vidaza
100 mg mannitol/vial

ANTINEOPLASTIC, Nucleoside Metabolic Inhibitor (Myelodysplastic Syndrome)
Parenteral (SC or IV)

Nutr: Anorexia, ↓ wt.
Oral/GI: Dysphagia, oral bleeding, stomatitis, glossitis, NAUSEA/VOMITING, dyspepsia, abdominal pain, CONSTIPATION, hemorrhoids, diarrhea.
S/Cond: Not c̄ lactation. Do dental care cautiously, see p 11 & 15.
Caution c̄ ↓ hepatic func.
Pregnancy: Category D. Man should not father child during treatment.
Other: FEVER, JOINT PAIN, muscle pain/cramps, edema, chest/back/limb pain, fatigue, lethargy, headache, weakness, dizziness, insomnia, anxiety, confusion, pallor, ↑ sweating, shivering, dyspnea, cough, URTI, pneumonia, bruising, cellulitis, rash, hypotension, syncope, tachycardia, cardiac murmur. IV- petechiae, rigors.
Blood/Serum: Anemia, ↑ crea, ↓ K, ↓ WBC, ↓ PLATELETS. **Urinary:** Dysuria, UTI.
Monitor: Baseline & at least prior to each treatment cycle- CBC c̄ diff, renal func. Baseline hepatic func.

Azactam

ANTIBIOTIC, Monobactam   See **aztreonam p 49**

azathioprine
Imuran
Tab- lactose,
  potato starch
Azasan
Tab- lactose,
  starch, cornstarch

IMMUNOSUPPRESSANT (Renal Transplants),
ANTIARTHRITIC (Rheumatoid arthritis)   Oral or Parenteral (IV)
Drug: May take c̄ food to ↓ GI upset. **Nutr:** Anorexia.
Oral/GI: Stomatitis, esophagitis, N/V, diarrhea, steatorrhea.
S/Cond: Not c̄ lactation. Do dental care cautiously, see p 11 & 15.
Caution c̄ ↓ renal or ↓ hepatic func. **Pregnancy:** Category D.
Other: Bone marrow suppression (may be delayed), rash, ↑ infection, neoplasia, hepatotoxicity (↑ risk c̄ transplants). Acute pancreatitis (↑ risk c̄ Crohn's disease).[95]
Blood/Serum: ↓ WHITE BLOOD CELLS, ↓ PLATELETS, macrocytic anemia, ↑ MCV, ↑ AST, ↑ ALT, ↑ bil, ↑ alk phos, ↓ uric acid, ↑ amylase, ↓ alb.
Urinary: ↓ uric acid. **Monitor:** CBC weekly X 1 month, then 2X/month, then 1X/month. Hepatic func.

Azilect PARKINSON'S TREATMENT, MAO-B Inhibitor   See **rasagiline p 275**

azithromycin ANTIBIOTIC, Macrolide   Oral or Parenteral (IV)
Zithromax
Tab- lactose, starch
Pwd for Susp- sucrose,
xanthan gum
Zithromax IV
Z-Pak
(pack of 6, 250 mg tabs)
Zmax (SR)
microspheres for
oral susp- sucrose,
xanthan gum

Drug: May take all forms s̄ regard to food, except **Zmax**- take on empty
stomach ≥ 1 hr before or ≥ 2 hr after food.
Take **Zithromax** or **Z-Pak** c̄ food if GI distress occurs.
Do not take c̄ Al or Mg antacids or suppl.
Oral/GI: Stomatitis c̄ IV, N/V, abdominal pain, <u>diarrhea</u>.
Rare- pseudomembranous colitis.
S/Cond: Caution c̄ lactation. Caution c̄ ↓ hepatic or severe ↓ renal func.
Pregnancy: Category B. **Other:** Fever, joint pain, vaginitis.
Rare- photosensitivity, allergic reaction, SJS, TEN.
IV- Dizziness, headache, dyspnea.
Blood/Serum: ↑ CPK, ↑ AST, ↑ ALT, ↑ GGT, ↑ K.
< 1%- dyscrasias, ↑ BUN, ↑ crea, ↑ P, ↑ LDH, ↑ alk phos, ↑ bil, ↑ glucose.
Monitor: Possibly hepatic func c̄ LT oral use or IV.[26]

Azmacort ANTIASTHMA, Inhalant   See **triamcinolone p 322**

Azor ANTIHYPERTENSIVE
amlodipine & **olmesartan**   Combination drug   See **Angiotensin II Receptor Antagonists p 38**
Tab- starch   See **amlodipine p 32**

aztreonam ANTIBIOTIC, Monobactam   Parenteral (IM or IV)[a], Inhalation soln[b]
Azactam[a]
Pwd- Na free
Cayston[b]
Vial- sterile lyophilized
pwd
Ampule- sterile diluent

Drug: Use inhalation soln immediately after reconstitution.
Administer only c̄ Altera Nebulizer System
Oral/GI: Altered taste (IV only), N/V[a, b], diarrhea[a].
< 1%- pseudomembranous colitis.[a]
S/Cond: Not c̄ lactation. Caution c̄ ↓ renal func or ↓ hepatic func.
Pregnancy: Category B. **Other:** Rash[a], wheezing[b], <u>fever</u>[b], cough[b],
nasal congestion[b], pharyngolaryngeal pain[b], abdominal pain[b].
Blood/Serum: <u>Eosinophilia</u>, ↑ crea, ↑ PT/INR, ↑ platelets, ↑ PTT.
< 1%- dyscrasias, ↑ <u>AST</u>, ↑ <u>ALT</u>, ↑ <u>alk phos</u>, ↑ LDH.[7]
Urinary: False glucose results c̄ CuSO₄. **Monitor:** Hepatic & renal func.

A

Bacid	BIOTHERAPEUTIC AGENT	See **lactobacillus p 186**

baclofen
   Lioresal
   Tablets- generic only
   Lioresal Intrathecal
   preservative free

SKELETAL MUSCLE RELAXANT, ANTISPASMODIC   Oral & Intrathecal
Intrathecal form used to treat spinal cord origin spasticity, eg brain injury, MS.
Oral/GI: Dry mouth, altered taste, <u>N/V</u>, <u>constipation</u>.
S/Cond: Avoid alcohol. Not c̄ lactation. Caution c̄ diabetes- may ↑ glucose.
Caution c̄ seizures or psychotic disorder. Caution c̄ ↓ renal func.
Pregnancy: Category C.
Other: <u>DROWSINESS</u>, <u>dizziness</u>, <u>weakness</u>, <u>confusion</u>, <u>headache</u>,
depression, insomnia, ↓ BP, edema. Rare- seizures, psychosis.
↓ alcohol craving/intake in alcoholics.[88]
Blood/Serum: ↑ alk phos, ↑ AST, ↑ ALT, ↑ glucose.
Urinary: ↑ frequency, retention.

Bactrim	ANTIBIOTIC	See **trimethoprim c̄ sulfamethoxazole p 324**

balsalazide
   Colazal- 86 mg Na/Cap

ANTI-INFLAMMATORY, pro-drug of **mesalamine**
   S/Cond: 99% serum pro bound.   See listing for **mesalamine p 209**

Baraclude	ANTIVIRAL, Hepatitis B Treatment	See **entecavir p 124**

Bayer Aspirin Tab- cornstarch	ANALGESIC, ANTIINFLAMMATORY ANTITHROMBOTIC, ANTIPYRETIC	See **aspirin p 44**

Bayer Extra Strength   ANALGESIC   See **aspirin p 44**
   Tab- starch, propylene glycol
Bayer Extra Strengh Back and Body   Combination drug   See **aspirin p 44**
   Tab- cornstarch   See **caffeine p 67**
Bayer Quick Release Crystals
   Aspartame, sucralose, isomalt

belimumab
Benlysta

TO TREAT ADULT PATIENTS WITH ACTIVE AUTOANTIBODY POSITIVE-SYSTEMIC LUPUS ERYTHEMATOSIS ON STANDARD THERAPY,
Monoclonal Antibody   Parenteral only (IV)

Drug: Administer IV over period of 1 hr c̄ prophlaxis for infusion & hypersensitivity reactions.
Oral/GI: Nausea, diarrhea, viral gastroenteritis.
S/Cond: Not c̄ lactation. Not c̄ live vaccines.
Pregnancy: Category C.
Other: Infusion reactions, (bradycardia, muscle pain, headache, rash, urticaria, hypotension, nausea, skin reactions), hypersensitivity reactions, depression, nasopharyngitis, pharyngitis, fever, bronchitis, insomnia, extremity pain, migraine, serious infection.
<1%- anaphylaxis, suicidal thinking and behavior, death.
Blood/Serum: ↓ WBC.
Urinary: UTI.
Monitor: S/S of hypersensitivity, infusion reactions. S/S of infection.

beclomethasone
Beconase- Nasal Inhaler
Beconase AQ- Nasal Spray

QVAR Oral Inhalant-
CFC-free

ANTIASTHMA (Oral inhaler), ANTIALLERGIC RHINITIS (Nasal)
Drug: Rinse mouth after use of oral inhaler. Do not swallow rinse water.
Oral/GI: ↓ sense of taste, <u>sore throat</u>, N/V.
Oral only- <u>OROPHARYNGEAL</u> <u>FUNGAL</u> <u>INFECTION</u>.
S/Cond: Nasal- Caution c̄ lactation. Oral- Not c̄ lactation.
Pregnancy: Category C.
Other: <u>NASOPHARYNGEAL</u> <u>IRRITATION</u>, nose bleed, cough, dizziness, headache.
Corticosteroid effects, especially c̄ LT high dose, see p 94.
Rare- cataracts, glaucoma, ↑ intraocular pressure.

B

belatacept
 Nulojix
 Vial- lyophilized pwd

IMMUNOSUPPRESSANT, Prophylaxis of Organ Rejection in Kidney Transplant
Parenteral (IV only)

Drug: Dose is based on actual body wt. Dose must be evenly divisible by 12.5 mg in order to prepare dose accurately using reconstituted soln and silicone free disposable syringe.

Oral/GI: DIARRHEA, CONSTIPATION, NAUSEA, VOMITING, abdominal pain, stomatitis.

S/Cond: Not c̄ lactation. Not c̄ live vaccines. Not in seronegative pts. Not c̄ liver transplants.

Pregnancy: Category C.

Other: HEADACHE, HYPERTENSION, COUGH, PERIPHERAL EDEMA, FEVER, ↓ BP, dyspnea, graft dysfunction, joint/back pain, renal tubular necrosis, URTI, nasopharyngitis, CMV infection, influenza, bronchitis, dizziness, tremor, acne, insomnia, anxiety, herpes viral infection, atrial fibrillation, polyoma viral infection, TB.
Rare- progressive multi focal leukoencephalopathy.

Blood/Serum: ↓ HEMOGLOBIN, ↓ HEMATOCRIT, ↓ WBC, ↓ neutrophils, ↑ or ↓ POTASSIUM, ↓ P, ↑ glucose, ↓ Ca, ↑ chol, ↑ crea, ↓ Mg, uric acid.

Urinary: UTI, hematuria, pro.

Monitor: Test for Epstein Barr Virus serostatus and latent TB prior to initiation of therapy. Monitor for new or worsening neurological, cognitive or behavioral S/S of lymphoproliferative disorder.
S/S of infection.

| Benadryl | ANTIHISTAMINE, Sleep Aid | See **diphenhydramine p 112** |
| **benazepril**
    Lotensin/Lotensin HCT | ANTIHYPERTENSIVE | See **Angiotensin Converting**
Enzyme Inhibitors p 36 |

Lotensin HCT also contains **hydrochlorothiazide**, see **p 166**

| **Benefiber** | LAXATIVE, Bulk Forming | See **wheat dextrin p 345** |
| **Benicar/Benicar HCT**
    olmesartan | ANTIHYPERTENSIVE | See **Angiotensin II Receptor Antagonists p 38** |

Benicar HCT also contains **hydrochlorothiazide,** see **p 166**

| **Bentyl/Bentylol** | ANTISPASMOTIC | See **dicyclomine p 108** |

Benzodiazepines   ANTIANXIETY (a), SKELETAL MUSCLE RELAXANT (b), ANTIEPILEPTIC (c), ANTIPANIC (d), SLEEP AID (e), ACUTE ALCOHOL WITHDRAWAL (f), ANESTHESIA ADJUNCT (Parenteral) (g)

Drug: May take c̄ food if GI distress occurs. Mix intensol c̄ $\geq$ 30 mL water, juice, soda or c̄ semi-solid food. Dissolve ODT on tongue c̄ or s̄ liquid, swallow saliva. **Clobazam** tab may be swallowed whole c̄ or s̄ food or crushed & put into applesauce.

Diet: Limit caffeine to < 400-500 mg/day,[9b] see p 379. Caution c̄ grapefruit/related citrus c̄ oral **clobazam diazepam**, **triazolam** or **midazolam**,[9b] see p 390. Caution c̄ sedative herbal products, eg chamomile or kava (↑ sedative effect) or stimulant products, eg caffeine, guarana, mate (↓ sedative effect).[4] Caution c̄ echinacea c̄ **midazolam**- ↓ drug levels.[4] Avoid SJW c̄ **alprazolam**, **clobazam**, **clonazepam**, **diazepam** or **midazolam**.[3]

Nutr: Anorexia, ↓ wt. ↑ appetite, ↑ wt c̄ **alprazolam** or **chlordiazepoxide**. ↑ thirst.

Oral/GI: Dry mouth, ↑ salivation, N/V, constipation, diarrhea.

S/Cond: Avoid alcohol. Not c̄ lactation. May be habit forming c̄ LT use. Caution c̄ geriatric,[84] debilitated, ↓ hepatic func or ↓ renal func. Caution c̄ soy or egg allergy c̄ parenteral. ↑ drug effect c̄ **clobazam** in CYP2C19 poor metabolizers.

Chlordiazepoxide, **diazepam**, **flurazepam**, **midazolam**, **oxazepam**, **temazepam** are > 94% serum pro bound- hypoalbuminemia (< 3 g/dL) may ↑ drug effects.

Caution c̄ obesity c̄ **diazepam**, **lorazepam**, **midazolam**, **oxazepam**- ↑ time for drug clearance.[91]

Pregnancy: Category D.[13] **Clobazam**- Category C. **temazepam**, **triazolam** & **flurazepam**- Category X.[23]

Other: SOMNOLENCE (**clobazam**) drowsiness, sedation, ataxia, fatigue, dizziness, confusion, slurred speech, headache, tremor, blurred vision, depression, hypotension, tachycardia, palpitations. Anterograde amnesia (↑ c̄ **triazolam**).[13] Rare- rash, jaundice, photosensitivity, paradoxical reaction, suicidal thinking & behavior c̄ **clobazam**.

flurazpam, temazepam & **triazolam** - rare- parasomnias c̄ amnesia (eg sleep walking).

Blood/Serum: ↑ AST, ↑ ALT, ↑ LDH, ↑ bil, ↑ alk phos. Rare- dyscrasias. **diazepam**[7]- ↓ T4.

Urinary: Retention, incontinence. **diazepam** only- False negative glucose c̄ Clinistix or Diastix.[6]

Monitor: CBC c̄ diff, hepatic & renal func c̄ LT use.

alprazolam [a d]	**Xanax** Tab- lactose, cornstarch **Xanax XR** [d] Tab- lactose **Alprazolam Intensol** conc
	Niravam ODT- cornstarch, mannitol, sucralose, sucrose
chlordiazepoxide [a f g]	**Librium** Cap- lactose, cornstarch Parenteral (IM or IV)- 1.5% benzyl alcohol
clobazam [c]	**Onfi** (Antiepileptic for Lennox Gastaut Syndrome) Tab- corn starch, lactose

clonazepam [c d (also as a)]	**Klonopin** Tab- lactose, cornstarch **Klonopin Wafer** (ODT)- gelatin, mannitol
clorazepate [a c f]	**Tranxene** SD Tab- lactose
diazepam [a b c f g]	**Valium** Tab- lactose, cornstarch, starch

clonazepam [c d (also as a)]
clorazepate [a c f]
diazepam [a b c f g]

Klonopin Tab- lactose, cornstarch   **Klonopin Wafer** (ODT)- gelatin, mannitol
Tranxene SD Tab- lactose
Valium Tab- lactose, cornstarch, starch
Parenteral (IM or IV)- 10% ethyl alcohol, 1.5% benzyl alcohol
Diazepam Intensol- 19% alcohol   **Diastat Rectal**- 10% ethyl alcohol,
1.5% benzyl alcohol
Parenteral (IV)- may contain soybean oil, egg yolk phospholipids

flurazepam [e]
lorazepam [a c g (also as e f)]

Dalmane Cap
Ativan Tab- lactose   **Intensol**- alcohol free
Parenteral (IM or IV)- 2% benzyl alcohol

midazolam [g]
oxazepam [a f (also as e)]
temazepam [e]
triazolam [e]

Versed Oral Syrup- sorbitol, saccharin Parenteral (IV)- 1% benzyl alcohol
Cap- lactose   Tab- tartrazine, lactose. **Serax** brand discontinued.
Restoril Cap- lactose, may contain benzyl alcohol
Halcion Tab- lactose, docusate Na

benzphetamine
  Didrex

APPETITE SUPPRESSANT   See **amphetamines p 33**

benztropine
  Cogentin generic equivalents
  Tab- lactose,
  Na starch glycolate-potato
  Parenteral
    4 mg (0.17 mEq) Na/mL

ANTIPARKINSON, ANTI-EPS, Anticholinergic   Oral or Parenteral (IM or IV)
Drug: May take c̄ food to ↓ GI upset.
Oral/GI: <u>DRY MOUTH</u>, N/V, epigastric distress, <u>constipation</u>, paralytic ileus.
S/Cond: Avoid alcohol. May inhibit lactation.
↑ risk of dental problems, see p 11 & 15. Caution in hot weather.
Will not improve & may aggravate tardive dyskinesia.[7]
Caution c̄ geriatrics- ↑ CNS effects. Caution c̄ BPH, glaucoma.
Pregnancy: Category C.
Other: <u>CONFUSION</u>, <u>DEPRESSION</u>, <u>drowsiness</u>, <u>blurred vision</u>, ↓ <u>sweating</u> &
hyperthermia, dizziness, photosensitivity, memory impairment,
hallucinations, dry eyes, weakness, muscle cramps, hand or foot
numbness, tachycardia, hypotension.[17]
Urinary: <u>Retention</u>, pain.

B

beta carotene

PROVITAMIN (precursor of Vitamin A) ANTIOXIDANT   See **vitamin A p 336**

Used to ↓ photosensitivity in erythropoietic protoporphyria.

Diet: Pectin ↓ abs of beta carotene- generally not clinically significant.[3a]

Nutr: No known toxicity.[93] Very low fat diet ↓ abs of beta carotene.[47c]

Pregnancy: Category C. No problems documented up to 30 mg/day (5,000 RE).[13]

Other: Yellow/orange skin c̄ high dose (> 30 mg/day for at least 2-6 wk).[6, 10b]

Betapace/Betapace AF

ANTIARRHYTHMIC, Non-selective Beta Blocker   See **sotalol p 296**

Betaseron

MULTIPLE SCLEROSIS TREATMENT   See **interferon beta-1b p 178**

bevacizumab
  Avastin
  preservative free

ANTINEOPLASTIC, Angiogenesis Inhibitor (Colon CA, Renal Ca)

Also used to Treat Breast Ca   Parenteral only (IV)

Nutr: <u>Anorexia</u>, ↓ <u>wt</u>.

Oral/GI: <u>Dry</u> <u>mouth</u>, <u>stomatitis</u>, <u>taste</u> <u>changes</u>, <u>dyspepsia</u>, <u>N/V</u>, <u>abdominal pain</u>, <u>colitis</u>, <u>constipation</u>, <u>diarrhea</u>, <u>GI</u> <u>hemorrhage</u>/perforation (may be fatal), flatulence.

S/Cond: Not c̄ lactation. Suspend use c̄ proteinuria, uncontrolled HTN, nephrotic syndrome or surgery. Do dental care cautiously, see p 11 & 15.

Pregnancy: Category C.

Other: <u>Deep</u> <u>vein</u> <u>thrombosis</u>, <u>hypertension</u>, <u>hypotension</u>, <u>dizziness</u>, <u>headache</u>, <u>nosebleed</u>, <u>URTI</u>, <u>dyspnea</u>, ↑ <u>tearing</u>, <u>skin ulcer</u>, <u>slow</u> <u>wound</u> <u>healing</u>, <u>voice</u> <u>changes</u>, <u>hair</u> <u>loss</u>, syncope, weakness, muscle pain, edema, stroke, CHF, MI, angina.

Blood/Serum: ↓ <u>WBC</u>, ↓ <u>platelets</u>, ↓ K, ↑ bil.

Urinary: <u>Proteinuria</u>, ↑ frequency.

Monitor: BP, CBC c̄ diff, platelets, electrolytes, urinalysis.

Beyaz

ORAL CONTRACEPTIVE   See **Oral Contraceptives p 237**

Biaxin/Biaxin XL

ANTIBIOTIC, Macrolide   See **clarithromycin p 87**

bicalutamide
  Casodex
  Tab- lactose,
  Na starch glycolate

ANTINEOPLASTIC (Prostate Cancer), Antiandrogen, used in combo c̄ LHRH analog

Diet: Take s̄ regard to food.

Nutr: <u>Anorexia</u>, ↓ <u>wt</u>.

Oral/GI: Dry mouth, <u>N/V</u>, <u>dyspepsia</u>, <u>abdominal pain</u>, <u>flatulence</u>, <u>diarrhea</u>,

CONSTIPATION.
S/Cond: Avoid alcohol. Not for women.
Caution c̄ moderate to severe ↓ hepatic func.
Pregnancy: Category X.
Other: HOT FLASHES, WEAKNESS, PAIN, BACK PAIN, dyspnea, ↑ BP,
gynecomastia, breast pain, bone pain, infection, headache, rash,
sweating, dizziness, paresthesia, anxiety, insomnia, edema, cough,
flu syndrome, rhinitis, bronchitis, pharyngitis, depression, pneumonia,
hair loss. Rare- jaundice, neuropathy.
Blood/Serum: ↑ AST, ↑ ALT, ↑ bil, ↑ alk phos, ↑ glucose, ↑ BUN,
↑ crea, anemia, ↓ WBC.
Urinary: Hematuria, retention, ↑ frequency.
Monitor: Hepatic func, PSA.

bicillin L-A/bicillin CR	ANTIBIOTIC	See **penicillin p 249**
BiCNU	ANTINEOPLASTIC, Alkylating Agent	See **carmustine p 249**
Bidil	CHF TREATMENT ADJUNCT for Black Patients	See **hydralazine p 166**
Tab- lactose, Na starch glycolate	Combination drug	See **isosorbide p 180**

bisacodyl LAXATIVE, Stimulant Oral Tab or Rectal Suppository
  Dulcolax Enteric-Coated
  Tab- lactose,
  sucrose, cornstarch
  Rectal Suppository
  Ex-Lax Ultra
  Tab- alcohol, lactose
  Fleet Stimulant Laxative
  Enteric-Coated
  Tab- lactose, gelatin,
  cornstarch, sucrose,
  Na starch glycolate

Drug: Take PM on empty stomach c̄ 8 oz water or juice. Swallow tab
whole. Do not crush or chew. Do not take within 1 hr of milk/milk products,
Ca or Mg suppl (to protect enteric coating).
Diet: High fiber c̄ 1500-2000 mL fluid/day to prevent constipation.
Nutr: ↓ wt.
Oral/GI: ↑ INTESTINAL PERISTALSIS. Nausea, belching,
abdominal cramps, diarrhea.
LT use- laxative dependence, malabsorption, steatorrhea.
S/Cond: Not c̄ lactation. ↓ K in dialysis patients.
Pregnancy: Stimulant laxatives should be avoided.[2]
Blood/Serum: LT use- ↓ K, ↓ Ca.

bismuth subsalicylate
  Pepto-Bismol
  $\leq$ 12 mg Na/dose
  Liquid- saccharin
  Chew Tab & Caplet-
   mannitol, saccharin
  Kaopectate- Liquid, Cap
  Maalox Total Stomach Relief
  Liquid- xanthan gum,
   sorbitol, sucralose,
   propylene glycol

ANTIDIARRHEAL, ANTINAUSEANT   See also **aspirin p 44**
  Drug: Chew chewable tabs well.
  Oral/GI: Temporary darkening of tongue, mouth & stool.
  Constipation. Impaction (debilitated geriatric & children).
  S/Cond: Caution $\bar{c}$ lactation $\bar{c}$ chronic use.
  Bismuth > 90% serum pro bound, but < 1% abs.[13]
  Not $\bar{c}$ salicylate/aspirin allergy. Caution $\bar{c}$ diabetics on insulin or
  oral agents- large doses ↑ risk of hypoglycemia.
  Avoid $\bar{c}$ children- aspirin ↑ risk of Reyes syndrome.
  Pregnancy: aspirin- Category D.[7]
  Blood/Serum: ↑ or ↓ uric acid, ↓ K, ↓ T_4, ↓ T_3, ↑ alk phos, ↑ AST,
  ↑ ALT.
  Urinary: False + glucose ($CuSO_4$).

bisoprolol
  Zebeta
  Tab- cornstarch
  Ziac
  also contains
  hydrochlorothiazide,
  see **p 166**
  Tabs- cornstarch
  2.5 mg Tab also
  contains starch

ANTIHYPERTENSIVE, Cardioselective Beta-Blocker
  Drug: Take $\bar{s}$ regard to food.
  Diet: Possible ↓ Na, ↓ cal. Avoid natural licorice, see p 374.
  Oral/GI: N/V, diarrhea.
  S/Cond: Caution $\bar{c}$ lactation. Caution $\bar{c}$ diabetes- may mask signs of
  hypoglycemia. May reduce insulin release in response to hyperglycemia.
  Caution $\bar{c}$ ↓ renal func or severe ↓ hepatic func or cirrhosis.
  Caution $\bar{c}$ asthma/bronchospasm.
  Pregnancy: Category C.
  Other: ↓ _BP_ $\bar{c}$ possible hypotension. <u>Fatigue</u>, rash, weakness.
  Blood/Serum: ↑ <u>AST</u>, ↑ <u>ALT</u>, + <u>ANA</u>, ↑ TG.
  Monitor: BP.

Bisphosphonates, Oral OSTEOPOROSIS TREATMENT[a] or PREVENTION[b],
PAGET'S DISEASE TREATMENT[c] HETEROTOPIC OSSIFICATION TREATMENT or PREVENTION[d]

Drug: Swallow c̄ 6-8 oz <u>plain</u> <u>water</u> <u>only</u>. (Avoid water c̄ high mineral content). Do not chew or break.
Take **alendronate** or **risedronate** at least 30 minutes or **ibandronate** at least 60 minutes before first food,
beverage or other medication/suppl of the day. Abs optimal if taken 2 hours before food.
Take **risedronate** DR (**Atelvia**) once a week after breakfast. Do not take antacids, Ca, Mg, or
Fe suppl concurrently c̄ **risedronate DR** (**Atelvia**). Do not lie down for at least 30 minutes (60 minutes c̄
ibandronate) & until after the first food of the day. Do not take HS. Take **alendronate** or **risedronate**
35 or 70 mg tab once a week on the same day of the week. Take **ibandronate** 150 mg tab once a
month on the same day of the month. Take **risedronate 75** mg Tab- twice a month, 2 days in a row.
Take **etidronate** 2 hr before or 2 hr after food or mineral suppl c̄ full glass of water. May take at HS.
Follow package schedule (**Didrocal**).
Diet: Adequate Ca & Vit D intake essential. Suppl may be needed (total 1500 mg Ca & 800 IU Vit D in divided doses).
Oral/GI: Dysphagia, esophageal ulcer &/or erosions, esophagitis, abdominal pain, constipation,
diarrhea, flatulence. **S/Cond:** Avoid alcohol. Not c̄ lactation. Caution c̄ dysphagia or upper GI disease.
Limit or stop smoking. Not c̄ hypocalcemia- must be corrected before use of drug. Not c̄ severe ↓ renal func.
Pregnancy: Category C.
Other: ↓ <u>BONE</u> <u>RESORPTION</u>. ↑ <u>BONE</u> <u>MINERAL</u> <u>DENSITY</u>. Headache, musculoskeletal pain (may be severe).
Rare- jaw osteonecrosis, blurred vision, eye pain/inflammation.
Blood/Serum: <u>TRANSIENT</u> <u>MILD</u> ↓ <u>Ca</u>, mild ↓ P. **etidronate** - Rare- ↓ WBC, ↓ RBC, ↓ platelets.
Monitor: Possibly alk phos level.[13] Bone density. Dental exam prior to use.

alendronate	etidronate	ibandronate	risedronate
Fosamax [a][b][c] (daily)	**Didronel** [c][d]	**Boniva** [a][b]	**Actonel** [a][b][c]
Tab- lactose	Tab- lactose free, starch	Tab- lactose	Tab- lactose
5 or 10 mg (daily)	200 mg (daily for Paget's)	2.5 mg (daily)	5 mg (daily)
35 mg (once weekly)	400 mg (cyclical therapy)	150 mg	35 mg (once weekly)
40 mg (daily for Paget's)		(once monthly)	30 mg (daily for Paget's)
Fosamax 70 [a] (once weekly)	**Didrocal** [a][b]- 90 day pack c̄ 14 days **etidronate**,		**Actonel 75**[a] (monthly-2 days)
Tab- lactose	then 76 days **Ca Carbonate** 500 mg Ca/day.		Tab- does not contain lactose
Soln- saccharin Na	**Ca Carbonate** tab- starch		**Actonel 150**[a] once monthly Tab
Fosamax Plus D [a] (once weekly)			Tab- does not contain lactose
Tab- lactose, sucrose, gelatin, modified food starch			**Atelvia DR** 35 mg weekly tab
70 mg **alendronate** + 2800 IU or 5600 IU			Tab- simethicone,
cholecalciferol, see also **vitamin D p 340**			polyethylene glycol, EDTA

Bisphosphonates, Parenteral OSTEOPOROPSIS TREATMENT[a], PAGET'S DISEASE TREATMENT[b],
HYPERCALCEMIA OF MALIGNANCY THERAPY[c],
ADJUNCT TO TREATMENT OF BONE METASTASES[d],
Ca Regulator   Parenteral only (IV)

Drug: To treat hypercalcemia- insure adequate fluid intake/hydration for urine output of 2 L/day,
but avoid overload. For **Reclast** drink $\geq$ 2 glasses fluids within a few hr of infusion.

Diet: To treat hypercalcemia- Avoid Ca or Vit D suppl. Maintain well balanced diet c̄ adequate, not
excessive Ca & Vit D. May need ↑ P or P suppl.[7]
To treat osteoporosis- adequate Ca/Vit D intake or suppl- 1200 mg Ca & 400-800 IU Vit D in divided doses.
To treat Paget's 1500 mg Ca & 800 IU Vit D in divided doses.

Nutr: Anorexia. **Oral/GI:** N/V, abdominal pain, GI bleeding, constipation, diarrhea.

S/Cond: Not c̄ lactation. Caution c̄ moderate ↓ renal func, ↓ alb or dyscrasias. Not c̄ severe ↓ renal func.
Avoid invasive dental surgery.

Pregnancy: Category D.

Other: ↓ BONE RESORPTION. FEVER, musculoskeletal pain (may be severe), fatigue, headache, edema, rash.
c̄ high dose- HTN, drowsiness, syncope, tachycardia, hypothyroidism.
Rare- jaw osteonecrosis, visual problems - including scleritis.[1]

Blood/Serum: ↓ CALCIUM, ↓ phosphate, ↓ Mg, ↓ K, ↓ WBC, ↑ BUN, ↑ crea. Anemia c̄ high dose.

Monitor: Ca (correct for ↓ alb), P, electrolytes, Mg, CBC c̄ diff, renal func. Dental exam prior to use.

ibandronate[a]	**Boniva Injection** (once q 3 mo)
pamidronate[b c d]	**Aredia** Pwd in vial- mannitol
zoledronic acid	**Zometa**[c d] Vial- 220 mg mannitol/5mL
	Reclast[a b] mannitol (one dose for Paget's or once a year for osteoporosis)

Bladder Control Agents   ANTIMUSCARINIC, ANTISPASMODIC, ANTICHOLINERGIC

Drug: Swallow SR forms whole c̄ liquid- do not chew, crush or divide. **Darifenacin, fesoterodine, oxybutynin, solifenacin, tolteradine-** take s̄ regard to food. May take c̄ food or milk to ↓ GI distress. **trospium-** Take on empty stomach 1 hr before meals.

Diet: Darifenacin, fesoterodine, solifenacin, tolteradine, oral **oxybutynin-** Theoretical interaction c̄ grapefruit/related citrus, see p 390.

Oral/GI: DRY MOUTH & throat, ↓ salivation causing dysphagia, reflux, dyspepsia, abdominal pain, N/V, flatulence, diarrhea, constipation.

S/Cond: Avoid alcohol. Drug ↓ lactation. **Darifenacin, oxybutynin, trospium-** caution c̄ lactation. **Fesoterodine, solifenacin** & **tolteradine-** not c̄ lactation.

↑ risk of dental problems, see p 11 & 15.

Not c̄ urinary or gastric retention, uncontrolled narrow angle glaucoma.

Caution c̄ ↓ hepatic func or ↓ renal func, HTN, controlled glaucoma, GERD, GI obstruction, colitis, myasthenia gravis.

Caution c̄ geriatric.[84]

Darifenacin, solifenacin, tolteradine- 96-98% serum pro bound.

Pregnancy: Category C, except **oxybutynin-** Category B.

Other: Drowsiness, dizziness, palpitations, tachycardia, dry eyes, ↑ BP, blurred vision, ↓ sweating, weakness, fatigue, hallucinations, insomnia, restlessness, headache, flushing, rash.

Urinary: ↓ URGENCY, ↓ FREQUENCY, ↑ CAPACITY. RETENTION, hesitancy.

(Note- less anticholinergic side effects c̄ patch vs. oral forms).

darifenacin	fesoterodine	oxybutynin	solifenacin	tolterodine	trospium
Enablex (SR)	**Toviaz (SR)**	**Ditropan**	**Vesicare** (SR)	**Detrol**	**Sanctura**
Tab- lactose	Tab- lactose	Tab- lactose, cornstarch	Tab- lactose, cornstarch	Tab- Na starch glycolate	Tab- sucrose, lactose,
	Syrup- sorbitol, sucrose			**Detrol LA** (SR)	wheat starch,
		Ditropan XL (SR)		Tab- Na starch glycolate,	$CaCO_3$
		Tab- lactose		sucrose,	**Sanctura SR**
		Oxytrol Patch		sugar spheres	Cap
		Gelnique 10% Topical Gel- alcohol, gelatin			

bleomycin
Blenoxane

ANTINEOPLASTIC, Antibiotic   Parenteral only (IM, IV, SC or intrapleural)
(used in many different malignancies- see PI)
Diet: Insure adequate fluid intake/hydration.
Nutr: <u>ANOREXIA</u>, ↓ <u>wt</u>. **Oral/GI:** <u>STOMATITIS</u>, <u>NAUSEA/VOMITING</u>.
S/Cond: Not c̄ lactation. Caution c̄ ↓ renal func.
Pregnancy: Category D.
Other: <u>SKIN TOXICITY</u>, <u>HAIR LOSS</u>, <u>RASH</u>, <u>FEVER</u>, <u>CHILLS</u>, pulmonary toxicity
(↑ <u>IN SMOKERS</u>, [26] ↑ <u>IN GERIATRIC ≥ 70</u>), pulmonary fibrosis (can be fatal), <u>dyspnea</u>.
Blood/Serum: Rare- renal & hepatic toxicity, ↓ WBC.
Monitor: Hepatic & renal func, CBC, pulmonary x-rays.

Blocadren previous brand name ANTIHYPERTENSIVE, ANTIMIGRAINE, POST MI TREATMENT
timolol   Tab (IR)- starch Nonselective Beta-Blocker See listing for **propranolol p 267**

boceprevir
Victrelis
Cap- glatin,
lactose,
pre-gelatinized starch

TREATMENT FOR CHRONIC HEPATITIS C, Protease inhibitor
Drug: Take c̄ food.
Diet: Not c̄ SJW, see p 286.
Nutr: ↓ <u>APPETITE</u>.
Oral/GI: <u>DIARRHEA</u>, <u>DYSGEUSIA</u>, <u>N/V</u>, <u>dry mouth</u>.
S/Cond: Not as monotherapy. Not c̄ lactation. Caution c̄ geriatrics.
Caution c̄ moderate to severe ↓ hepatic func. Not in solid organ
transplant recipients. Not with concurrent HIV or HBV infection.
Pregnancy: Category X (when used c̄ peginterferon alfa and ribavirin).
Contraindicated in men whose female partners are pregnant.
Negative pregnancy test required before starting treatment
Other: <u>ASTHENIA</u>, <u>FATIGUE</u>, <u>INSOMNIA</u>, <u>IRRITABILITY</u>, <u>ARTHRALGIA</u>, <u>CHILLS</u>,
<u>dizziness</u>, <u>rash</u>, <u>dry skin</u>, <u>exertional dyspnea</u>.
Blood/Serum: ↓ <u>HEMOGLOBIN</u>, ↓ <u>HEMATOCRIT</u>, ↓ <u>NEUTROPHILS</u>.
Monitor: HCV-RNA levels at weeks 4, 8, 12, 24 & at the end of
treatment & during follow-up & as clincally indicated.
CBC c̄ diff prior to & at weeks 4, 8, 12, & as clinically indicated.
Females- routine monthly pregnancy test during treatment & for 6 mos
after DC of treatment.

| **Bonine** | ANTINAUSEANT, ANTIVERTIGO | See **meclizine p 205** |

| **Boniva**
    ibandronate | OSTEOPOROSIS TREATMENT | See **Bisphosphonates, Oral p 59** |

| **Boniva Injection**
    ibandronate | OSTEOPOROSIS TREATMENT | See **Bisphosphonates, Parenteral p 60** |

bortezomib
    Velcade
        35 mg mannitol/vial

ANTINEOPLASTIC (Multiple Myeloma), Proteasome Inhibitor   Parenteral only (IV)
Nutr: ↓ APPETITE, dehydration.
Oral/GI: Dysgeusia, dyspepsia, NAUSEA/VOMITING, DIARRHEA, CONSTIPATION, hemorrhage.
S/Cond: Not c̄ lactation. Caution c̄ ↓ hepatic func.
Pregnancy: Category D.
Other: FATIGUE, WEAKNESS, PERIPHERAL NEUROPATHY, FEVER, HEADACHE, INSOMNIA, MUSCLE/JOINT PAIN, EDEMA, DIZZINESS, DYSPNEA, RASH, hypotension, URTI, blurred vision, intracerebral hemorrhage.
Blood/Serum: ↓ PLATELETS, ANEMIA, ↓ WHITE BLOOD CELLS.
Monitor: CBC c̄ diff.

Brilinta

ACUTE CORONARY SYNDROME TREATMENT, REDUCTION OF MI, CVA, CV DEATH, platelet aggregation inhibitor   See **ticagrelor p 314**

bromocriptine
Parlodel
Tab & Cap-
lactose, starch
Cycloset
Tab- lactose, corn starch

ANTIPARKINSON, GROWTH HORMONE & PROLACTIN SUPPRESSANT,
ANTIDIABETIC AGENT TYPE 2 DIABETES MELLITUS (**Cycloset** only)
Dopamine Agonist, ergot derivative. Also used to treat Restless Leg Syndrome.
Drug: Take c̄ food or milk to ↓ GI irritation. Take HS to ↓ nausea.
Nutr: Anorexia.
Oral/GI: Dry mouth, metallic taste,[6] dysphagia, dyspepsia,
<u>NAUSEA</u>/vomiting, abdominal cramps, <u>constipation</u>, diarrhea, GI bleeding.
S/Cond: Avoid alcohol. Will inhibit lactation. > 90% serum albumin bound.
Caution c̄ hepatic impairment. **Pregnancy:** Category B.
Other: <u>Drowsiness</u>, <u>fatigue</u>, <u>headache</u>, <u>dizziness</u>, <u>fainting</u>, ↓ <u>BP</u> c̄ <u>possible</u>
<u>hypotension</u>, <u>hallucinations</u>, <u>confusion</u>, depression, nasal stuffiness.
Blood/Serum: ↓ <u>*PROLACTIN*</u>, ↓ <u>*GH*</u>.
Transient ↑ BUN, ↑ AST, ↑ ALT, ↑ alk phos, ↑ GGPT, ↑ CPK, ↑ uric acid.
Monitor: BP. LT use- Hepatic, renal & cardiovascular func. CBC c̄ diff.

brompheniramine

ANTIHISTAMINE, Alkylamine   See listing for **chlorpheniramine p 82**
Dimetapp Cold & Allergy also contains **phenylephrine**
See listing for **pseudoephedrine p 269**

Brovana
arformoterol

COPD TREATMENT, Beta-2 Agonist   See listing for **salmeterol p 286**
Inhalation Soln, long acting

budesonide
Entocort EC
Cap- sugar spheres
(sucrose & starch)
Pulmicort
Respules susp- EDTA
Flexhaler- lactose
Rhinocort Aqua
Nasal spray- EDTA

TO TREAT MILD TO MODERATE CROHN'S DISEASE, Corticosteroid,
ANTIASTHMA (Oral Inhaler), ALLERGIC RHINITIS (Spray)
See also **corticosteroids p 94**
Drug: Swallow caps whole- do not break, crush or chew.
Take once a day before breakfast.[13] High fat meal ↓ time to peak conc.
Rinse mouth after using inhaler.
Diet: Ca/Vit D suppl recommended.[13]
Cap only- avoid grapefruit/related citrus, see p 390. **Nutr:** ↑ appetite, ↑ wt.
Oral/GI: Glossitis, tooth disorder, tongue edema, dyspepsia, nausea,
GI fistula, enteritis, hemorrhoids.
S/Cond: Not c̄ lactation. Do dental care cautiously.
Caution c̄ ↓ hepatic func. 85-90% serum pro bound.

Pregnancy: Category C. **Rhinocort Aqua**- Category B.
Other: Headache, HTN, edema, moon face, respiratory infection, flu-like disorder, bronchitis, dizziness, weakness, chest pain, tachycardia, palpitations, dyspnea, dermatitis, acne, eczema, bruising, paresthesia, tremor, hyperkinesias, muscle cramps/pain, aggravated arthritis, agitation, confusion, insomnia, nervousness, drowsiness, ↑ sweating, abnormal vision. Corticosteroid effects, especially c̄ LT high dose.
Blood/Serum: ↑ C-Reactive Pro[10], ↑ WBC, ↓ K.
Urinary: Dysuria, ↑ frequency.

Bufferin	ANALGESIC, ANTIPYRETIC, NSAID　　See **aspirin p 44** 325 mg aspirin, $CaCO_3$, $MgCO_3$, Mg Oxide
bumetanide 　**Bumex**	DIURETIC　　　　　　　　　　　　See **Diuretics, Loop p 114**

bupropion
　Wellbutrin
　Tab
　Wellbutrin SR (12 hr)
　Tab
　Wellbutrin XL (24 hr)
　Tab
　Zyban (SR)
　Tab

ANTIDEPRESSANT (**Wellbutrin**), Aid to smoking cessation (**Zyban**)
　Drug: May take c̄ food to ↓ GI irritation.
　Swallow SR/XL forms whole, do not break, crush or chew.
　Diet: Avoid SJW, see p 286.
　Nutr: Anorexia, ↓ wt, ↑ appetite, ↑ wt, ↓ chocolate craving reported.[6]
　Oral/GI: Dry mouth, stomatitis, taste changes, dysphagia, pharyngitis, dyspepsia, N/V, abdominal pain, constipation, diarrhea.
　S/Cond: Minimize or avoid alcohol. Not c̄ lactation.
　Not c̄ seizures, anorexia or bulimia. > 80% albumin bound.
　↑ risk of dental problems, see p 11 & 15.
　Caution c̄ ↓ hepatic func or ↓ renal func. **Pregnancy:** Category C.
　Other: Tremor, dizziness, agitation, sweating, insomnia (> 20% c̄ **Zyban**), seizures, confusion, anxiety, memory impairment, drowsiness, paresthesia, HTN, cough, infection, fever, weakness, muscle/joint pain, twitch, blurred vision, rash, headache, tachycardia, suicidal thinking & behavior. Rare- pancreatitis, hepatotoxicity, SJS, akathisia, ↓ *tobacco dependence*.
　Blood/Serum: ↓ WBC.[13] **Urinary:** ↑ frequency/urgency c̄ SR form.

buspirone
BuSpar
Tab- lactose,
 Na starch glycolate

ANTIANXIETY
Drug: Food ↑ bioavailability, always take c̄ or s̄ food.
Diet: Avoid grapefruit/related citrus,[3] see p 390. Avoid **SJW** see p 286.
Oral/GI: Sore throat, nausea, diarrhea.
S/Cond: Avoid alcohol. Not c̄ lactation. 95% serum pro bound.
Caution c̄ ↓ hepatic funcor ↓ renal func.
Pregnancy: Category B.
Other: <u>Dizziness</u>, drowsiness, confusion, nervousness, tremor, ataxia,
sweating, weakness, blurred vision, headache, rash.
Blood/Serum: < 1%- ↑ AST, ↑ ALT.

butalbital
Fioricet
Tab- starch
 50 mg butalbital
 40 mg caffeine
 325 mg acetaminophen
Fiorinal
Cap- starch
 50 mg butalbital
 40 mg caffeine
 325 mg aspirin
May contain benzyl alcohol

ANALGESIC, SEDATIVE, Barbituate
See also **acetaminophen p 22** or **aspirin p 44** & **caffeine p 67**
butalbital is combined c̄ aspirin <u>or</u> acetaminophen & caffeine.
Drug: Aspirin form- take c̄ food. Acetaminophen form- take s̄ regard to food.
Oral/GI: Dyspepsia, N/V, flatulence.
S/Cond: Avoid alcohol. Not c̄ lactation. May be habit forming c̄ LT use.
For aspirin form- not c̄ aspirin allergy & not for children.
Pregnancy: Category C. (aspirin- Category D[7]).
Other: <u>Drowsiness</u>, <u>dizziness</u>.
Blood/Serum: See **acetaminophen p 22** or **aspirin p 44**
                    See **caffeine p 67**
Fioricet c̄ codeine & **Fiorinal** c̄ codeine also contain
15 or 30 mg **codeine** see **p 91**.

Byetta   ANTIHYPERGLYCEMIC   See **exenatide p 134**

Bystolic   ANTIHYPERTENSIVE   See **nebivolol p 226**

Caduet   ANTIHYPERTENSIVE, ANTIANGINA   See **amlodipine p 32**
Tab- CaCO3, starch   13.26mg Ca/10 mg **atorvastatin**   See **HMG-CoA**
multiple strength tabs   Combination drug **amlodipine** & **atorvastatin**   **Reductase Inhibitors p 164**

caffeine

Cafcit (caffeine citrate)
Oral Soln & IV- 10 mg
  caffeine/mL,
  preservative free

Caffedrine
Tab- Extended Release
  200 mg caffeine,
  lactose, starch

NoDoz Maximum Strength
Tab- 200 mg caffeine,
  sucrose, cornstarch

Vivarin
Tab/Caplet- 200 mg
  caffeine, dextrose,
  cornstarch

STIMULANT, Methylxanthine, Diuretic   Oral or Parenteral (IV)
Also an ingredient in pain & migraine formulations.
To treat APNEA OF PREMATURITY (**Cafcit**)
Drug: Swallow SR form whole. Do not take HS to avoid insomnia.
Diet: Limit dietary & natural product caffeine sources, see p 379.
Take Fe suppl separately by 2 hr.[13]
High cruciferous vegetable intake ↑ caffeine metabolism.[106]
Nutr: May ↓ Fe abs. ↑ glycogenolysis & lipolysis.[7] Anorexia c̄ high
dose.[17] Minor interaction c̄ grapefruit, not clinically significant, see p 390.
Possible slight ↓ Ca abs.[107] ↓ glucose tolerance.[83]
Oral/GI: N/V, GI DISTRESS, dyspepsia, ↑ GASTRIC ACID, ↑ PEPSIN, diarrhea.
S/Cond: Not c̄ lactation.[13] Caution c̄ diabetes- ↑ glucose. Caution c̄ HTN.
Not c̄ peptic ulcer, GERD, irritable bowel[7] or symptomatic arrhythmia.
Caution c̄ ↓ hepatic func (↑ half-life of caffeine).
Dependence may develop c̄ LT use of dose ≥ 130 mg[24] (withdrawal
symptoms = headache, fatigue, irritability, anxiety, dizziness).
Pregnancy: Category C.[13]
Other: 100 to 200 mg cause CNS stimulation.[6]
150-200 mg/kg body weight can be fatal.[2] INSOMNIA, ↑ HEART RATE,
↑ GLOMERULAR FILTRATION RATE, MILD DIURETIC EFFECT, tremor, nervousness,
irritability, hyperactivity,[17] headache.
Blood/Serum: ↑ GLUCOSE.[83] ↑ homocysteine, ↓ K, ↓ Na.
False ↑ uric acid c̄ Bittner method.
Urinary: ↑ Na, ↑ water, ↑ K, ↑ VMA, ↑ catecholamines,
↑ 5-hydroxyindolacetic acid.[2]
Monitor: Possibly caffeine & glucose serum levels c̄ **Cafcit** in infants.[10]

Calan/Calan SR	ANTIARRHYTHMIC, ANTIHYPERTENSIVE	See **verapamil p 332**
Calcijex	Ca REGULATOR	See **calcitriol p 68**

calcitonin
  Fortical[a]
   Nasal Spray-
   benzyl alcohol,
   phenylethyl alcohol
  Miacalcin
   Parenteral[a b c] or
   Nasal Spray[a]

Ca REGULATOR, OSTEOPOROSIS TREATMENT[a],
PAGET'S DISEASE TREATMENT[b], HYPERCALCEMIA TREATMENT[c]

   Polypeptide Hormone   Parenteral (IM or SC) & Nasal
   Bone Resorption Inhibitor
   Drug: Use HS to ↓ N/V.
   Diet: <u>To treat post-menopausal bone loss</u>- Adequate Vit D ($\geq$ 400 IU)[10]
   & Ca ($\geq$ 1000 mg)[10] intake essential.
   <u>To treat hypercalcemia</u> (parenteral)- May need ↓ Ca, ↓ Vit D diet.
   Avoid Ca & Vit D suppl.
   Nutr: Anorexia.
   Oral/GI: Metallic or salty taste, epigastric discomfort, <u>nausea/vomiting</u> c̄
   <u>parenteral</u> (< 3% c̄ nasal form), diarrhea.
   S/Cond: Not c̄ lactation. **Pregnancy:** Category C.
   Other: <u>Flushing</u>, edema of feet, headache, rash, eye pain, feverish
   sensation. Rare- allergic reaction. <u>Rhinitis</u>, nasal <u>irritation/ulceration</u>, <u>back</u>
   or muscle pain c̄ nasal spray.[10]
   Blood/Serum: ↓ *ALK PHOS*, slightly ↓ Ca, ↓ P.
   Urinary: ↑ <u>frequency</u>, ↑ P, ↑ or ↓ Ca, ↓ *HYDROXYPROLINE*, ↑ Mg, ↑ K, ↑ Cl.
   Transient ↑ Na, ↑ water. Urine sediment c̄ parenteral in subjects on bed rest.[13]
   Monitor: Serum alk phos & Ca. Lumbar vertebral bone mass.
   Nasal exams c̄ spray. Possibly urinalysis for urine sediment.[13]

calcitriol
  Rocaltrol
   Cap- sorbitol,
   fractionated TG of
   coconut oil
   Soln- fractionated TG of
   palm seed oil
  Calcijex
   Parenteral (IV)
  Zemplar
   (paricalcitol)

Ca REGULATOR, Active Vit D_3 (1,25 $[OH]_2$—D_3)   Oral or Parenteral (IV)
                               See also **Vitamin D p 340**
   Used to treat hypocalcemia in hypoparathyroid or dialysis patients.
   Also to manage secondary hyperparathyroidism in predialysis patients.
   Paricalcitol is synthetic **calcitriol.**
   (note- effects in outline type are S/S of Vit D toxicity).
   Drug: May mix soln with food or fruit juice. Take cap s̄ regard to food.
   Diet: Not c̄ Vit D or Mg suppl.
   With dialysis- adequate, but not excessive Ca, low P diet.
   To treat Rickets or Osteomalacia- add Ca suppl.
   Nutr: ↑ *CALCIUM ABS*, anorexia, ↓ wt, ↑ thirst.

IV- propylene glycol 30%, alcohol 20% Cap- alcohol, fractionated TG from coconut or palm kernel oil	**Oral/GI:** Dry mouth, metallic taste, N/V, constipation, diarrhea. **S/Cond:** Not c̄ lactation. Not c̄ hypercalcemia. **Pregnancy:** Category C. **Other:** Weakness, ataxia, headache, bone pain, muscle pain. **Blood/Serum:** ↓ _PTH_. Slightly ↑ Ca, ↑ P, ↓ alk phos, ↑ Mg. Hypercalcemia, hyperphosphotemia, ↑ BUN, ↑ crea, ↑ AST, ↑ ALT, ↑ chol. **Urinary:** ↑ Ca, ↑ P. ↑ alb. Hypercaliuria. **Monitor:** Serum Ca, P, (Ca x P should be < 70 recommended c̄ **calcitriol**), Mg, alk phos, renal func, PTH. Urinary Ca & P.
calcitriol ointment **Vectical** mineral oil, dl-alpha-tocopherol (Vit E)	PLAQUE PSORIASIS TREATMENT (mild to moderate psoriasis for > 18 yr old) **Drug:** Topical use only, not on eyes, lips or face. Maximum weekly dose should not exceed 200 g. **Nutr:** Caution c̄ Ca or Vit D suppl. **S/Cond:** Caution c̄ lactation. Avoid excessive natural or artificial sunlight. **Pregnancy:** Category C. **Other:** Skin discomfort. **Blood/Serum:** ↑ CALCIUM (< 10% above ULN). **Urinary:** Hypercalcemia. **Monitor:** Possibly serum Ca.
calcium acetate **PhosLo** Gelcap- contains 25% Ca[7] 169 mg Ca/Cap **Eliphos** Tab- contains 25% Ca[7] 169 mg Ca/Tab **Phoslyra** Soln- maltitol, glycerin, Magnasweet 110, sucralose	PHOSPHATE BINDER for use in renal failure <div align="center">See also listing for **calcium carbonate p 70**</div>**Drug:** Take c̄ meals. **Diet:** Avoid Ca suppl/antacid. Take Fe suppl separately. **Nutr:** ↓ Fe abs, anorexia. Does <u>not</u> promote Al abs. **Oral/GI:** N/V, constipation. **S/Cond:** Not c̄ hypercalcemia. **Pregnancy:** Category C. **Other:** Kidney stones c̄ LT high dose. **Blood/Serum:** Slightly ↑ Ca & ↓ P, ↓ PTH in ESRD. Hypercalcemia. **Monitor:** Serum Ca, P. (Ca x P should be < 66).

calcium carbonate ($CaCO_3$) ANTACID, MINERAL SUPPLEMENT, PHOSPHATE BINDER Also used as antidiarrheal

Contains 40% Ca   Also used in treating Osteomalacia, Rickets, Chronic hypoparathyroidism, Latent tetany, Hypocalcemia secondary to anticonvulsant drugs

Caltrate 600

600 mg Ca/tab, cornstarch   **Drug:** Take c̄ meals as suppl or P binder. Take 1-3 hr after meals as antacid. Chew chew tab well.

Caltrate 600 + D

600 mg Ca, 200 IU Vit D, starch, sucrose   **Diet:** Insure adequate fluid intake/hydration.

Take separately from large amounts high fiber, high oxalate or high phytate foods, see p 381 & 382.

Os-Cal 250 + D

250 mg Ca + 125 IU Vit D   Take Fe, Zn, Mg or F separately by 1-2 hr (may ↓ abs of Fe, Zn, Mg or F).[2, 9b]

Os-Cal 500- 500 mg Ca   Adequate Vit D essential to normal Ca/bone metabolism. Vit D- ↑ Ca abs.

Os-Cal 500 + D   Caffeine does not significantly affect Ca abs,[107] but slightly ↑ excretion.[47b]

500 mg Ca + 200 IU Vit D   **Nutr:** Anorexia. **AI** (mg/day) = Ages 0-6 mo - **210**. 7-12 mo - **270**.

Os-Cal Chewable 500   1-3 yr - **500**. 4-8 yr - **800**. 9-18 yr - **1300**. 19-50 yr - **1000**.

Chew Tab- 500 mg Ca, dextrose   51-70+ yr - **1200**. Lactation **AI** = **1300** for ages ≤18.

1000 for ages 19-50. **UL** = **2500** mg/day.

Tums Tab- Na-free, sucrose, cornstarch, 200 mg Ca/tab   **Oral/GI:** Chalky taste, dry mouth, ↓ diarrhea.

Excessive dose- N/V, abdominal pain, bloating, constipation, flatulence.

S/Cond: Not c̄ hypercalcemia. Not c̄ kidney stones.

Tums EX 300 mg Ca/tab   Caution c̄ achlorhydria or steatorrhea- ↓ Ca abs.[6]

Tums Ultra Tab- 400 mg Ca/tab, 1.5 g sucrose, cornstarch   **Pregnancy: AI** (mg/day) **1300** for ages ≤18. **1000** for ages 19-50.

Other: Kidney stones c̄ LT high dose. Rare- milk-alkali syndrome

Tums Smooth Dissolve   (hypercalcemia, metabolic alkalosis, renal insufficiency) c̄ LT high dose

Tab- 300 mg Ca, sorbitol, dextrose, 2.0 g sucrose   (>12 g $CaCO_3$/day = 5g Ca).[10b]

Blood/Serum: Slightly ↑ Ca & ↓ P, ↓ PTH in ESRD. Hypercalcemia.

Urinary: ↑ Ca. Polyuria c̄ excessive dose.

Tums Quikpak-   **Monitor:** Serum Ca, P.

400 mg Ca/pak, 1 g sugar/pak

Generic Susp- 500 mg Ca/5 mL

calcium citrate   MINERAL SUPPLEMENT, PHOSPHATE BINDER See **calcium carbonate above**

Citracal 250 mg + D   Contains 21% Ca.

Tab- 250 mg Ca, 200 IU Vit D   **Drug:** Take s̄ regard to food. Food does not affect abs. Take c̄ full glass of water.

Other: ↓ risk of kidney stones than c̄ calcium carbonate.

Citracal+D Petite Caplets- 200 mg Ca, 200 IU Vit D
Citrical Plus Heart Health- 315 mg Ca, 250 IU, Vit D 200 mg, phytosterols
Citrical Plus Bone Density Builder- 300 mg Ca, 200 IU Vit D, 25 mg Mg, 13.5 mg Genistein
Citracal Creamy Bites- 500 mg Ca, 200 IU Vit D- sugar, wheat flour, palm & soybean oil, non-fat milk, cornstarch, salt.

calcium gluconate   MINERAL SUPPLEMENT Contains 9% Ca See **calcium carbonate above**

calcium   LAXATIVE, Bulk Forming, ANTIDIARRHEAL
polycarbophil   **Drug:** Do not take dry, tab can swell & cause choking <u>unless</u> <u>taken</u> c̄
  FiberCon   adequate fluid. Take c̄ 8 oz water or other non-alcoholic liquid.
  140 mg Ca/tab,   **Diet:** High fiber c̄ 1500-2000 mL fluid/day to prevent constipation.
  Na Free   Take Fe, Zn, Ca or F suppl separately by 1-2 hr.
          Nutr: Ca is about 30% absorbed. Provides significant dietary Ca.
          Oral/GI: ↑ *PERISTALSIS & BOWEL MOTILITY*. ↓ *DIARRHEA*. Rare- bowel obstruction.

Caldolor (IV)   ANTIARTHRITIC, ANALGESIC, NSAID   See **ibuprofen p 170**

CaloMist   VITAMIN, ANTIANEMIC   See **vitamin B$_{12}$ p 338**
  cyanocobalamin Nasal Spray
  benzyl alcohol

Caltrate   MINERAL SUPPLEMENT, PHOSPHATE BINDER
Caltrate + D   See **calcium carbonate above**   See also **Vitamin D p 340**

Cambia   ANALGESIC for acute migraine attacks, oral soln   See **diclofenac p 107**
  potassium bicarbonate

Campral   ALCOHOL ABUSE DETERRENT   See **acamprosate p 20**

Camptosar   ANTINEOPLASTIC, Topoisomerase I Inhibitor   See **irinotecan p 179**

Canasa   ANTI-INFLAMMATORY   See **mesalamine p 209**

Cancidas caspofungin	ANTIFUNGAL	See **echinocandins p 120**

candesartan
  Atacand/Atacand HCT

ANTIHYPERTENSIVE   See **Angiotensin II Receptor Antagonists p 38**
  Atacand HCT also contains **hydrochlorothiazide**, see **p 166**

capecitabine
  Metabolized to **5-FU**
  Xeloda
  Tab- lactose

ANTINEOPLASTIC, Antimetabolite (metastatic breast or colorectal cancer)
  Drug: Swallow c̄ water within 1/2 hr of the end of a meal.
  Dose based on body surface area.
  Nutr: <u>ANOREXIA</u>, <u>dehydration</u>.
  Oral/GI: Candidiasis, <u>STOMATITIS</u>, <u>NAUSEA</u>, <u>VOMITING</u>, <u>dyspepsia</u>,
  <u>ABDOMINAL PAIN</u>, intestinal obstruction, <u>severe DIARRHEA</u> (interrupt
  treatment if ≥ grade 2 diarrhea), <u>constipation</u>.
  S/Cond: Not c̄ lactation. Do dental care cautiously, see p 11 & 15.
  Caution c̄ ↓ hepatic func or ↓ renal func. Not c̄ severe ↓ renal func.
  Caution c̄ geriatrics, especially ≥ 80 yr. **Pregnancy:** Category D.
  Other: <u>HAND</u> & <u>FOOT SYNDROME</u>, <u>FATIGUE</u>, <u>DERMATITIS</u>, <u>PARESTHESIA</u>, <u>fever</u>,
  <u>eye irritation</u>, <u>edema</u>, <u>headache</u>, <u>dizziness</u>, <u>nail disorder/fungus</u>, insomnia,
  limb or muscle pain, ↑ or ↓ BP, photosensitivity, ataxia, hepatitis.
  Blood/Serum: ↓ <u>WHITE BLOOD CELLS</u>,
  ↓ <u>NEUTROPHILS</u>, ↓ <u>PLATELETS</u>, <u>ANEMIA</u>, ↑ <u>BIL</u>, ↑ <u>AST</u>, ↑ <u>ALT</u>, ↑ <u>alk phos</u>, ↑ TG.
  Monitor: Hepatic func. CBC c̄ diff.

captopril **Capoten**	ANTIHYPERTENSIVE	See **Angiotensin Converting Enzyme Inhibitors p 36**
Carafate	ANTIULCER	See **sucralfate p 298**

carbamazepine
  Tegretol
  Chewable Tab-
  sucrose,
   Na starch glycolate
  Susp- sucrose,

ANTIEPILEPTIC, To Treat TRIGEMINAL NEURALGIA PAIN
  ANTIMANIC (**Equetro**), Also used as antipsychotic
  Drug: Take tab, chew tab or susp c̄ food or milk to ↓ GI distress.
  Take SR form s̄ regard to food. Chew chew tab well. Do not chew or
  crush XR tab. May open SR cap & sprinkle beads on small amount
  soft food- do not chew. For NG tube- mix susp c̄ equal amount diluent.

sorbitol
Tab- starch
Tegretol XR (SR)
Tab- mannitol
Carbatrol (SR)
Cap- lactose
Equetro (SR)
Cap- lactose

Diet: Caution c̄ grapefruit/related citrus,[49] see p 390.
Caution c̄ star fruit or pomegranate juice- may ↑ drug level/toxicity.[112]
Limit or avoid quinine- may ↑ drug level.[3a]
Possible Ca-Vit D suppl c̄ **carbamazepine** use > 6 mo.[93]
Nutr: Anorexia. ↓ biotin, Fol, Vit D, Ca.
Oral/GI: Dry mouth, stomatitis, glossitis, N/V, abdominal pain, constipation, diarrhea.
S/Cond: Avoid alcohol.[13] Not c̄ lactation. ↑ risk of dental problems, see p 11 & 15. Caution c̄ ↓ hepatic func. Caution c̄ Asian pt c̄ HLA-B*1502 gene- ↑ risk of severe skin reactions.
Pregnancy: Category D.
Other: Hyponatremia, confusion, dizziness, ataxia, drowsiness, blurred vision, double vision, rash, SIADH, edema, water intoxication, photosensitivity, ↑ or ↓ BP. Rare- CHF, jaundice/hepatitis, peripheral neuropathy, bone marrow suppression, lens opacities. SJS, TEN (↑ in Asian pt).
Rare- suicidal thinking & behavior.
Blood Serum: ↓ WBC, ↓ FOLATE, ↑ HOMOCYSTEINE, dyscrasias, ↑ BUN, ↑ AST, ↑ ALT, ↑ alk phos, ↑ bil, ↓ T_3, ↓ T_4, ↓ Na, ↑ chol, ↑ HDL, ↑ TG, ↓ biotin.[11] ↓ Ca & ↓ Vit D c̄ use > 6 mo,[93] ↓ carnitine.[93]
Aplastic anemia (rare, can be fatal).
Urinary: ↑ frequency. Pro, sediment. Glucose in diabetics.
Monitor: Drug levels. Eye exams. Baseline & periodic[21]- renal & hepatic func, CBC c̄ diff, serum Fe, Ca, electrolytes, thyroid func, urinalysis. Possibly Vit D levels. Prior to use- genetic testing for Asian pt.

carbidopa
 Lodosyn
 Tab- starch

ANTIPARKINSON adjunct   See **levodopa & carbidopa p 193**
Prescribed c̄ **levodopa** or c̄ **carbidopa-levodopa** (eg **Sinemet**), particularly to ↓ **levodopa** induced N/V or c̄ Pyr suppl ≥ 10-25 mg/day.

carboplatin
platinum coordination
 complex
Generic brands only
pwd- mannitol

ANTINEOPLASTIC (Ovarian or Lung Cancer)   Parenteral only (IV)
Diet: Insure adequate fluid intake/hydration to ↑ urinary output.
Nutr: <u>ANOREXIA</u>. **Oral/GI:** Altered taste, <u>MUCOSITIS</u>, <u>STOMATITIS</u>,
<u>NAUSEA/VOMITING</u>, <u>GI pain</u>, diarrhea, <u>constipation</u>.
S/Cond: Not c̄ lactation. Do dental care cautiously, see p 11 & 15.
Caution c̄ ↓ renal func. **Pregnancy:** Category D. **Other:** <u>BONE MARROW</u> <u>SUPPRESSION</u>,
<u>WEAKNESS</u>, <u>PAIN</u>, <u>infections</u>, <u>peripheral</u> <u>neuropathy</u>, ototoxicity, ↓ or ↑ BP,
blurred vision, allergic reaction. **Blood/Serum:** ↓ <u>PLATELETS</u>, ↓ <u>NEUTROPHILS</u>,
↓ <u>WHITE</u> <u>BLOOD</u> <u>CELLS</u>, <u>ANEMIA</u>, ↓ <u>MAGNESIUM</u>, ↓ <u>CALCIUM</u>, ↓ <u>POTASSIUM</u>, ↓ <u>SODIUM</u>,
↑ <u>BUN</u>, ↑ <u>crea</u>, ↑ <u>ALK</u> <u>PHOS</u>, ↑ <u>bil</u>, ↑ <u>AST</u>. **Urinary:** ↓ <u>output</u>.
Monitor: Renal func & CBC c̄ diff, platelets, before each dose. Electrolytes, Mg.

Cardizem/Cardizem LA
Cardizem CD

ANTIANGINA, ANTIHYPERTENSIVE, Ca Channel Blocker
See **diltiazem p 111**

Cardura/Cardura XL
doxazosin

ANTIHYPERTENSIVE, BPH TREATMENT
See **Alpha₁-Adrenergic Blockers p 28**

carmustine
BiCNU (IV)
10% alcohol
Gliadel Wafer
placed in surgical
resection cavity after
brain tumor resection

ANTINEOPLASTIC, Alkylating Agent   Parenteral (IV) or Polymer Wafer
Diet: Insure adequate fluid intake/hydration. **Nutr:** Anorexia.
Oral/GI: Stomatitis, dysphagia, <u>NAUSEA/VOMITING</u>, diarrhea.
S/Cond: Not c̄ lactation. Do dental care cautiously, see p 11 & 15.
Caution c̄ ↓ hepatic func or ↓ renal func. **Pregnancy:** Category D.
Other: Drowsiness, dizziness, ataxia, <u>flushing</u>, <u>bone</u> <u>marrow</u> <u>suppression</u>
<u>(often</u> <u>delayed)</u>, <u>MILD</u> <u>HEPATOTOXICITY</u>, jaundice, rash, ocular toxicity,
pulmonary toxicity/fibrosis- can be fatal or delayed for years (↑ c̄ smoking).
Nephrotoxicity c̄ LT high dose. **Blood/Serum:** ↑ <u>AST</u>, ↑ <u>ALT</u>, ↑ <u>bil</u>,
↑ alk phos, ↓ <u>WBC</u>, ↓ <u>PLATELETS</u>, anemia, ↑ BUN.
Monitor: Weekly CBC c̄ diff & platelets for ≥ 6 weeks after last dose.
Hepatic, renal & pulmonary func.

carnitine/Carnitor

NUTRITIONAL SUPPLEMENT, Amino Acid Derivative   See **levocarnitine p 192**

Cartia XT

ANTIANGINA, ANTIHYPERTENSIVE, Ca Channel Blocker   See **diltiazem p 111**

carvedilol
  Coreg
    Tab- lactose,
    sucrose
  Coreg CR
    Cap- castor oil,
    hydrogenated vegetable
    oil

CHF TREATMENT, ANTIHYPERTENSIVE, Non-selective Beta-Blocker & Alpha$_1$ Blocker
  Drug: Tab- take c̄ food to ↓ orthostatic hypotension.
  CR Cap- take c̄ food to ↑ drug level, but not within 2 hr of alcohol.[1]
  May open cap & sprinkle beads on cool applesauce. Do not chew or crush.
  Diet: ↓ Na, ↓ cal may be recommended. Avoid natural licorice, see p 374.
  Nutr: ↑ wt. **Oral/GI:** N/V, diarrhea.
  S/Cond: Not c̄ lactation. Caution c̄ diabetes- may mask symptoms of
  or prolong hypoglycemia. May reduce insulin release in response
  to hyperglycemia. Caution c̄ ↓ renal func. 98% serum pro bound.
  Hypoalbuminemia (< 3 g/dL) may ↑ drug effects.
  Not c̄ severe ↓ hepatic func. Not c̄ asthma/bronchospasm.
  Pregnancy: Category C.
  Other: ↓ *BP* c̄ possible hypotension, bradycardia, dizziness
  (↑ in CYP2D6 poor metabolizers), chest pain, edema, fever, muscle pain,
  bronchitis, vision abnormalities, insomnia, headache, weakness, URTI.
  Rare- hepatotoxicity, worsening CHF.
  Blood/Serum: ↑ glucose, ↑ BUN, ↑ crea, ↑ NPN, ↑ chol, ↑ TG,
  ↑ uric acid, ↓ Na, ↑ K, ↑ AST, ↑ ALT, ↑ alk phos, ↓ platelets, ↑ GGT.
  < 1%- ↓ K, ↑ bil, anemia, ↓ WBC.
  Urinary: Glucose, alb, RBC.
  Monitor: BP, hepatic func, renal func, glucose, heart rate.[13]

Casodex	ANTINEOPLASTIC, Antiandrogen	See **bicalutamide p 56**
caspofungin **Cancidas**	ANTIFUNGAL	See **echinocandins p 120**
Cataflam	ANTIARTHRITIC, ANALGESIC, NSAID	See **diclofenac potassium p 107**
Catapres	ANTIHYPERTENSIVE	See **clonidine p 88**
Cayston	ANTIBIOTIC, Monobactam, Inhalation soln	See **aztreonam p 49**
Ceclor/Ceclor CD previous brand name	ANTIBIOTIC, Cephalosporin	See **cefaclor p 76**

C

cefaclor
   Ceclor generic equivalent
   Susp- 3 g
   sucrose/5mL,
   cornstarch
   Cap- cornstarch
   Ceclor CD (SR)
   generic equivalent
   Tab- mannitol
   Raniclor
   Chew Tab-
   aspartame, mannitol

ANTIBIOTIC, Cephalosporin, 2nd generation   Oral only
   Drug: Take cap or susp s̄ regard to food. Take CD tab c̄ food.
   Do not cut, chew or crush CD tab.
   Diet: Take CD tab 1 hr before Al or Mg antacid or Mg suppl.
   Oral/GI: Oral candidiasis & sore mouth & tongue c̄ LT use,
   pharyngitis, N/V, cramps, diarrhea, pseudomembranous colitis.
   Nutr: Mg or Al ↓ abs of CD Tab.
   S/Cond: Caution c̄ lactation. Caution c̄ ↓ renal func. **Pregnancy:** Category B.
   Other: Allergic reaction, headache, rash, rhinitis, vaginal candidiasis, cough.
   Rare- SJS, anaphylaxis, TEN, serum sickness-like reactions,
   hepatitis, jaundice, interstitial nephritis.
   Blood/Serum: ↑ alk phos, ↑ AST, ↑ ALT, eosinophilia.
   Rare- ↓ platelets, ↓ neutrophils. **Urinary:** False + glucose ($CuSO_4$).

cefadroxil
   Duricef

ANTIBIOTIC, Cephalosporin, First Generation See listing for **cephalexin p 79**
   Susp- 2 g sucrose/5mL, xanthan gum

cefazolin sodium
   Ancef

ANTIBIOTIC, Cephalosporin   See **cephalosporins p 80**

cefdinir
   Omnicef
   Susp- sucrose, guar gum,
   xanthan gum
   Cap

ANTIBIOTIC, Cephalosporin, 3rd generation   Oral only
   Drug: Take s̄ regard to food.
   Diet: Take 2 hr before or after antacid, Mg suppl, Fe suppl or MVI c̄ Fe.
   Nutr: Fe, Mg or Al ↓ abs of drug.
   Oral/GI: N/V, abdominal pain, _diarrhea_. Rare- pseudomembranous colitis.
   S/Cond: Caution c̄ ↓ renal func.
   Pregnancy: Category B.
   Other: Allergic reaction, rash, headache, fungal overgrowth.
   Rare- anaphylaxis, SJS, TEN, hepatitis, jaundice.
   Blood/Serum: ↑ GGT, ↑ or ↓ WBC.
   < 1%- ↑ AST, ↑ ALT, ↑ alk phos, ↑ LDH, ↑ BUN, ↑ or ↓ glucose, ↑ or ↓ P,
   dyscrasias, eosinophilia.
   Urinary: Pro, WBC, RBC, ↑ pH, glucose. False + ketones.

cefditoren	ANTIBIOTIC, Cephalosporin, 3rd generation Oral only
Spectracef	**Drug:** Take $\bar{c}$ meals. ↑ abs $\bar{c}$ moderate - high fat meals.
Tab- mannitol,	(test meals = 648-825 cal, 27-64 g fat)
Na Caseinate	**Nutr:** Carnitine def $\bar{c}$ LT use. **Oral/GI:** N/V, dyspepsia, abdominal pain, <u>diarrhea</u>.
	Rare- pseudomembranous colitis.
	S/Cond: Caution $\bar{c}$ lactation. 88% serum pro bound.
	Hypoalbuminemia (<3 g/dL)- may ↑ drug effect.
	Caution $\bar{c}$ moderate to severe ↓ renal func. Not $\bar{c}$ carnitine def or
	inborn error of carnitine metabolism. Not milk protein allergy.
	Pregnancy: Category B. **Other:** Vaginal candidiasis, headache.
	Blood/Serum: ↓ carnitine, ↑ glucose, ↑ HCT.
	<1%- ↑ platelets, ↓ WBC, ↑ AST, ↑ ALT.
	Urinary: Hematuria, ↑ carnitine. False + glucose ($CuSO_4$).
cefepime	ANTIBIOTIC, Cephalosporin, See **cephalosporins p 80**
Maxipime	4th generation
Cefizox	ANTIBIOTIC, **ceftizoxime sodium** See **cephalosporins p 80**
cefotaxime sodium	ANTIBIOTIC, Cephalosporin See **cephalosporins p 80**
Claforan	
cefoxitin	ANTIBIOTIC, Cephalosporin See **cephalosporins p 80**
Mefoxin	
cefprozil	ANTIBIOTIC, Cephalosporin, 2nd generation Oral only
Cefzil	**Drug:** Take $\bar{s}$ regard to food.
Susp- aspartame =	**Oral/GI:** Oral candidiasis & sore mouth & tongue $\bar{c}$ LT use, N/V,
28 mg phenylalanine/	diarrhea. Rare- pseudomembranous colitis.
5 mL, NaCl, sucrose	**S/Cond:** Caution $\bar{c}$ lactation. Caution $\bar{c}$ ↓ renal func. **Pregnancy:** Category B.
Tab- Na starch glycolate	**Other:** Dizziness, rash, vaginal candidiasis.
	Rare- anaphylaxis, SJS, angioedema, serum sickness.
	Blood/Serum: ↑ AST, ↑ ALT, eosinophilia. False negative glucose $\bar{c}$
	ferricyanide test. **Urinary:** False + glucose ($CuSO_4$).

C

ceftazidime **Fortaz, Tazicef**	ANTIBIOTIC, Cephalosporin	See **cephalosporins p 80**

Ceftin	ANTIBIOTIC, Cephalosporin	See **cefuroxime axetil below**

ceftriaxone sodium **Rocephin**	ANTIBIOTIC, Cephalosporin	See **cephalosporins p 80**

cefuroxime axetil
  Ceftin- Tab-
    hydrogenated vegetable oil
    Susp- sucrose,
    aspartame, xanthan gum
  cefuroxime sodium
    Zinacef- Parenteral
    54 mg Na/g

ANTIBIOTIC, Cephalosporin, 2nd generation   Oral or Parenteral (IM or IV)
    Drug: Take susp $\bar{c}$ food to ↑ abs. May take tab $\bar{s}$ food, but food ↑ abs.
    Swallow tab whole- strong, bitter taste when crushed.
    Diet: Take separately from antacids, Ca or Mg suppl.
    Oral/GI: Oral candidiasis & sore mouth & tongue $\bar{c}$ LT use, <u>bitter taste</u>,
    <u>N/V</u>, <u>diarrhea</u>. Rare- pseudomembranous colitis.
    S/Cond: Tab- Not $\bar{c}$ lactation. IV- Caution $\bar{c}$ lactation. Caution $\bar{c}$ ↓ renal func.
    Pregnancy: Category B. **Other:** <u>Jarisch-Herxheimer reaction</u> in Lyme
    disease (acute fever, muscle pain, headache).[6] < 1%- rash, seizures,[6]
    vaginal candidiasis. Rare- anaphylaxis, interstitial nephritis, angioedema, TEN.
    Blood/Serum: (↑ incidence $\bar{c}$ Parenteral) ↓ <u>Hb</u>, ↓ <u>HCT</u>, <u>eosinophilia</u>,
    ↑ AST, ↑ ALT, ↑ LDH, ↑ alk phos. False + Coombs' test.
    False negative glucose $\bar{c}$ ferricyanide test
    Urinary: False + glucose ($CuSO_4$).

Cefzil	ANTIBIOTIC, Cephalosporin	See **cefprozil above**

celecoxib
  Celebrex
  Cap- lactose

ANALGESIC (acute pain, primary dysmenorrhea),
ANTIARTHRITIC (osteo or rheumatoid arthritis, JRA in children > 2 yr,
  ankylosing spondylitis),
ADJUNCT TO ↓ POLYPS IN FAMILIAL ADENOMATOUS POLYPOSIS, NSAID
    Drug: Take ≤ 200 mg BID $\bar{s}$ regard to meals
    (risk of GI distress is ↓ if taken $\bar{c}$ food or ≥ 8 oz milk).
    Take higher dose (eg 400 mg BID) $\bar{c}$ food to ↑ abs.
    Diet: High fat meal delays peak conc, but ↑ total abs.
    Limit caffeine to ↓ GI effect.

Nutr: ↑ wt.
Oral/GI: Taste changes, dyspepsia, nausea, abdominal pain, diarrhea, flatulence. Rare- sudden, serious GI bleeding, colitis.
S/Cond: Not c̄ lactation. 97-98% serum pro bound.
Caution c̄ cardiac disease, HTN or edema. Caution c̄ geriatric, especially if **BW** < 50 kg. Caution c̄ gastritis/ulcer. Caution c̄ moderate ↓ hepatic or ↓ renal func, not c̄ serious dysfunction. Not c̄ dehydration. Not c̄ aspirin or NSAID allergy or sulfonamide allergy.
Pregnancy: Category C, but not recommended in pregnancy.
Category D in 3rd trimester due to ↑ risk to fetus & mother, including death.
Other: Edema, ↑ <u>BP</u>, headache, pharyngitis, rhinitis, URTI, back pain, rash. Risk of CV problems, eg HTN, CHF, MI, CVA.
Blood/Serum: ↑ AST, ↑ ALT, ↑ CPK. < 1%- ↑ alk phos, anemia, ↑ BUN, ↑ crea, ↑ Cl, ↓ P, ↓ K, ↑ glucose, ↑ chol. **Urinary:** Alb.
Monitor: BP. Hepatic func- baseline & periodically.[1]

Celexa	ANTIDEPRESSANT, SSRI	See **citalopram p 86**
CellCept	IMMUNOSUPPRESSANT	See **mycophenolate p 222**
Cenestin	HORMONE, Estrogen	See **Hormone Therapy p 165**

cephalexin
Keflex- Cap
generic Susp- 3 g
sucrose /5 mL
Panixine DisperDose
Disperible Tab for Susp-
aspartame, mannitol

ANTIBIOTIC, Cephalosporin, first generation   Oral only
Drug: May be taken s̄ regard to food.
Oral/GI: Oral candidiasis & sore mouth/ tongue c̄ LT use.
Dyspepsia, gastritis, <u>diarrhea</u>. < 1%- pseudomembranous colitis.
S/Cond: Caution c̄ lactation. Caution c̄ ↓ renal func.
Pregnancy: Category B.
Other: Dizziness, headache, fatigue, rash, genital candidiasis, agitation, confusion. Rare- hepatitis, jaundice, interstitial nephritis, joint pain, anaphylaxis, angioedema, SJS, TEN.
Blood/Serum: ↑ AST, ↑ ALT, eosinophilia, ↓ WBC, ↑ BUN, ↑ crea.
False + Coombs' test. **Urinary:** False + glucose ($CuSO_4$).

C

cephalosporins (parenteral)   ANTIBIOTIC   Parenteral Only (IM or IV)
Diet: Consider Na content c̄ ↓ Na diet. May need ↑ Vit K or supplement c̄ **cefoperazone,** to prevent
bleeding due to hypoprothrombinemia. **Nutr:** Anorexia.
Oral/GI: Oral candidiasis & sore mouth & tongue c̄ LT use. N/V, diarrhea. < 1%- pseudomembranous colitis.
S/Cond: No alcohol c̄ **cefoperazone**- disulfiram-like reaction.
Caution c̄ lactation. LT use in malnourished- ↓ Vit K synthesis. Caution c̄ ↓ renal func. Caution c̄ ↓ hepatic
func c̄ **cefoperazone**.[7] Do not mix **ceftriaxone** c̄ Ca or Ca containing products for > 48 hr.
Cefazolin, cefoperazone & **ceftriaxone** are ≥ 85% serum pro bound.
Pregnancy: Category B. **Other:** Allergic reaction, rash, genital candidiasis. < 1%- headache, dizziness,
seizures. Rare- gallbladder sludge c̄ **ceftriaxone**. Rare- anaphylaxis, SJS, TEN, angioedema, serum sickness.
Blood/Serum: Dyscrasias, eosinophilia. (Rare- anemia, hemolytic anemia, ↓ alb, ↓ TP,[6]
hypoprothrombinemia & ↑ PT/INR). Transient ↑ AST, ↑ ALT, ↑ bil, ↑ LDH, ↑ alk phos, ↑ GGT, ↑ BUN,
↑ crea, (possible false ↑ crea c̄ Jaffe method c̄ **cefoxitin**), false + Coombs' test.
Urinary: False + glucose ($CuSO_4$). **Monitor:** PT/INR, CBC c̄ diff if used > 10 days.

cefazolin sodium	**cefoxitin**	**ceftriaxone sodium**
Ancef*	**Mefoxin***	**Rocephin***
cefepime (L-arginine 725 mg/g)	**ceftaroline** Teflaro	
Maxipime (Na free)	**ceftazidime**	
cefoperazone sodium	**Fortaz***	
Cefobid*	**Tazicef***	
cefotaxime sodium	**ceftizoxime sodium**	*Contains Na- 34-83 mg
Claforan*	**Cefizox***	(1.48-3.61 mEq)/g

Ceptaz   ANTIBIOTIC, **ceftazidime**   See **cephalosporins above**

Cerebyx   ANTIEPILEPTIC, Parenteral only   See **fosphenytoin** p 151
                         Water-soluble **phenytoin** prodrug c̄ better safety profile than **phenytoin**

certolizumab   TNF Inhibitor for treatment of Rheumatoid Arthritis and Crohn's disease
  Cimzia   Parenteral only (SC)
  Prefilled syringe-   **Drug:** Injection q 2 or 4 wks.
   sodium chloride 7.31 mg,   **Oral/GI:** Abdominal pain, diarrhea, intestinal obstruction.

sodium acetate 1.36 mg
Lyophilized pwd for
reconstitution-
  sucrose 100 mg,
  lactic acid 0.9 mg,
  polysorbate 0.1 mg

S/Cond: Not c̄ lactation. Not c̄ untreated active infection eg TB, HBV. Caution c̄ demyelinating disorders. Caution c̄ hematologic disorders. Caution c̄ CHF.
Pregnancy: Category B.
Other: <u>URTI</u>, <u>rash</u>, <u>UTI</u>, headache, HTN, back pain, fever, fatigue, TB, cellulitis, pneumonia, pyelonephritis, lupus like syndrome. Rare- angioedema, allergic dermatitis, dyspnea, SJS, TEN, syncope, malignancies (eg lymphoma), serious infection (can be fatal).
Blood/Serum: ↓ WBC, ↓ platelets, pancytopenia, aplastic anemia (rare). Possibly false ↑ APTT.
Monitor: monitor for active TB prior to & during treatment.

cetirizine
  Zyrtec
  Tab- lactose
  Syrup- sugar, propylene glycol
  Chew Tab- acesulfame K,
    lactose, mannitol

ANTIHISTAMINE
Drug: Take s̄ regard to food (food ↓ rate, but not extent of abs).
Diet: No interaction c̄ grapefruit/related citrus, see p 390.
Oral/GI: Dry mouth. N/V in children.
S/Cond: Avoid alcohol. Not c̄ lactation. 93% serum pro bound. Caution c̄ ↓ hepatic func or ↓ renal func.
Pregnancy: Category B.
Other: <u>Drowsiness</u>, fatigue, headache.

cetuximab
  Erbitux
  preservative free

ANTINEOPLASTIC (Colorectal Cancer, Head & Neck Cancer)
  Epidermal Growth Factor Inhibitor   Parenteral IV
Nutr: <u>ANOREXIA</u>, ↓ <u>wt</u>, <u>dehydration</u>.
Oral/GI: <u>Stomatitis</u>, <u>NAUSEA/VOMITING</u>, <u>ABDOMINAL</u> <u>PAIN</u>, dyspepsia, <u>DIARRHEA</u>, <u>CONSTIPATION</u>. **S/Cond:** Not c̄ lactation. **Pregnancy:** Category C.
Other: <u>ACNEFORM</u> <u>RASH</u>, <u>WEAKNESS</u>, <u>FEVER</u>, <u>INFUSION REACTION</u>, <u>HEADACHE</u>, <u>DYSPNEA</u>, <u>HAIR LOSS</u>, cough, pain, infection, insomnia, depression, conjunctivitis, nail disorder. Rare- pulmonary toxicity.
Blood/Serum: <u>Anemia</u>, ↓ WBC. ↓ <u>MAGNESIUM</u>, ↓ Ca, ↓ K.
Monitor: Electrolytes, Ca, Mg. BP, infusion reaction.

C

Chantix	SMOKING CESSATION AIDE, Nicotinic Receptor Agonist

See varenicline p 330

chlordiazepoxide
  Librium   ANTIANXIETY   See **Benzodiazepines p 54**

chlorothiazide   ANTIHYPERTENSIVE, DIURETIC (K-depleting)   Oral or Parenteral (IV)
  All Tabs- starch, gelatin   250 mg Tab- also contains lactose
  Susp- saccharin, sucrose, alcohol 0.5%
  Pregnancy: Category C.   See listing for **hydrochlorothiazide p 166**

chlorpheniramine   ANTIHISTAMINE, Alkylamine
  Chlor-Trimeton 4 hr   **Drug:** Take c̄ food to ↓ GI distress. Do not crush SR form- swallow whole.
  Tab- lactose   **Nutr:** Anorexia.
  Chlor-Trimeton   **Oral/GI:** <u>Dry mouth</u>, ↓ salivation, N/V, GI distress, constipation.
   8 & 12 hr (SR)   **S/Cond:** Avoid alcohol. Not c̄ lactation. Caution c̄ geriatric.[84]
  Tab- lactose, sugar,   ↑ risk of dental problems, see p 11 & 15.
  cornstarch, potato starch   **Pregnancy:** Category B.
  8 hr tab- 63 mg sugar   **Other:** <u>Drowsiness</u>, dizziness, paradoxical excitability in children or
  12 hr tab- 55 mg sugar   geriatric, blurred vision, ↑ sweating, flushing.
                                   Blood/Serum: Dyscrasias, anemia.
                                   Urinary: Retention.

chlorpromazine   ANTIPSYCHOTIC, ANTIEMETIC   See **Phenothiazines p 254**
  Thorazine previous brand name

chlorthalidone   ANTIHYPERTENSIVE, DIURETIC (K-depleting)
  Tab- cornstarch,   See listing for **hydrochlorothiazide p 166**
  Na starch glycolate   Structurally & pharmacologically similar to thiazides.
                                 Drug: Take c̄ food in AM. Longer duration of action than thiazides.

Chlor-Trimeton   ANTIHISTAMINE, Alkylamine   See **chlorpheniramine above**

cholecalciferol (D₃)   Vitamin, Ca REGULATOR, ANTIRICKETS   See **vitamin D p 340**

cholestyramine
  Questran
    3.8 g sucrose/9 g

  Questran Light
    aspartame =
    28 mg phenylalanine/6.4g
    0.9 g sucrose/6.4 g

ANTIHYPERLIPIDEMIC, ANTIDIARRHEAL, Bile Acid Sequestrant
  Drug: Take before meals. Mix pwd in 4-6 oz water, non-carbonated beverage, fluid soup or pureed fruit. NEVER TAKE POWDER DRY.
  Diet: ↓ fat, ↓ chol, ↑ fluids, ↑ fiber, ↓ cal if needed. Fat soluble Vit in water miscible form & Fol suppl recommended c̄ LT use.[1]
Take suppl at least 1 hr before or 4 hr after drug.
  Nutr: May ↓ abs of fat, Ca, Fe, Zn, Mg,[11] beta-carotene, Vits A, D, E, & K, Fol. Anorexia, ↑ or ↓ wt.
  Oral/GI: Tongue irritation,[7] belching, N/V, dyspepsia, pain, CONSTIPATION, flatulence, diarrhea. Rare- GI bleeding, steatorrhea.
  S/Cond: Caution c̄ lactation- ↓ abs of Vits may ↓ Vit content of breast milk.
  Pregnancy: Category C.
  Other: Drowsiness, dizziness, headache, osteomalacia/osteoporosis c̄ LT use, ↑ thyroid hormone degradation. Rare- bleeding due to Vit K def.
  Blood/Serum: ↓ CHOL, ↓ LDL, ↑ HDL, stable or ↑ TG & VLDL. ↓ Ca, ↓ K, ↓ Na, ↑ P, ↑ Cl, ↓ Fol, ↑ PT/INR, ↓ T_4. Transient ↑ alk phos, ↑ AST, ↑ ALT.
  Urinary: ↑ Ca, ↑ Mg.
  Monitor: Chol, TG, PT/INR, Ca, electrolytes.

chondroitin
  multiple brands
  (note many brands
  do not meet content
  claims)[75]

NATURAL PRODUCT (Not FDA approved), ANTIARTHRITIC (Osteoarthritis)
  Nutr: Not c̄ chitosan (possible chelation reaction).
  Oral/GI: Epigastric distress, nausea, diarrhea, constipation.
  S/Cond: Not c̄ lactation. Not for children.
  Pregnancy: Do not use.
  Other: Eyelid edema, lower limb edema, extra systoles.

Cialis
  tadalafil

ERECTILE DYSFUNCTION TREATMENT
  Tab- lactose   See listing for **sildenafil p 292**

ciclesonide
  Omnaris

ANTIALLERGIC RHINITIS   See **beclomethasone p 51**
  Nasal Spray

cilostazol
  Pletal
  Tab- cornstarch
	PERIPHERAL VASCULAR DISEASE TREATMENT
	  (Reduction of Symptoms of Intermittent Claudication)
	  Phosphodiesterase III Inhibitor Platelet Aggregation Inhibitor
	  Drug: High fat meal ↑ abs of drug.
	  Take 1/2 hr before or 2 hr after breakfast & supper.
	  Diet: Avoid grapefruit/related citrus, see p 390.
	  Oral/GI: Dyspepsia, nausea, abdominal pain, <u>abnormal stool</u>, <u>diarrhea</u>, flatulence.
	  S/Cond: Not c̄ lactation. 95-98% serum pro bound. Not c̄ CHF of any severity.
	  Pregnancy: Category C.
	  Other: <u>HEADACHE</u>, <u>palpitations</u>, tachycardia, dizziness, cough, rhinitis, infection, edema. **Blood/Serum:** ↓ *PLATELET AGGREGATION*, ↓ <u>TG</u>, ↑ <u>HDL</u>.

Ciloxan	ANTIBIOTIC, Fluoroquinolone Eye Drops	See **ciprofloxacin** p 85

cimetidine **Tagamet/Tagamet HB** (OTC)	ANTIULCER, ANTIGERD, ANTISECRETORY	See **Histamine H$_2$ Receptor Antagonists** p 162

Cimzia	RHEUMATOID ARTHRITIS OR CROHN'S DISEASE TREATMENT, TNF Inhibitor	See **certolizumab** p 80

cinacalcet
  Sensipar
  Tab- starch
	SECONDARY HYPERPARATHROIDISM TREATMENT IN DIALYSIS,
	ANTIHYPERCALCEMIA IN PARATHYROID CARCINOMA
	  Drug: Take c̄ meals to ↑ abs. (High fat meal ↑ drug C$_{max}$ 82%).
	  Take tab whole, do not divide.
	  Diet: Theoretical interaction c̄ grapefruit/related citrus, see p 390.
	  Nutr: Anorexia.
	  Oral/GI: N/V, diarrhea.
	  S/Cond: Not c̄ lactation. 93-97% serum pro bound. Caution c̄ ↓ hepatic func.
	  Pregnancy: Category C.
	  Other: Weakness, dizziness, HTN, muscle pain, chest pain.
	  Blood/Serum: ↓ *HYPERCALCEMIA*, ↓ *PTH*. Hypocalcemia.
	  Monitor: PTH, Ca.

ciprofloxacin
  Cipro
  Tab- cornstarch
  Microcapsule Susp
  (5 & 10 %)- sucrose,
  lecithin,
  medium chain triglycerides
  Cipro XR (SR)
  Tab
  Cipro I.V.
  Ciloxan eye drops
  Soln or ointment
  Proquin XR (SR)
  Tab

ANTIBIOTIC, Fluoroquinolone   Oral, Parenteral (IV) or Eye Drops

Drug: Food delays, but does not ↓ abs. Do not take c̄ dairy products or Ca fortified foods alone, but may take c̄ a meal that contains these products. Do not chew microcapsules in susp. Do not crush or chew XR tab.

Diet: Insure adequate fluid intake/hydration. Take drug at least 2 hr before or 6 hr after milk, yogurt, Ca fortified foods (eg OJ), antacids, Mg, Ca, Fe or Zn suppl or MVI + minerals. Take separately from oral enteral product.[39] Avoid or limit caffeine/xanthine- drug causes ↑ caffeine effect.

Nutr: Divalent or trivalent cations, milk, yogurt, enteral product or Ca fortified food ↓ drug abs & bioavailability.[3, 9b]

Oral/GI: Bad taste, <u>N</u>/V, abdominal pain, diarrhea.
Rare- oral candidiasis, pseudomembranous colitis.

S/Cond: Not c̄ lactation. Do not use susp c̄ TF- clogs tube.[1]
May crush tab for TF, but separate from enteral product by ≥ 2 hr.[39]
Caution c̄ ↓ renal func. Caution c̄ seizures.

Pregnancy: Category C.

Other: Headache, dizziness, restlessness, drowsiness, rash, photosensitivity. Rare- CNS toxicity, confusion, tendon rupture, tendonitis, joint or muscle pain, seizures, allergic reaction, anaphylaxis, angioedema, SJS, TEN, pancreatitis, hepatic necrosis.

Blood/Serum: ↑ AST, ↑ ALT, ↑ BUN, ↑ crea, ↑ CPK, ↑ TG, ↑ uric acid.
< 1%- dyscrasias, ↑ alk phos, ↑ LDH, ↑ GGT, ↑ bil, ↑ chol, ↑ TG,
↑ or ↓ glucose, ↑ or ↓ K.[7]

Urinary: False positive opiate tests.[9c]

Monitor: Renal & hepatic func, CBC c̄ diff.[6]

cisplatin
  Platinol-AQ

ANTINEOPLASTIC (testicular, ovarian, bladder or lung cancers)
    alkylating agent   Parenteral only (IV)

Drug: Pretreatment IV hydration c̄ 1-2 L normal saline recommended.[4, 26]
Diet: Insure adequate fluid intake/hydration to produce
100-200 mL urine/hr for ≥ 24 hr after infusion.[26] May need mineral suppl.
Mg & K may be added to pre & post treatment hydration fluids.[26]
Vit E suppl ↓ peripheral neuropathy.[110]
Nutr: Anorexia, ↓ wt.
Oral/GI: <u>Altered</u> <u>taste</u>, stomatitis, SEVERE PROLONGED <u>N/V</u> (up to 1 week),
<u>diarrhea</u>.
S/Cond: Not c̄ lactation. Do dental care cautiously, see p 11 & 15.
90% serum pro bound. Not c̄ ↓ renal func.
Pregnancy: Category D.
Other: <u>RENAL TOXICITY</u>, <u>WEAKNESS</u>, <u>OTOTOXICITY</u>, <u>PERIPHERAL NEUROPATHY</u>,
<u>INFECTIONS</u>, <u>BONE MARROW SUPPRESSION</u>, <u>HAIR LOSS</u>. Rare- SIADH.
Blood/Serum: ↓ <u>WBC</u>, ↓ <u>PLATELETS</u>, <u>ANEMIA</u>, ↑ <u>BUN</u>, ↑ <u>URIC</u>
<u>ACID</u>, ↑ <u>ALK PHOS</u>, ↑ <u>AST</u>, ↑ bil, ↓ <u>MAGNESIUM</u>, ↓ <u>K</u>, ↓ <u>Na</u>, ↓ Zn, ↓ <u>Ca</u>, ↓ P.
Urinary: ↑ <u>Mg</u>, ↑ Ca, ↑ K, ↑ Zn, ↑ Cu, ↑ amino acids.
Monitor: Weekly CBC c̄ diff.
Renal & hepatic func, electrolytes, Mg, uric acid.
Hearing & neurological func.

citalopram
  Celexa
  Tab- cornstarch,
    lactose
  Soln- sorbitol

ANTIDEPRESSANT, SSRI   Also used as an antianxiety or antipanic agent
Drug: Take s̄ regard to food.
Diet: Avoid tryptophan suppl- may ↑ drug side effects.[3] Avoid SJW, see p 286.
Nutr: ↑ <u>weight</u>, ↑ <u>appetite</u>. Anorexia, ↓ wt.
Oral/GI: <u>Dry mouth</u>, taste changes, ↑ salivation, dyspepsia, <u>nausea</u>,
vomiting, abdominal pain, diarrhea, flatulence.
S/Cond: Avoid alcohol. Caution c̄ lactation.
Caution c̄ ↓ hepatic func, severe ↓ renal func or geriatric.
Pregnancy: Category C.
Other: Drowsiness, tremor, ↑ sweating, fatigue, muscle/joint pain,
insomnia, anxiety, agitation, rhinitis, sinusitis, URTI, tachycardia, ↓ BP,

paresthesia, migraine, confusion, coughing, rash.
Rare- SIADH, serotonin syndrome, suicidal thinking & behavior.
Blood/Serum: Rare- ↓ Na. **Urinary:** ↑ frequency.

Citracal	MINERAL SUPPLEMENT	See **calcium citrate p 70**
Citrucel	LAXATIVE, Bulk Forming	See **methylcellulose p 212**
Claforan	ANTIBIOTIC, **cefotaxime sodium**	See **cephalosporins p 80**

Clarinex ANTIHISTAMINE See lising **for loratadine p 199**
  desloratadine metabolite of **loratadine** < 90% serum pro bound.
  Tab- cornstarch, lactose **Drug:** Dissolve ODT on tongue c̄ or s̄ liquid, swallow saliva.
  ODT- mannitol, aspartame, starch, Na starch glycolate
  Syrup- sorbitol, propylene glycol, granulated sugar

clarithromycin ANTIBIOTIC, H-PYLORI TREATMENT, ANTI-MAC (tab or susp), Macrolide
  Biaxin (Note: XL tab is not indicated to treat or prevent MAC)
  250 mg Tab- **Drug:** Take tab or susp s̄ regard to food. XL tab should be taken c̄ food.
  starch, **Oral/GI:** Abnormal taste, dyspepsia, N/V, abdominal pain, diarrhea.
  propylene glycol Rare- oral candidiasis, pseudomembranous colitis.
  500 mg Tab-propylene glycol **S/Cond:** Caution c̄ alcohol- ↑ sedative effect of alcohol.
  Susp- sucrose, Caution c̄ lactation. Caution c̄ severe ↓ renal func.
  castor oil **Pregnancy:** Category C. **Other:** Headache, rash.
  Biaxin XL (SR) Rare- hepatotoxicity, pancreatitis, allergic reaction, anaphylaxis, SJS, TEN.
  XL Tab- lactose, **Blood/Serum:** ↑ BUN, ↑ PT/INR. < 1%- ↑ AST, ↑ ALT, ↑ LDH, ↑ alk phos,
  propylene glycol ↑ bil, ↑ GGT, ↑ crea, ↓ WBC.

Claritin ANTIHISTAMINE See **loratadine p 199**

Claritin-D ANTIHISTAMINE, DECONGESTANT See **loratadine p 199**
  12 hr Tab- lactose, Combination drug See **pseudoephedrine p 269**
    30 mg Ca **loratadine** & **pseudoephedrine**
  24 hr Tab- sugar, 25 mg Ca **Drug:** Swallow whole- do not crush, chew or divide.

Cleocin	ANTIBIOTIC	See **clindamycin below**
Climara	HORMONE, Estrogen	See **Hormone Therapy p 165**

clindamycin ANTIBIOTIC Oral or Parenteral (IM or IV)
  Cleocin
  Cap- lactose, cornstarch
  75 & 150 mg Cap-
  tartrazine
  Pediatric Soln- sucrose

  Parenteral- Vial- benzyl
  alcohol 9.45 mg/mL
  IV Soln- 5% dextrose

> **Drug:** May take oral forms c̄ food or 8 oz water to ↓ esophageal irritation.
> **Nutr:** Anorexia, ↓ wt, ↑ thirst.
> **Oral/GI:** Metallic taste (c̄ IV), esophagitis, N/V, cramps, severe
> pseudomembranous colitis, flatulence, bloating, DIARRHEA.
> **S/Cond:** Not c̄ lactation. 93% serum pro bound.
> Caution c̄ severe ↓ hepatic func or ↓ renal func.
> Caution c̄ history of GI disease, especially colitis.
> **Pregnancy:** Category B.
> **Other:** RASH, hypotension c̄ rapid IV, jaundice, SJS.
> **Blood/Serum:** Transient dyscrasias, ↑ ALT, ↑ AST, ↑ alk phos, ↑ bil.
> **Monitor:** Renal func, hepatic func & CBC c̄ LT use.

clomipramine ANTI-OCD, ANTIDEPRESSANT See **Tricyclic Antidepressants p 323**
  Anafranil

clonazepam ANTIEPILEPTIC, ANTIPANIC See **Benzodiazepines p 54**
  Klonopin

clonidine ANTIHYPERTENSIVE, ANALGESIC
  Catapres
  Tab- lactose, gelatin,
  cornstarch
  Catapres TTS
  Transdermal patch
  Duraclon
  epidural infusion
  for cancer/intractable pain
  (used c̄ opiates)

> Also Treatment of ADHD, withdrawal symptoms of opiate, alcohol or
> nicotine addiction. Oral, Transdermal patch (TTS) & Epidural Infusion
> **Duraclon-** Used epidurally c̄ opiates to treat intractable pain
> **Drug:** Take last dose HS.[6]
> **Diet:** for HTN- ↓ Na & ↓ cal may be recommended.
> Avoid natural licorice, see p 374. Insure adequate fluid intake/hydration.
> **Nutr:** ↑ wt due to edema. Anorexia.
> **Oral/GI:** DRY MOUTH, N/V, constipation.
> **S/Cond:** Avoid alcohol- drug ↑ sensitivity to alcohol. Caution c̄ lactation.

↑ risk of dental problems, see p 11 & 15. Caution $\bar{c}$ ↓ renal func.
Pregnancy: Category C.
Other: ↓ *BP* $\bar{c}$ possible hypotension, <u>DROWSINESS</u>, <u>dizziness</u>, <u>sedation</u>, <u>weakness</u>, fatigue, insomnia, depression, agitation, headache, transient edema, rash. ECG abnormalities, tachycardia, bradycardia, arrhythmias. [7] Rebound HTN if stopped suddenly.
Blood/Serum: Mild transient ↑ AST, ↑ ALT, ↑ GH.
Transient ↑ glucose $\bar{c}$ single high dose.[6]
Urinary: ↓ <u>Na</u>, ↓ <u>Cl</u>, ↓ <u>water</u>.
Monitor: BP with all forms. $\bar{c}$ infusion- monitor heart rate, temp, respiration.

clopidogrel
  Plavix
    Tab- lactose,
    castor oil,
    mannitol

ACUTE CORONARY SYNDROME TREATMENT, PREVENTION OF REPEAT MI, CVA, OR VASCULAR EVENT, Platelet Aggregation Inhibitor, Thienopyridine Prodrug
To ↓ rate of new ischemic stoke, MI or other vascular death
Drug: Food significantly ↑ bioavailability.[117] Take $\bar{c}$ food if GI distress occurs.[7]
Oral/GI: <u>Dyspepsia</u>, N/V, <u>abdominal pain</u>, <u>GI bleeding</u>/hemorrhage, diarrhea, constipation.
S/Cond: Not $\bar{c}$ lactation. Caution $\bar{c}$ ↓ hepatic func.
Not $\bar{c}$ conditions which ↑ bleeding risk, e.g. peptic ulcer.
Do dental care cautiously, ↑ risk of bleeding. ≥ 94% serum pro bound.
Pregnancy: Category B.
Other: <u>Pain</u>, <u>flu-like symptoms</u>, <u>URTI</u>, <u>dizziness</u>, <u>headache</u>, <u>purpura</u>, <u>HTN</u>, hypotension, fatigue, edema, depression, nosebleed, gout, cough, dyspnea, syncope, palpitations, bradycardia, atrial fibrillation, insomnia, paresthesia, leg cramps, fever, rash, bleeding (can be fatal), bruising.
Blood/Serum: ↑ <u>BLEEDING TIME</u>, ↓ <u>PLATELETS</u>, anemia, ↓ neutrophils, ↑ bil, ↑ AST, ↑ ALT, ↑ <u>chol</u>, ↑ NPN, ↑ uric acid.
Urinary: UTI.

clorazepate
  Tranxene

ANTIANXIETY, ANTIEPILEPTIC   See **Benzodiazepines p 54**
RELIEF OF ACUTE ALCOHOL SYMPTOMS

C

Clorpres
  Tab

ANTIHYPERTENSIVE, DIURETIC
  Combination drug

See **chlorthalidone** p 82
See **clonidine** p 88

clotrimazole
  Mycelex
  Troche (oral lozenge)-
    dextrose

ANTIFUNGAL (Anti-Oropharyngeal Candidiasis)
  Drug: Dissolve slowly in mouth over 15-30 minutes, swallow saliva.
  <u>Do not chew.</u>
  Oral/GI: <u>Unpleasant</u> <u>mouth</u> <u>sensations</u>, <u>N/V</u>, cramps, diarrhea.
  Pregnancy: Category C.
  Blood/Serum: ↑ <u>AST</u>.
  Monitor: Hepatic func.

clozapine
  Clozaril
  Tab- lactose,
    cornstarch
  Fazaclo
  ODT- mannitol,
    aspartame
    phenylalanine/Tab
  12.5 mg tab- 0.87 mg
  25 mg tab- 1.74 mg
  50 mg tab- 3.48 mg
  100 mg tab- 6.69 mg

ANTIPSYCHOTIC (Second Generation) Dibenzothiazepine Derivative
Also TO PREVENT RECURRENT SUICIDAL BEHAVIOR
  Drug: Take s̄ regard to food.
  Dissolve ODT on tongue c̄ or s̄ liquid, swallow saliva.
  Diet: Caution c̄ caffeine, see p 67.
  Caffeine inhibits drug metabolism & ↑ drug levels.[62]
  Nutr: ↑ <u>APPETITE</u>, ↑ <u>WT</u>, <u>obesity</u>, anorexia.
  Oral/GI: <u>Dry mouth</u>, ↑ OR ↓ <u>SALIVATION</u>, sore tongue, <u>reflux</u> <u>esophagitis</u>,[21]
  <u>N/V</u>, dyspepsia, severe <u>CONSTIPATION</u>,[21] impaction, diarrhea.
  S/Cond: Avoid alcohol. Not c̄ lactation. 97% serum pro bound.
  Hypoalbuminemia (< 3 g/dL) may ↑ drug effects. ↑ risk of dental
  problems, see p 11 & 15. Caution c̄ ↓ hepatic func or ↓ renal func.
  Caution c̄ seizures/history of seizures.
  Caution c̄ Asian pt- may need ↓ dose.[21]
  Pregnancy: Category B.
  Other: <u>DROWSINESS</u>, <u>TACHYCARDIA</u>, <u>DIABETES</u>,[1] <u>dizziness</u>, <u>headache</u>,
  <u>sedation</u>, <u>tremor</u>, <u>fever</u>, <u>visual</u> <u>changes</u>, <u>orthostatic</u> <u>hypotension</u>, <u>syncope</u>,
  <u>sweating</u>, <u>seizures</u>, ↑ BP, ataxia, agitation, confusion, rigidity, weakness,
  muscle pain/spasm, insomnia, EPS, rash.
  Rare- (can be fatal) pulmonary embolism, cardiomyopathy, myocarditis,
  nephritis, NMS. ↑ mortality in geriatrics c̄ dementia-related psychosis.[10]
  Blood/Serum: ↑ <u>TRIGLYCERIDES</u>.[21] ↑ <u>GLUCOSE</u>,[1] agranulocytosis
  (↓ WBC- rare, can be fatal), eosinophilia.

Mild transient ↑ AST, ↑ ALT, ↑ LDH, ↑ alk phos.[6]
Urinary: INCONTINENCE,[21] retention.
Monitor: Baseline WBC, ANC, weekly WBC, ANC, for 6 mo, then q 2 wk for 6 mo, then q 4 wk. Baseline wt then monthly X 3, then quarterly. Possibly waist circumference. Baseline BP, FBS, HbA1$_c$ & lipids then at 12 wk, then at least annually.[1, 21]

codeine
Parenteral-
sulfites

ANTITUSSIVE, ANALGESIC, Narcotic, Opioid   Oral or Parenteral (IM or SC)
Drug: Take c̄ food or milk to ↓ GI distress.
Nutr: Anorexia. Delays digestion.
Oral/GI: Dry mouth, N/V, CONSTIPATION.
S/Cond: Avoid alcohol. Caution c̄ lactation- infants at ↑ risk of overdose if mother is CYP 2D6 ultra-rapid metabolizer.
↑ risk of dental problems, see p 11 & 15. Caution c̄ ↓ pulmonary func or mild-moderate ↓ renal func.[58] Not c̄ severe ↓ hepatic func or ↓ renal func. May be habit forming c̄ LT use.
Pregnancy: Category C.
Other: ↓ COUGH, drowsiness, sedation, dizziness, confusion, headache, blurred vision, palpitation, itching, euphoria, respiratory depression.
Blood/Serum: ↑ amylase, ↑ lipase. **Urinary:** Retention.

coenzyme Q-10
CoQ10
ubiquinone

ANTIOXIDANT, Enzymatic Cofactor, Antioxidant
        (FDA approved only as orphan drug to treat mitochondrial disorders)
Used for treatment of cardiovascular disease (eg CHF, angina, HTN), Parkinson's disease, to stimulate immune system in HIV.
Used to treat adverse reactions of statin drugs, eg muscle pain.
Drug: Take c̄ meal containing fat to ↑ abs.
Formulations in soybean oil have ↑ bioavailability.[93]
Nutr: Prolongs antioxidant effect of Vit E. < 1%- ↓ appetite.
Oral/GI: < 1%- gastritis, nausea, diarrhea.
S/Cond: Not c̄ lactation. Caution c̄ diabetics on insulin- ↓ insulin requirements. Caution c̄ ↓ hepatic func- ↑ CoQ10 blood levels.
Pregnancy: Safety not established. Use not recommended.
Other: Insomnia c̄ doses > 100 mg in the evening.

Cogentin generic equivalents	ANTIPARKINSON	See **benztropine p 55**

Colace — STOOL SOFTENER — See **docusate sodium p 115**

Colazal
balsalazide — ANTI-INFLAMMATORY — See listing for **mesalamine p 209**
pro-drug of **mesalamine** — Cap- 86 mg Na/cap

colchicine
Colchicine
Tab- sucrose
or lactose
Colcrys
Tab- lactose,
starch

ANTIGOUT, Anti-inflammatory
TREATMENT OF FAMILIAL MEDITERANEAN FEVER (**Colcrys** only)
Diet: ↓ purine diet during acute attack.
Avoid grapefruit/related citrus, see p 390.
Nutr: Anorexia, ↓ wt. May ↓ abs of Vit B$_{12}$.
Oral/GI: Sore throat, NAUSEA/VOMITING, STOMACH PAIN, DIARRHEA.
S/Cond: Avoid alcohol. Caution c̄ lactation. Caution c̄ ↓ hepatic func or
severe ↓ renal func, cardiac disease, GI disorder, geriatric or debilitated.
Not c̄ combined ↓ renal func & ↓ hepatic func.[7]
Do not use IV c̄ severe ↓ hepatic func or renal func.
Pregnancy: Category C.
Other: Peripheral neuritis, ↑ BP, weakness, rash, renal damage,
bone marrow suppression c̄ LT use.
Blood/Serum: Dyscrasias, ↓ platelets, ↓ Vit B$_{12}$, ↑ alk phos, ↑ AST,
↑ CPK, ↓ chol. **Urinary:** False + RBC or Hb. **Monitor:** CBC c̄ diff c̄ LT use.

colesevelam
Welchol
Tab

ANTIHYPERLIPIDEMIC, Bile Acid Sequestrant
Drug: Take c̄ meal(s) & liquid 1-2X per day.
Diet: Adjunct to ↓ fat, ↓ chol diet.
Nutr: Does not affect abs of fat soluble Vit.[9a]
Oral/GI: Dyspepsia, constipation.
S/Cond: Not c̄ bowel obstruction. Not abs from GI tract.
Pregnancy: Category B. **Other:** Weakness, pharyngitis.
Blood/Serum: ↓ CHOL, ↓ LDL, ↑ HDL, SLIGHTLY ↑ TG.
Monitor: Chol, LDL, TG.

CombiPatch — HORMONE, Estrogen plus Progestin Patch — See **Hormone Therapy p 165**

Combipres (generics only) ANTIHYPERTENSIVE, DIURETIC See **chlorthalidone p 82**
Tab- lactose, cornstarch See **clonidine p 88**

Combivent ANTI-COPD, BRONCHODILATOR See **albuterol p 25**
Inhaler- soy lecithin See **ipratropium p 178**
Combivent Respimat
Inhalation spray- EDTA, CFC free

Combivir ANTIRETROVIRAL (HIV/AIDS), NRTI See **lamivudine p 181**
Tab- starch Combination drug See **zidovudine p 348**

Compazine ANTIEMETIC, ANTINAUSEANT, ANTIPSYCHOTIC
prochlorperazine See **Phenothiazines p 254**

Complera ANTIRETROVIRAL (HIV/AIDS), Combination drug
See **emtricitabine p 123**
See **rilpivirine p 280**
See **tenofovir p 306**

Comtan ANTIPARKINSON, COMT Inhibitor See **entacapone p 124**

Concerta PSYCHOSTIMULANT, ANTI-ADHD See **methylphenidate p 214**

Constulose LAXATIVE (Hyperosmotic), To Treat ↑ AMMONIA LEVEL
See **lactulose p 186**

Copegus ANTIVIRAL, use with **Pegasys** to treat Hepatitis C
See **ribavirin p 228**

Cordarone ANTIARRHYTHMIC See **amiodarone p 31**

Coreg/Coreg CR CHF TREATMENT, ANTIHYPERTENSIVE, Non-selective Beta-Blocker
See **carvedilol p 75**

Corgard ANTIHYPERTENSIVE, ANTIANGINA, Beta-Blocker See **nadolol p 223**

corticosteroids   ANTI-INFLAMMATORY, IMMUNOSUPPRESSANT, Hormone, Glucocorticoid
Oral or Parenteral (IM, IV, SC, Intralesional, Intra-articular)

Drug: Take c̄ food to ↓ GI effects. Dissolve ODT on tongue c̄ or s̄ liquid, swallow saliva.
Diet: ↓ Na, ↑ Ca, ↑ Vit D, ↑ pro.[7] May need ↑ K, ↑ Vits A, C, ↑ P, (or suppl).
Ca-Vit D suppl recommended c̄ LT use. Caution c̄ grapefruit/related citrus c̄ **methylprednisolone,** see p 390.
Limit caffeine to ↓ GI effects.
Oral/GI: Esophagitis, N/V, dyspepsia, peptic ulcer, bloating, GI bleeding/perforation.
Nutr: ↑ APPETITE, ↑ WT, except ANOREXIA c̄ **triamcinolone.**[13] Negative N balance due to pro catabolism.
C̲A̲ WASTING c̄ LT use. Cr def may ↑ risk for steroid induced diabetes.[93]
S/Cond: Avoid alcohol. Not c̄ lactation. Not c̄ peptic ulcer.[6] Caution c̄ diabetes - ↑ glucose. Highly pro bound.
Hypoalbuminemia (< 3 g/dL)- may ↑ drug effects.[6] Caution c̄ ↓ renal func or seizures.
Pregnancy: Category C.
Other: EDEMA, ↑ BP, insomnia, masking of infection, slow healing, diabetes, bruising, hypogonadism,
weakness, dizziness, headache, seizures, psychological disturbances, acne, rash.
LT use of > 1 g for 6 mo- OSTEOPOROSIS/NECROSIS, FRACTURES, MUSCLE WASTING, cataracts, pancreatitis,
adrenocortical insufficiency, Cushing's syndrome, ↓ growth in children.
Blood/Serum: ↑ Na, ↓ K, ↓ Ca, ↑ glucose, ↓ Zn,[11] ↓ uric acid, ↓ Vit C,[6] ↓ Vit A,[6] ↑ TG, ↓ T_3, ↓ T_4,[7] ↑ Hb,[4]
↑ RBC,[4] dyscrasias, ↑ chol (↑ c̄ **cortisone**).[6]
Urinary: ↓ Na, ↑ K, ↑ Ca, ↑ uric acid, glucose, ↑ N, ↑ Zn, ↑ Vit C, ↑ Cr.
Monitor: LT use- Electrolytes, adrenal func, glucose, BP, wt, children's growth. Bone density c̄ use > 6 mo.

cortisone acetate- Cortone Acetate Tab- lactose, starch. Parenteral- benzyl alcohol.
dexamethasone - Low mineralocorticoid effects - less Na retention, edema, K loss, or HTN.
  Tab- lactose, starch, sucrose. Soln- propylene glycol, sorbitol. Intensol - 30% alcohol
  Parenteral- Na sulfite, benzyl alcohol.
hydrocortisone (cortisol)-Cortef Tab- lactose, sucrose. Susp- sucrose. **Solu-Cortef** Parenteral- benzyl alcohol.
methylprednisolone- Low mineralocorticoid effects- less Na retention, edema, K loss, or HTN.
  Depo-Medrol/Solu-Medrol Parenteral- benzyl alcohol. **Medrol** Tab- lactose, sucrose. 24 mg Tab- tartrazine.
prednisolone- Orapred - Soln- 2% alcohol, fructose, sorbitol. ODT- mannitol, sucralose, sucrose.
  Prelone- Syrup- 5% alcohol, saccharin, sucrose.
prednisone- Tab- lactose, sucrose.
triamcinolone- Kenalog Parenteral- benzyl alcohol.

cortisol   CORTICOSTEROID, **hydrocortisone**   See **corticosteroids above**

Corzide	ANTIHYPERTENSIVE	See **nadalol p 223**
Tab- lactose, starch	Combination drug	See listing for **hydrochlorothiazide p 166**
Pregnancy: Category C.	**nadalol/bendroflumethiazide** 40 mg/5 mg & 80 mg/5 mg tabs	

Cosmegen ANTINEOPLASTIC, Antibiotic See **dactinomycin p 100**

Coumadin ANTICOAGULANT See **warfarin p 344**

Covera-HS ANTIANGINA, ANTIHYPERTENSIVE See **verapamil p 332**

Cozaar ANTIHYPERTENSIVE See **Angiotensin II Receptor Antagonists p 38**
  losartan

Crestor ANTIHYPERLIPIDEMIC, **rosuvastatin** See **HMG-CoA Reductase Inhibitors p 164**

Crixivan ANTIRETROVIRAL (HIV/AIDS), Protease Inhibitor See **indinavir p 173**

Cubicin ANTIBIOTIC, Cyclic Lipopeptide See **daptomycin p 102**

cyanocobalamin B-COMPLEX VITAMIN, ANTIANEMIC See **vitamin B$_{12}$ p 338**

Cyclessa ORAL CONTRACEPTIVE See **Oral Contraceptives p 237**

cyclobenzaprine SKELETAL MUSCLE RELAXANT, Anticholinergic
  Flexeril   Also used as fibromyalgia treatment
  Tab- lactose,   Closely related to **tricyclic antidepressants**, See also p 323
    starch   **Drug:** Take s̄ regard to food, but food ↑ C$_{max}$ & AUC of Tab.
  Amrix (SR)   **Oral/GI:** <u>DRY MOUTH</u>, unpleasant taste, dyspepsia, nausea, constipation.
  Cap- sugar spheres   **S/Cond:** Avoid alcohol. Caution c̄ lactation. 93% serum pro bound.
    ↑ risk of dental problems, see p 11 & 15. Not c̄ CHF or hyperthyroidism.
    Tab- not c̄ moderate-severe ↓ hepatic func. Caution c̄ geriatric.[84]
    Cap- not c̄ any ↓ hepatic func or c̄ geriatric.[7] Caution c̄ hx of urinary
    retention, glaucoma, or ↑ intraocular pressure.
    Pregnancy: Category B.
    Other: <u>DROWSINESS</u>, <u>dizziness</u>, fatigue, weakness, blurred vision, headache,
    confusion, nervousness. Rare- SIADH, hepatitis. **Urinary:** Retention.

cyclophosphamide ANTINEOPLASTIC, Alkylating Agent Oral or Parenteral (IV)
  Cytoxan previous brand name (Hodgkin's, leukemia, multiple myeloma, other cancers)
  Tab- lactose **Drug:** Take tab on empty stomach.
  Parenteral- If GI distress occurs, may take c̄ meals in divided doses.[13]
   mannitol- **Diet:** ↑ fluid before dose & for ≥ 72 hr after dose.
   75 mg/100 mg drug, 2-3 L/day essential to induce frequent voiding.
   NaCl- **Nutr:** Anorexia, ↓ wt.
   45 mg/100 mg drug **Oral/GI:** Dry mouth, stomatitis, N/V, abdominal pain, diarrhea.
  S/Cond: Not c̄ lactation. Do dental care cautiously, see p 11 & 15.
  Caution c̄ ↓ hepatic or ↓ renal func. Not c̄ severe ↓ bone marrow func.
  Pregnancy: Category D.
  Other: BONE MARROW SUPPRESSION, HAIR LOSS, delayed wound healing,
  weakness, headache, pulmonary fibrosis, darkening of pigment/nail beds.
  Acute hemorrhagic cystitis (rarely can be fatal).
  Blood/Serum: ↓ WBC, ↓ PLATELETS, anemia, ↑ uric acid, ↑ AST, ↑ ALT,
  ↑ bil, ↑ LDH, ↑ BUN, ↑ crea.
  Urinary: Hematuria.
  Monitor: Hepatic & renal func, CBC c̄ diff, platelets, uric acid.
  Urine for RBC. Fluid intake & output.

Cycloset ANTIDIABETIC AGENT Type 2 Diabetes Mellitus See **bromocriptine p 64**

cyclosporine IMMUNOSUPPRESSANT (Prevent organ rejection, Antiarthritic (RA),
  Neoral To treat Psoriasis) Oral or Parenteral (IV)
  Oral Soln- **Drug: Neoral** Soln- mix in glass container c̄ orange or apple juice at
   9.5% alcohol room temp (unpalatable c̄ milk). **Sandimmune** Soln- mix in glass
  Cap- 9.5% alcohol container c̄ 1 cup milk, chocolate milk or orange juice at room temp.
  Sandimmune Drink mixtures immediately.
  Oral Soln- **Diet:** No K suppl or salt sub. Avoid grapefruit/related citrus, see p 390.
   12.5 % alcohol, Vit E may ↑ abs of drug.[65] Avoid SJW, see p 286. Caution c̄ red wine.[46]
   olive oil **Nutr:** Anorexia. Water soluble Vit E ↑ drug abs.[65]
  Cap- **Oral/GI:** Gum hyperplasia, N/V, diarrhea.
   12.7% alcohol, sorbitol **S/Cond:** Not c̄ lactation. 90-98% serum pro bound. Do dental care

Inj- 32.9% alcohol	cautiously, see p 11 & 15. Caution c̄ diabetes- ↑ glucose. Caution c̄ ↓ hepatic func or ↓ renal func. **Pregnancy:** Category C. **Other:** <u>NEPHROTOXICITY</u>, <u>TREMOR</u>, <u>HYPERTENSION</u>, <u>headache</u>, <u>hepatotoxicity</u>, confusion, flushing, sinusitis, conjunctivitis, muscle pain, edema, convulsions, infections, fever. **Blood/Serum:** ↑ <u>BUN</u>, ↑ <u>CREA</u>, ↑ <u>ALT</u>, ↑ <u>AST</u>, ↑ <u>alk phos</u>, ↑ <u>bil</u>, ↑ <u>GGT</u>, ↑ <u>K</u>, ↓ <u>Mg</u>, ↓ <u>bicarb</u>, ↑ uric acid, ↑ glucose, anemia, ↓ WBC, ↑ amylase. ↑ <u>TG</u>, ↑ chol.[6] **Urinary:** ↑ <u>MAGNESIUM</u>, ↓ K.[66] **Monitor:** <u>Renal</u> & hepatic func, BP, CBC, Mg, K, drug level.
Cymbalta	ANTIDEPRESSANT, ANTIANXIETY, FYBROMYALGIA TREATMENT ANALGESIC for Diabetic Peripheral Neuropathy, SSNRI See **duloxetine p 119**
cyproheptadine **Periactin** previous brand name Tab- lactose, starch	ANTIHISTAMINE, ANTIPRURITIC (also used as an appetite stimulant) **Drug:** Take c̄ food or milk to ↓ GI distress. **Nutr:** ↑ <u>APPETITE</u>, ↑ <u>WT</u>. **Oral/GI:** <u>Dry mouth/throat</u>, N/V, constipation, diarrhea. **S/Cond:** Avoid alcohol. Not c̄ lactation. ↑ risk of dental problems, see p 11 & 15. Caution c̄ geriatric.[84] **Pregnancy:** Category B. **Other:** <u>DROWSINESS</u>, <u>SEDATION</u>, dizziness, ataxia, blurred vision, confusion, tremor, edema, hypotension, headache, rash, photosensitivity, restlessness, insomnia, irritability, euphoria, hallucinations, paresthesia, palpitations, tachycardia, hepatic func abnormality. **Blood/Serum:** Dyscrasias. **Urinary:** ↑ frequency, retention.

cytarabine (ara-C)
Cytosar-U
benzyl alcohol
DepoCyt (liposome form)
(intrathecal use)
preservative free
cholesterol 4.1 mg/mL

ANTINEOPLASTIC, Antimetabolite (leukemias) Parenteral only (IV, Intrathecal or SC)
Diet: ↑ fluid intake/hydration essential.
Nutr: <u>ANOREXIA</u>, ↓ wt.
Oral/GI: <u>STOMATITIS</u>, esophagitis, sore throat, <u>NAUSEA/VOMITING</u>, diarrhea, <u>anal inflammation</u> or <u>ulceration</u>.
S/Cond: Not c̄ lactation. Do dental care cautiously, see p 11 & 15.
Caution c̄ ↓ hepatic func or ↓ renal func.[7]
Pregnancy: Category D.
Other: <u>BONE MARROW SUPPRESSION</u>, <u>INFECTION</u>, <u>fatigue</u>, hepatotoxicity, dizziness, headache, fever, rash, renal toxicity, muscle/bone pain, conjunctivitis, chest pain, neural toxicity, pneumonia.
Blood/Serum: <u>DYSCRASIAS</u>, ↓ <u>WBC</u>, anemia, ↑ <u>uric acid</u>, ↑ alk phos, ↑ AST, ↑ ALT, ↑ bil, ↓ K, ↓ Ca.
Urinary: ↑ uric acid. Retention.
Monitor: Daily <u>leukocytes</u>, <u>platelets</u> during <u>induction</u>.
<u>Bone aspiration</u> q <u>2</u> wks.[26] Renal & hepatic func, uric acid.

Cytovene
ANTIVIRAL, ANTI-CMV
See **ganciclovir** p 154

Cytoxan previous brand name ANTINEOPLASTIC, Alkylating Agent
See **cyclophosphamide** p 96

dabigatran
Pradaxa
cap- tartaric acid

PREVENTION NON STROKE/SYSTEMIC EMBOLISM in NON VALVULAR ATRIAL FIBRILLATION, oral anticoagulant, direct thrombin inhibitor
Drug: Do not break, chew, open or empty pellets from cap. Swallow cap whole. Bioavailability ↑ 75% if pellets are removed from intact shell. Take s̄ regard to food. Take c̄ food if GI distress
Diet: Not c̄ supplements, anticoagulants or antiplatelet activity. SJW ↓ drug level, see p 286.
Oral/GI: <u>DYSPEPSIA</u>, abdominal pain, GERD, esophagitis, erosive gastritis, gastric hemorrhage, GI ulcer, diarrhea.
S/Cond: Avoid or limit alcohol/other GI irritants which may cause bleeding. Caution c̄ lactation. Caution c̄ pts > 75 yrs, bleeding ↑ age. Not c̄ severe ↓ renal func (CrCl < 15 ml/min). Do dental care cautiously, ↑ risk of bleeding.

Pregnancy: Category C.
Other: Bleeding (can be fatal), dizziness, dyspnea, peripheral edema, fatigue, cough, arthralgia, nasopharyngitis, URTI.
< 1%- ischemic stroke, hemorrhagic stroke, systemic embolism, hypersensitivity reaction.
Blood/ Serum: ↑ ALT, ↑ AST, ↑ aPTT ↑ ECT, ↑ TT (no blood testing required).
Urinary: UTI.
Monitor: For S/S of bleeding/blood loss.

dacarbazine
DTIC-Dome
Vial- mannitol

imidazole

ANTINEOPLASTIC, Alkylating Agent   Parenteral Only (IV)
(Metastatic malignant melanoma, Hodgkin's lymphoma, Kaposi sarcoma)
Drug: Restrict oral food/fluids 4-6 hr prior to IV to ↓ N/V. **Nutr:** ANOREXIA.
Oral/GI: Stomatitis, SEVERE NAUSEA/VOMITING, diarrhea.
S/Cond: Not c̄ lactation. Caution c̄ ↓ hepatic func or ↓ renal func.[26]
Pregnancy: Category C.
Other: BONE MARROW SUPPRESSION, hair loss, flu-like syndrome.
Rare- facial flushing, paresthesia, photosensitivity.
Rare- hepatotoxicity- can be fatal.
Blood/Serum: Anemia, ↓ WHITE BLOOD CELLS, ↓ PLATELETS.
Rare- ↑ alk phos, ↑ AST, ↑ ALT, ↑ BUN.
Monitor: CBC, platelets. Possibly renal & hepatic func.[13]

Dacogen
decitabine

ANTINEOPLASTIC, Pyrimidine Analog

See listing for **azacitidine p 48**

dactinomycin (ACT)
  (actinomycin-D)
  Cosmegen
  20 mg mannitol/ vial

ANTINEOPLASTIC, Antibiotic   Parenteral Only (IV)
  (Wilm's tumor, rhabdomyosarcoma, Ewing's sarcoma, testicular cancer,
  gestational trophoblastic neoplasia)
  Note - toxic effects, except N/V, often are delayed 2-14 days.
  Diet: Insure adequate fluid intake/hydration. **Nutr:** <u>Anorexia</u>, ↓ wt.
  Oral/GI: <u>Dry mouth</u>, STOMATITIS, <u>taste changes</u>, <u>glossitis</u>,
  <u>SEVERE ESOPHAGITIS</u>, <u>dysphagia</u>, SEVERE <u>NAUSEA/VOMITING</u>, <u>dyspepsia</u>, <u>pain</u>,
  GI ulceration, <u>diarrhea</u>.
  S/Cond: Not c̄ lactation. Do dental care cautiously, see p 11 & 15.
  Obese patient may need ↓ dose/kg body wt.
  Caution c̄ geriatric or ↓ hepatic func.[13] Not c̄ chickenpox or herpes zoster.
  Pregnancy: Category D.[10]
  Other: <u>FATIGUE</u>, <u>BONE MARROW SUPPRESSION</u>, <u>hair loss</u>, rash, acne.
  Rare- hepatotoxicity, ascites, anaphylaxis,[7] uric acid nephropathy.[13]
  Blood/Serum: ↓ <u>WHITE BLOOD CELLS</u>, ↓ <u>PLATELETS</u>, <u>ANEMIA</u>, ↑ uric acid, ↓ Ca.
  Rare- ↑ AST, ↑ ALT, ↑ LDH, ↑ bil. **Urinary:** ↑ uric acid.
  Monitor: Daily platelets & WBC. Hepatic & renal func, uric acid.

dalfampridine
  Ampyra
  Tab- polyethelene glycol

MULTIPLE SCLEROSIS TREATMENT
  Broad spectrum potassium blocker to improve walking in MS pts
  Drug: Take c̄ or s̄ food. Swallow tab whole. Do not divide, chew crush
  or dissolve tab.
  Oral/GI: <u>Nausea</u>, constipation, diarrhea, dyspepsia, throat pain.
  S/Cond: Not c̄ lactation, not c̄ Hx of seizures.
  Not c̄ moderate to severe ↓ renal func (CrCl ≤ 50 mL/min).
  Pregnancy: Category C.
  Other: <u>Insomnia</u>, <u>dizziness</u>, <u>headache</u>, <u>weakness</u>, <u>back pain</u>,
  <u>balance disorder</u>, MS relapse, parasthesia, nasopharyngitis. Rare- seizure.
  Urinary: <u>UTI</u>.
  Monitor: Renal func.

Daliresp

COPD Treatment, Selective Phosphodiesterase 4 Inhibitor
See **roflumilast p 284**

| **Dalmane** | SLEEP AID | See **Benzodiazepines p 54** |
| flurazepam | | |

dalteparin   ANTICOAGULANT   Parental only (SC)   See **heparin p 161**

Fragmin
prefilled syringe-
  preservative free
multi-dose vial-
  benzyl alcohol 14 mg/mL

low molecular weight **heparin**
S/Cond: Not c̄ pork allergy- derived from porcine intestinal mucosa.
Pregnancy: Category B.
Monitor: CBC, platelet count, UA, fecal occult blood,
possibly Anti-Factor Xa.
Unlike **heparin**, APTT monitoring is not recommended.

dapsone (DDS)   ANTIBACTERIAL, ANTILEPROSY, ANTI-PCP, toxoplasmosis

Dapsone
Tab- cornstarch
Avlosulfon
 Canada only

Diet: Prophylactic administration of Vit C, Fol & Fe may prevent some
adverse hematologic effects.[6]
Nutr: Anorexia.
Oral/GI: N/V, abdominal pain.
S/Cond: Not c̄ lactation. Not c̄ severe anemia. Caution c̄ G6PD or
methemoglobin reductase deficiency- ↑ risk of hemolytic anemia.
70-90% serum pro bound. Hypoalbuminemia (< 3.0 g/dL) may ↑ drug effects.
Caution c̄ ↓ hepatic func.[13]
Pregnancy: Category C.
Other: Dizziness, blurred vision, headache, tachycardia, insomnia, fever,
rash, paresthesia, toxic hepatitis, cholestatic jaundice, tinnitus,
photosensitivity, pancreatitis, psychosis.
Rare- peripheral neuropathy, renal toxicity, lupus erythematosus,
hypersensitivity.
Blood/Serum: <u>Dyscrasias</u>, <u>hemolytic anemia</u>, ↑ <u>methemoglobin</u>, ↑ <u>K</u>,
↓ <u>Hb</u>, ↓ alb, ↑ AST, ↑ ALT, ↑ bil (more common c̄ G6PD def), ↑ glucose.
Rare- ↑ BUN, ↑ crea.
Urinary: Alb, pro.
Monitor: CBC q wk x 1 mo; q mo x 6 mo, then 2X/yr.
Hepatic func- baseline & during treatment.

daptomycin
  Cubicin
  Preservative free

ANTIBIOTIC (To Treat Complicated Skin Infections), Cyclic Lipopeptide
Parenteral (IV)

  Nutr: ↓ appetite.
  Oral/GI: <u>Nausea</u>/vomiting, abdominal pain, <u>constipation</u>, <u>diarrhea</u>.
  Rare- pseudomembranous colitis.
  S/Cond: Caution c̄ lactation. 92% serum pro bound. Caution c̄ ↓ renal func.
  Pregnancy: Category B.
  Other: <u>Headache</u>, insomnia, dizziness, ↑ or ↓ BP, rash, limb/back pain,
  fungal infections, dyspnea, fever, anxiety, cough, sore throat, confusion,
  chest pain, cardiac failure. Rare- neuropathy, myopathy.
  Blood/Serum: ↑ CPK, anemia, ↑ alk phos, ↑ or ↓ glucose, ↓ K.
  < 1%- ↓ Mg, ↑ bicarb, electrolyte disturbance, ↑ INR, dyscrasias.
  Urinary: UTI, renal failure.
  Monitor: Baseline & weekly CPK.

darbepoetin alfa
  Aranesp

ANTIANEMIC, To Treat Anemia of Renal Failure or Chemotherapy
long acting **erythropoietin**
Parenteral only (SC or IV)
See **epoetin alfa p 126**

darifenacin
  Enablex

ANTIMUSCARINIC
See **Bladder Control Agents p 61**

darunavir
  Prezista
  Tab

ANTIRETROVIRAL (HIV/AIDS), Protease Inhibitor
Must be taken c̄ **ritonavir**, see also p 281 (Effects may be due to **ritonavir**)
  Drug: Must be taken c̄ food. Do not chew tab.
  Nutr: Anorexia, ↓ wt, polydipsia.
  Oral/GI: Dry mouth, dyspepsia, <u>nausea</u>/V, abdominal pain, constipation,
  <u>diarrhea</u>, flatulence. **S/Cond:** Not c̄ lactation. Caution c̄ ↓ hepatic func.
  Caution c̄ diabetes- ↑ glucose. Caution c̄ sulfa allergy.
  Pregnancy: Category B.
  Other: <u>Rash</u>, <u>headache</u>, <u>nasopharyngitis</u>, cough, fever, insomnia,
  drowsiness, peripheral neuropathy, lipoatrophy, muscle/joint pain,
  edema, fatigue, HTN, tachycardia, confusion, anxiety, dizziness,

↓ renal func, hepatotoxicity.
Blood/Serum: ↑ <u>amylase</u>, ↑ <u>lipase</u>, ↑ <u>GGT</u>, ↑ <u>AST</u>, ↑ <u>ALT</u>, ↑ bil, ↑ chol, ↑ TG, ↓ Na. **Urinary:** Polyuria.
Monitor: Baseline & periodic- hepatic func. Possibly lipid panel, glucose.

daunorubicin	ANTINEOPLASTIC, ANTILEUKEMIA, Antibiotic Parenteral Only (IV) 100 mg mannitol/vial See listing for **doxorubicin p 117**
Daypro **oxaprozin**	ANTIARTHRITIC (Rheumatoid or Osteoarthritis) See listing for **ibuprofen p 170** NSAID Tab- starch
Daytrana	ANTI-ADHD, Stimulant Transdermal system See **methylphenidate p 214**
DDAVP	ANTIDIURETIC, ANTIHEMORRHAGIC See **desmopressin p 106**
Decadron	CORTICOSTEROID, **dexamethasone** See **Corticosteroids p 94**

degarelix
  Firmagon
    80 mg vial-
     200 mg mannitol
    120 mg vial-
     500 mg mannitol

ANTINEOPLASTIC, TREATMENT OF ADVANCED PROSTATE CANCER, GnRH RECEPTOR ANTAGONIST   Parenteral only (SC)
    Drug: Initial dose followed by maintenance dose q 28 days.
    Nutr: ↑ wt. **Oral/GI:** Constipation, diarrhea, nausea.
    S/Cond: Not c̄ lactation. Caution in congenital long QT syndrome, electrolyte abnormalities, CHF, or c̄ use of class 1A or class III antiarrhythmic drugs (↑ QT interval from prolonged androgen deprivation). Caution c̄ moderate to severe ↓ renal func.
    Caution c̄ moderate ↓ hepatic func. 90% serum pro bound.
    Pregnancy: Category X.
    Other: <u>Injection</u> <u>site</u> <u>reactions</u>, <u>HOT</u> <u>FLASHES</u>, fatigue, chills, HTN, dizziness, headache, insomnia, testicular atrophy, sweating, gynecomastia, asthenia, night sweats, back & joint pain.
    Blood/Serum: ↓ <u>*TESTOSTERONE*</u>, ↑ <u>ALT</u>, ↑ <u>AST</u>, ↑ <u>GGT</u>. **Urinary:** Infection.
    Monitor: PSA. Testosterone levels if PSA increases.
    Monitor testosterone levels in pt c̄ severe ↓ hepatic func.

Demadex
  torsemide

ANTIHYPERYTENSIVE, DIURETIC   See **Diuretics, Loop p 114**

Demerol

ANALGESIC, Narcotic, Opioid   See **meperidine p 208**

denosumab
  Prolia[a]
  SC solution
  Preservative free,
  single use prefilled
  syringe or vial,
  sorbitol
  Xgeva[b]
  SC solution
  Preservative free
  single use vial,
  sorbitol

TREATMENT OF POSTMENOPAUSAL WOMEN WITH OSTEOPOROSIS AT HIGH RISK FOR FRACTURE[a]. TREATMENT IN MEN AT HIGH RISK FOR FRACTURE RECEIVING ANDROGEN DEPRIVATION THERAPY FOR NONMETATSTATIC PROSTATE CANCER[a]. TREATMENT IN WOMEN RECEIVING ADJUVANT AROMATASE INHIBITOR THERAPY FOR BREAST CANCER[a]. PREVENTION OF SKELETAL RELATED EVENTS IN PATIENTS WITH BONE METASTASES FROM SOLID TUMORS[b].
RANK ligand inhibitor. Parenteral (SC only)
  Drug: Administer **Prolia** by healthcare professional SC q 6 mos
  Administer **Xgeva** SC q 4wks.
  Administer in upper arm, upper thigh or abdomen.
  Nutr: Correct hypocalcemia prior to first dose.
  Min 1000 mg Ca and 400 IU Vit D daily.
  Oral/GI: Osteonecrosis of the jaw, nausea[a], diarrhea[a] NAUSEA[b], DIARRHEA[b].
  S/Cond: Not c̄ lactation. Proper oral hygiene and routine dental care required. Caution c̄ moderate-severe ↓ renal func- ↑ risk of hypocalcemia.
  Pregnancy: Category C.
  Other: Angina pectoris, URTI, pneumonia, pharyngitis, herpes zoster, pain in extremities, back pain, vertigo, peripheral edema, pharyngitis, muscle/bone pain, myalgia, spinal osteoarthritis, sciatica, insomnia, rash, pruritis, dyspnea[a], fatigue/asthenia[a], headache[a], DYSPNEA[b], FATIGUE/ASTHENIA[b], headache[b], cough[b]. Rare- pancreatitis.
  Blood/Serum: ↓ Hgb, ↓ Hct, ↓ Ca[a], ↓ CA[b] ↓ P[b], ↑ chol.
  Urinary: Cystitis.
  Monitor: Ca, Mg, P levels especially in pts predisposed to low levels. Routine oral exam by prescriber and routine dental exam and preventative dentistry prior to first dose and periodically.
  S/S of osteonecrosis of the jaw. S/S of infection.

Depacon	ANTIEPILEPTIC, **valproate sodium**	See **valproic acid p 328**
Depakene	ANTIEPILEPTIC	See **valproic acid p 328**
Depakote/Depakote ER	ANTIEPILEPTIC, **divalproex sodium**	See listing for **valproic acid p 328**
DepoCyt	ANTINEOPLASTIC, Antimetabolite	See **cytarabine p 98**
DepoDur	ANALGESIC, Narcotic, Opioid extended release liposome injection	See **morphine p 221**
Depo-Medrol	CORTICOSTEROID, **methylprednisolone**	See **Corticosteroids p 94**
Depo-Provera (IM) **Depo-subQ Provera 104** (SC)	HORMONE, ANTINEOPLASTIC, CONTRACEPTIVE	Parenteral See **progesterone p 265**
desipramine **Norpramin**	ANTIDEPRESSANT	See **Tricyclic Antidepressants p 323**

desloratadine ANTIHISTAMINE See listing for **loratadine p 199**
  Clarinex A major metabolite of **loratadine** < 90% serum pro bound.
   Tab- cornstarch, lactose
   Syrup- sorbitol, propylene glycol, granulated sugar ODT- gelatin, mannitol, aspartame

desmopressin **DDAVP** Tab- lactose, potato starch	ANTIENURESIS (oral only), ANTIDIURETIC (diabetes insipidus), (oral or spray) ANTIHEMORRHAGIC (IV or SC) Oral, Parenteral (IV, SC) or Nasal Spray Synthetic hormone related to antidiuretic hormone - vasopressin **Diet:** Adjust fluid intake to avoid overhydration.[7] **Oral/GI:** Nausea, belching,[4] abdominal pain, cramps. **S/Cond:** Caution c̄ alcohol- ↓ antidiuretic effect.[6] Caution c̄ lactation. Caution c̄ HTN. Caution c̄ pt at risk for water intoxication or hyponatremia. Not c̄ Hx of hyponatremia. Not c̄ moderate to severe ↓ renal func. **Pregnancy:** Category B. **Other:** <u>Headache</u>, flushing, dizziness, chills, weakness, ↓ or ↑ BP, water intoxication. Rare- seizures due to hyponatremia. Nasal form- nosebleed, URTI, hyponatremia. **Blood/Serum:** ↓ <u>Na</u>. Rare- hyponatremia. Transient ↑ AST c̄ Tab. **Urinary:** ↓ <u>*OUTPUT*</u>, ↑ <u>*OSMOLALITY*</u>. **Monitor**: c̄ Diabetes insipidus- Urinary output & osmolality. Electrolytes c̄ use > 7 days.	
Desogen	ORAL CONTRACEPTIVE	See **Oral Contraceptives p 237**
desvenlafaxine **Pristiq**	ANTIDEPRESSANT, SNRI Tab 100 mg- lactose	See listing for **venlafaxine p 331**
Desyrel (previous brand name)	ANTIDEPRESSANT	See **trazodone p 321**
Detrol/Detrol LA **tolterodine**	ANTIMUSCARINIC	See **Bladder Control Agents p 61**
dexamethasone	CORTICOSTEROID	See **Corticosteroids p 94**
Dexedrine	ANTI-ADHD, ANTINARCOLEPSY	See listing for **Amphetamines p 33**
dexlansoprazole **Kapidex** (DR) Cap- sugar spheres, glucose	ANTIGERD, ANTISECRETORY *R*-enantiomer of lansoprazole Dual Action Release	See **Proton Pump Inhibitors p 268**

dexmethylphenidate	ANTI-ADHD, Stimulant	See listing for
Focalin	Tab- starch, lactose, Na starch glycolate	**methylphenidate p 214**
Focalin XR	Cap- sugar spheres (sucrose & starch)	

dextroamphetamine	STIMULANT	See listing for **Amphetamines p 33**

DiaBeta	ORAL HYPOGLYCEMIC	See **sulfonylureas p 299**
glyburide		

diazepam	ANTIANXIETY, SKELETAL MUSCLE RELAXANT, ANTIEPILEPTIC
Valium	See **Benzodiazepines p 54**

diclofenac potassium
Cambia
Pwd for soln
aspartame =
25 mg phenylalanine,
mannitol, saccharin Na
Cataflam (IR)
Tab- sucrose, Na starch
glycolate, maize starch
Zipsor Cap- liquid filled
sorbitol, mineral oil
diclofenac sodium
Voltaren (DR)
EC Tab (DR)-
lactose, Na starch glycolate
Voltaren XR (SR)
Tab- sucrose
Flector
Patch

ANTIARTHRITIC (Osteo or Rheumatoid Arthritis), ANALGESIC , ANKYLOSING
SPONDYLITIS Treatment, ACUTE MIGRAINE ATTACKS (**Cambia**) NSAID
Drug: Take c̄ food, milk or 8 oz water to ↓ GI irritation. Food delays rate,
but not extent, of abs. Swallow DR/SR Tab whole. Do not crush or chew.
Diet: Caution c̄ GI irritants eg K suppl (↑ risk of GI irritation).
Limit caffeine to ↓ GI side effects. Avoid or limit natural products which
affect coagulation (eg garlic, gingko, ginger, ginseng or horse chestnut).
Oral/GI: Dysgeusia, <u>nausea</u>, <u>dyspepsia</u>, GI ulcers & bleeding (may be
sudden & serious), <u>abdominal pain</u>, <u>constipation</u>, <u>diarrhea</u>, colitis, flatulence.
S/Cond: Avoid alcohol. Not c̄ lactation. 99% serum pro bound.
Caution c̄ HTN, CHF, ↓ renal func or edema.
Not c̄ aspirin or NSAID allergy. Not c̄ gastritis/ulcer.
Pregnancy: Category C, not recommended in pregnancy. Category D in
3rd trimester due to risk of premature closure of the ductus arteriosus.
Other: <u>Headache</u>, <u>edema</u>, dizziness, rash, arrhythmia.
Rare- jaundice, hepatitis, pancreatitis, skin conditions eg SJS/TEN.
Risk of CV problems, eg HTN, CHF, MI, CVA.
Blood/Serum: ↑ <u>AST</u>, ↑ <u>ALT</u>. Rare- ↑ BUN, ↑ crea, dyscrasias.[6]
Monitor: Hepatic & renal func c̄ LT use.

dicloxacillin
  Dynapen
  previous brand name
  Pwd for Susp-
  saccharin, sucrose,
  27 mg (1.18 mEq)
  Na/5 mL

ANTIBIOTIC, Penicillin (penicillinase resistant)
  Drug: Take c̄ 8 oz water 1 hr before or 2 hr after food to ↑ abs.
  Oral/GI: N/V, diarrhea, flatulence. Rare- pseudomembranous colitis.
  S/Cond: Caution c̄ lactation. 98% serum pro bound. Caution c̄ ↓ renal func.[13]
  Pregnancy: Category B.
  Other: Rash, fever.
  Rare- allergic reaction, hepatotoxicity, serum sickness, interstitial nephritis.
  Blood/Serum: EOSINOPHILIA, ↑ alk phos, ↑ AST, ↑ ALT.
  Rare- dyscrasias, ↑ PT/INR, ↑ BUN, ↑ crea.
  Monitor: CBC c̄ diff. Hepatic func. Renal func c̄ LT use.[6]

dicyclomine
  Bentyl/Bentylol
  Cap- lactose, cornstarch
  Tab- lactose, cornstarch,
  sucrose
  Syrup- glucose,
  saccharin Na,
  propylene glycol

GASTROINTESTINAL ANTISPASMODIC, Anticholineric
  (Used to treat Irritable Bowel Syndrome)   Oral or Parenteral (IM)
  Drug: Take 30 min to 1 hr before food.[6]
  Oral/GI: DRY MOUTH/THROAT, ↓ taste acuity, nausea, constipation.
  S/Cond: Limit alcohol. Not c̄ lactation. ↑ risk of dental problems,
  see p 11 & 15. Syrup causes TF to precipitate.[8] Caution c̄ ↓ hepatic func
  or ↓ renal func, HTN, CHF, BPH, ulcerative colitis, hiatal hernia,
  hyperthyroidism. Not c̄ GERD, GI or urinary obstruction, glaucoma,
  myasthenia gravis. Caution c̄ geriatric or pediatric pt.
  Pregnancy: Category B.
  Other: DIZZINESS (especially c̄ IM), BLURRED VISION, drowsiness, weakness,
  headache, nervousness, confusion, tachycardia, ↑ heat sensitivity.
  Urinary: Retention.

didanosine (ddI)
  Videx
  Buffered Pwd-
  1380 mg (60 mEq) Na/pkt,
  sucrose
  Pediatric Pwd-
  Na free
  Videx EC (DR)

ANTIRETROVIRAL (HIV/AIDS), NRTI
  Also used to treat AIDS dementia complex
  Drug: Dosage based on body wt. Take on empty stomach at least
  30 minutes before or 2 hr after food (food ↓ abs). Take EC tab whole.
  Do not swallow chew tab whole. Chew or crush & mix
  c̄ > 1 oz water- may dilute in clear apple juice for flavor.[10] Do not mix c̄
  acidic liquid. Pediatric pwd is mixed by pharmacist c̄ sterile water & antacid.
  Diet: Consider Na content c̄ ↓ Na diet. Do not take c̄ Mg suppl.

Cap- contains EC
beadlets,
Na starch glycolate-potato

Take Fe 1 hr before or 4 hr after drug.
Nutr- ANOREXIA, ↓ wt.
Oral/GI: Dry mouth, stomatitis, ↓ taste acuity, dyspepsia, NAUSEA/VOMITING, abdominal pain, bloating, DIARRHEA, constipation, flatulence.
S/Cond: Avoid alcohol. Not c̄ lactation.
Caution c̄ ↓ renal func or ↓ hepatic func.
Pregnancy: Category B.
Other: Pancreatitis (can be fatal) (↑ c̄ history of alcohol abuse), PERIPHERAL NEUROPATHY (especially feet), HEADACHE, WEAKNESS, INSOMNIA, RASH, arthritis, pain, dizziness, congestion, chills/fever, blurred vision, cough, confusion, anxiety, edema, ↑ BP, seizures, fat redistribution.
Rare- hepatic steatosis, lactic acidosis, retinal lesions, optic neuritis.
Blood/Serum: Dyscrasias, anemia, ↑ AST, ↑ ALT, ↑ alk phos, ↑ bil, ↑ uric acid, ↑ amylase (often due to salivary isoenzymes),[43] ↑ lipase, ↓ K,[13] ↑ TG, ↑ CPK, ↑ or ↓ glucose.
Monitor: Amylase, lipase, uric acid, K, TG, CBC, hepatic func, retinal exams.

Didrex benzphetamine	APPETITE SUPPRESSANT	See **Amphetamines p 33**
Didronel etidronate	PAGET'S DISEASE TREATMENT, ANTIBONE RESORPTION	See **Bisphosphonates, Oral p 59**

Didrocal (Canada) includes 14 days **etidronate** & 76 days **ca carbonate**

Dificid	ANTIBIOTIC macrolide	See **fidaxomicin p 142**
Diflucan	ANTIFUNGAL	See **fluconazole p 145**
Di-Gel	ANTACID	See **aluminum hydroxide &** **magnesium hydroxide p 29**

digoxin
  Digoxin
  Lanoxin
  Tab- lactose,
   corn & potato starch
  Elixir Pediatric-
   sucrose, 10% alcohol
  Lanoxicaps
  8% ethyl alcohol,
   sorbitol
  IV Vial- 10% alcohol,
   40% propylene glycol

CARDIOTONIC, ANTIARRHYTHMIC, CHF TREATMENT, Inotropic agent
Cardiac Glycoside   Oral or Parenteral (IV or IM)
Drug: Dosage based on IBW.
Diet: Maintain diet $\bar{c}$ ↑ K, ↓ Na & adequate Mg & Ca.
Take at least 2 hr before antacids or Mg suppl- may ↓ abs of drug.[3]
Caution $\bar{c}$ Ca &/or Vit D suppl- ↑ risk of arrhythmias.[13]
Caution $\bar{c}$ some herbal products, eg aloe, foxglove, hawthorn & others.[4]
Avoid **SJW**,[4] see p 286. Avoid natural licorice, see p 374. ↑ risk of
hypokalemia.[4] No significant interaction $\bar{c}$ bran or grapefruit.[53]
Nutr: <u>Anorexia</u>, ↓ <u>wt</u>. Ca & Vit D induced hypercalcemia may ↑ drug effects.
Oral/GI: <u>N/V</u>, <u>diarrhea</u>.
S/Cond: Caution $\bar{c}$ lactation. Caution $\bar{c}$ obesity- dose should be based on IBW.
Caution- hypokalemia, hypomagnesemia & hypercalcemia ↑ drug toxicity.
Hypocalcemia ↓ drug effects. Caution $\bar{c}$ ↓ renal func. Caution $\bar{c}$ thyroid disease.[13]
Pregnancy: Category C.
Other: Drowsiness, arrhythmias, blurred (yellow) vision, apathy, dizziness,
confusion, weakness, headache, depression, psychosis.
Blood/Serum: ↑ or ↓ K, ↓ Mg. Rare- eosinophilia, ↓ platelets.
Urinary: ↑ Mg.[11]
Monitor: Electrolytes especially K, Ca, Mg.
Renal & hepatic func. Drug levels. Heart rate.

dihydrotachysterol **Hytakerol**	VITAMIN D ANALOG	See listing for **calcitriol p 69**
Dilacor XR	ANTIANGINA, ANTIHYPERTENSIVE	See **diltiazem p 111**
Dilantin	ANTIEPILEPTIC	See **phenytoin p 256**
Dilatrate SR	ANTIANGINA, Vasodilator	See **isosorbide dinitrate p 180**
Dilaudid **hydromorphone**	ANALGESIC, ANTITUSSIVE, Narcotic, Opioid	See listing for **morphine p 221** Oral, Parenteral or Suppository

Tab- lactose. Liquid- sucrose. 8 mg Tab & Oral liquid- may also contain traces of Na metabisulfite

diltiazem   ANTIANGINA, ANTIHYPERTENSIVE, Ca Channel Blocker   Oral or
   Cardizem   Parenteral (IV)
   Tab- lactose   **Drug:** Take tab or XR form before meals. Swallow SR, CD or XR cap
   Cardizem LA (SR)   whole- do not crush, break or chew.
   Tab- starch, sucrose,   **Diet:** ↓ cal may be needed. Avoid natural licorice, see p 374.
   Na starch glycolate,   Strict ↓ Na diet may blunt antihypertensive effect of drug.[45]
   vegetable oil   No significant interaction c̄ grapefruit/related citrus, see p 390.
   Cardizem CD   **Nutr:** Anorexia.
   Cap- sucrose, starch   **Oral/GI:** Dry mouth, dyspepsia, N/V, constipation, diarrhea.
   Cartia XT Cap- sucrose   **S/Cond:** Not c̄ lactation. Caution c̄ ↓ hepatic func or ↓ renal func.
   Dilacor XR (SR)   **Pregnancy:** Category C.
   Cap all- mannitol, starch   **Other:** ↓ _BP_ c̄ possible hypotension, <u>edema</u>,
   Cap 120 mg only- starch   <u>dizziness</u>, headache, drowsiness, weakness, flushing, insomnia, rash, pain.
   Diltia XT (SR) Cap- lactose   **Blood/Serum:** < 1%- ↑ alk phos, ↑ AST, ↑ ALT, ↑ LDH, ↑ CPK.
   Tiazac (SR) Cap- sucrose   **Monitor:** BP.
   Taztia XT (SR) Cap- sucrose   **diltiazem IV**- sorbitol

dimenhydrinate   ANTIVERTIGO, ANTIEMETIC, ANTINAUSEANT, Antihistamine
   Dramamine Original   See **diphenhydramine p 112**
   Formula   **Drug:** As antivertigo take at least 1/2 hr, preferably 1-2 hr, before travel.
   Tab- lactose
   Chewable Tab-
aspartame (1.5 mg phenylalanine), starch, sorbitol

Diovan/Diovan HCT   ANTIHYPERTENSIVE   See **Angiotensin II Receptor Antagonists p 38**
   valsartan   **Diovan HCT** also contains **hydrochlorothiazide,** see **p 166**

Dipentum Cap   ANTI-INFLAMMATORY (in ulcerative colitis) See listing for **mesalamine p 209**
   olsalazine   **Pregnancy:** Category C.

diphenhydramine
  Benadryl
  Cap- sorbitol
  Fast Melt (ODT)-
  aspartame, dextrose
  Liquid- sucrose
  Tab- starch

  Nytol
  Tab- starch

ANTIHISTAMINE, SLEEP AID, ANTI-EPS, ANTIVERTIGO
                              Oral or Parenteral (IM or IV)
  Drug: Take c̄ food if GI distress occurs. For sleep- take 1/2 hr before bedtime.
  Nutr: Anorexia.
  Oral/GI: Dry mouth/throat, N/V, epigastric distress, constipation, diarrhea.
  S/Cond: Avoid alcohol. Not c̄ lactation. Caution c̄ geriatric.[84]
  Pregnancy: Category B.
  Other: *DROWSINESS, SEDATION*, dizziness, ataxia, blurred vision,
  paradoxical stimulation (especially in children), confusion (especially in
  geriatric), headache, tachycardia, palpitations, photosensitivity,
  ↓ BP c̄ hypotension.
  Blood/Serum: Rare- hemolytic anemia, dyscrasias.
  Urinary: Retention.

diphenoxylate
  c̄ atropine
  Lomotil
  Tab- sucrose,
   sorbitol, cornstarch
  Liquid- 15% alcohol,
   1.8 g sorbitol/5 mL

ANTIDIARRHEAL, Antiperistaltic agent
  Drug: Take c̄ food if GI distress occurs.
  Diet: Diarrhea may ↑ fluid & electrolyte needs. **Nutr:** Anorexia.
  Oral/GI: Dry mouth, sore/swollen gums, N/V, cramps, bloating,
  constipation. Rare- toxic megacolon, paralytic ileus.
  S/Cond: Avoid alcohol. Not c̄ lactation. Not c̄ pseudomembranous
  colitis, toxigenic E. coli, Salmonella, Shigella or ulcerative colitis.
  Caution c̄ children- may mask dehydration or electrolyte imbalance.
  May be habit forming c̄ LT high dose. Caution c̄ ↓ renal or ↓ hepatic func.
  Not c̄ severe ↓ hepatic func, dehydration or electrolyte imbalance.
  Pregnancy: Category C.
  Other: DROWSINESS, dizziness, blurred vision, confusion, depression,
  euphoria, restlessness, numbness of extremities, flushing, headache.
  Rare- pancreatitis, tachycardia.
  Blood/Serum: ↑ amylase.
  Urinary: Retention.
  Monitor: Fluid & electrolytes. Hepatic func c̄ LT use.

Diprivan   ANESTHESIA, SEDATIVE   See **propofol p 266**

dipyridamole
  Persantine
  Tab- lactose,
   sucrose, cornstarch

  Aggrenox (SR)
  Cap- cornstarch,
  lactose, sucrose,
  25 mg Tab **aspirin**

PLATELET AGGREGATION INHIBITOR
  Drug: Take c̄ 8 oz water on empty stomach 1 hr before or 2 hr after food
  for faster abs. May take c̄ food or milk to ↓ GI distress.
  Diet: Caffeine ↓ drug effect- avoid concurrent use,[9b] see p 67.
  Oral/GI: <u>GI distress</u>, N/V, cramps, diarrhea.
  S/Cond: Avoid alcohol. Caution c̄ lactation.
  > 90% serum pro bound. Caution c̄ hypotension or severe CAD.
  Pregnancy: Category B. **Aggrenox**- category D due to **aspirin.**
  Other: <u>Dizziness</u>, <u>headache</u>, weakness, flushing, rash,
  ↓ BP c̄ possible hypotension.[13] Rare- hepatic dysfunction, angina.

Dispermox

ANTIBIOTIC   See **amoxicillin** p 32

disulfiram
  Antabuse
  Tab- lactose,
  Na starch glycolate

ALCOHOL ABUSE DETERRENT, Aldehyde Dehydrogenase Inhibitor
  (blocks conversion of acetaldehyde to acetic acid)
  Drug: Tab may be crushed & mixed c̄ beverages.
  Diet: Limit caffeine- drug ↓ caffeine metabolism &
  ↑ caffeine effects, see p 67. No alcohol-containing products- sauces,
  vinegars, juice or cider, extracts, soups or baked goods c̄ alcohol.
  Oral/GI: Transient <u>garlic</u> or <u>metallic</u> <u>taste</u>, dyspepsia.
  S/Cond: <u>AVOID ALL ALCOHOL</u>, <u>cough syrups</u>, <u>elixirs</u> & <u>topical alcohol</u> for ≥ 12 hr
  before use, during drug therapy & for ≥14 days after discontinuation.
  Caution c̄ diabetes, hypothyroidism, nephritis or seizures. Caution c̄ hepatic
  cirrhosis or insufficiency.[10] Not c̄ cardiovascular disease or psychoses.
  Pregnancy: Safety not established.
  Other: Peripheral neuropathy. Transient <u>drowsiness</u>, headache, fatigue.
  Rare- hepatitis, rash, psychotic reaction, optic neuritis.
  Blood/Serum: ↑ chol[13] (dose-related). Rare- ↑ AST, ↑ ALT, dyscrasias.
  Monitor: Baseline AST & ALT, repeat in 10-14 days.
  CBC & blood chemistry q 6 mo.

Ditropan/Ditropan XL
  oxybutynin

ANTIMUSCARINIC   See **Bladder Control Agents** p 61

D

Diuretics, Loop ANTIHYPERTENSIVE, DIURETIC (K-depleting) Oral or Parenteral (IM or IV)
To treat edema associated $\bar{c}$ CHF, renal or hepatic disease

Drug: Take **furosemide** on empty stomach- food ↓ bioavailablity,[94] but may take $\bar{c}$ food/milk if GI distress occurs.

Diet: ↑ K, ↑ Mg (or K, Mg suppl.), ↓ cal, ↓ Na may be recommended- except $\bar{c}$ **ethacrynic acid** rigid ↓ Na <u>not</u> necessary. Discontinue Na restriction if hyponatremia occurs. Avoid natural licorice, see p 374.

Nutr: Anorexia, ↑ thirst. **ethacrynic acid** has ↑ effect on Na excretion, ↓ Na diet-↑ risk of hyponatremia.[13]

Oral/GI: Oral irritation, cramps, N/V, diarrhea, constipation.[6] Sorbitol in **furosemide** soln- diarrhea $\bar{c}$ high dose.

S/Cond: Limit alcohol. **torsemide** & **furosemide**- caution $\bar{c}$ lactation. **bumetanide** & **ethacrynic acid**- not $\bar{c}$ lactation. Caution $\bar{c}$ diabetes- ↑ glucose. 91-97% serum pro bound. Caution $\bar{c}$ ↓ hepatic func or severe ↓ renal func. Not $\bar{c}$ anuria, hepatic coma or severe electrolyte depletion.
Caution $\bar{c}$ sulfa allergy, except $\bar{c}$ **ethacrynic acid**.

Pregnancy: Category C- **bumetanide** & **furosemide**. Category B- **torsemide** & **ethacrynic acid**.

Other: ↓ *BP* $\bar{c}$ possible hypotension, dizziness, blurred vision, headache, rash, weakness, photosensitivity, muscle cramps, ototoxicity (↑ risk $\bar{c}$ parenteral). Rare- gout, pancreatitis, hyponatremia. Dehydration $\bar{c}$ IV. **ethacrynic acid** only- confusion, nervousness.

Blood/Serum: ↓ <u>K</u>, ↓ <u>Mg</u>, ↓ <u>Na</u>, ↓ <u>Cl</u>, ↓ <u>Ca</u>, ↑ <u>glucose</u>, ↑ BUN, ↑ crea, ↑ uric acid, dyscrasias, anemia. ↑ Chol, ↑ LDL, ↑ VLDL, ↑ TG.[6]

Urinary: ↑ <u>WATER</u>, ↑ <u>K</u>, ↑ <u>Na</u>, ↑ <u>CL</u>, ↑ <u>Mg</u>, ↑ <u>Ca</u>, glucose. ↑ P $\bar{c}$ **bumetanide**.

Monitor: BP, electrolytes, Mg, Ca, glucose, uric acid, CO_2, renal func. Hepatic func $\bar{c}$ LT use.[6]
Wt, especially $\bar{c}$ treatment for edema.

bumetanide
generic only was **Bumex** Tab- lactose, cornstarch **Bumetanide** Parenteral (IM or IV)- 1% benzyl alcohol
furosemide **Lasix** Tab- lactose, starch Generic only-Soln- propylene glycol, sorbitol. Generic only- IV/IM
ethacrynic acid **Edecrin** Tab- lactose, starch IV- mannitol 62.5 mg/vial
torsemide **Demadex** Tab- lactose. IV

Diuril previous brand name	ANTIHYPERTENSIVE, DIURETIC	See **chlorothiazide p 82**
divalproex	ANTIEPILEPTIC	See listing for **valproic acid p 328**
Divigel Topical Gel	HORMONE REPLACEMENT, Estradiol	See **Hormone Therapy p 165**
DNase	CYSTIC FIBROSIS MANAGEMENT	See **dornase alfa p 116**

docetaxel **Taxotere** diluent- 13% ethanol	ANTINEOPLASTIC for Breast, Lung, Ovarian or Prostate Cancer, Gastric Adenocarcinoma or Squamous Cell Carcinoma Parenteral only (IV) Antimitotic Agent See listing for **paclitaxel p 242** **Diet:** Caution c̄ grapefruit/related citrus, see p 390. **Monitor:** Frequent CBC c̄ diff. AST, ALT, bil & alk phos before each drug cycle.

docetaxel
Taxotere
diluent- 13% ethanol

ANTINEOPLASTIC for Breast, Lung, Ovarian or Prostate Cancer,
Gastric Adenocarcinoma or Squamous Cell Carcinoma Parenteral only (IV)
Antimitotic Agent   See listing for **paclitaxel p 242**
Diet: Caution c̄ grapefruit/related citrus, see p 390.
Monitor: Frequent CBC c̄ diff. AST, ALT, bil & alk phos before each drug cycle.

docusate calcium
Kaopectate Stool Softener
Cap- sorbitol
docusate sodium
Colace
Syrup- 3 g sucrose/5 mL,
 alcohol (< 1%)
Cap- 2.5 mg (0.11 mEq)
 Na/50 mg, sorbitol,
 propylene glycol
Liquid- no sweetener
Dulcolax soft gel cap-
sorbitol, propylene glycol

STOOL SOFTENER, LAXATIVE
Drug: Mix liquid c̄ 6-8 oz milk or juice to mask bitter taste &
prevent throat irritation. Swallow cap whole c̄ full glass liquid.
Not with mineral oil.
Diet: High fiber c̄ 1500-2000 mL fluid/day to prevent constipation.
Nutr: Alters intestinal abs of water & electrolytes.
Oral/GI: BITTER TASTE, throat irritation & nausea (liquid forms),
cramps, diarrhea, rash.
S/Cond: Not c̄ N/V or abdominal pain. Caution c̄ intestinal disorder eg
Crohn's disease or ulcerative colitis.
Pregnancy: Category C.[23]
Blood/Serum: ↑ glucose, ↑ K (LT use).[13]

dofetilide
Tikosyn
Cap- cornstarch

ANTIARRHYTHMIC, Selective Potassium Channel Blocker
Drug: Take s̄ regard to food.
Diet: Adequate K & Mg essential. K & Mg levels must be WNL.
Caution c̄ grapefruit/related citrus, see p 390.
Oral/GI: Nausea, abdominal pain, diarrhea.
S/Cond: Not c̄ lactation. Caution c̄ ↓ renal func- dosage based on CrCL.
Not c̄ severe renal or hepatic failure. **Pregnancy:** Category C.
Other: ↑ QT INTERVAL. Headache, dizziness, chest pain, insomnia, rash,
back pain, URTI, flu syndrome, dyspnea, ventricular arrhythmia.
Monitor: Baseline- ECG, electrolytes, renal func.
During use- follow manufacturer's recommendations.[10]

Dolophine   ANALGESIC, Narcotic, Opioid   See **methadone p 210**

Dona   NATURAL PRODUCT (Not FDA approved) See **glucosamine p 157**

D

donepezil ANTIALZHEIMER'S, Acetylcholinesterase Inhibitor
  Aricept   Also used to treat vascular & mixed dementia
  Tab- lactose,   **Drug:** Take HS $\bar{s}$ regard to food.
    cornstarch   Dissolve ODT on tongue $\bar{c}$ or $\bar{s}$ liquid, swallow saliva.
  Aricept ODT   **Nutr:** Anorexia, ↓ wt, dehydration.
    mannitol   **Oral/GI:** <u>N</u>/V, pain, GI bleeding, bloating, <u>diarrhea</u>.
    S/Cond: Not $\bar{c}$ lactation. 96% serum pro bound.
    Caution $\bar{c}$ seizures, asthma, obstructive pulmonary disease.
    Caution $\bar{c}$ peptic ulcer disease- drug may ↑ gastric acid secretion.
    Pregnancy: Category C.
    Other: ↓ *IRRITABILITY*, ↓ *AGITATION*. <u>Insomnia</u>, fatigue, muscle cramps,
    headache, dizziness, syncope, tremor, ataxia, depression,
    ↑ or ↓ BP $\bar{c}$ possible hypotension, blurred vision, rash, bruising.
    Blood/Serum: < 1% dyscrasias.
    Urinary: ↑ frequency.

Dopar previous brand name ANTIPARKINSON   See **levodopa p 192**

doripenem ANTIBIOTIC, Carbapenem (Intra-abdominal infections, UTI)
  Doribax   **Other:** Vaginitis.   Parenteral Only (IV)
  Preservative free   **S/Cond:** Not for pediatric.   See listing for **meropenem p 208**

dornase alfa CYSTIC FIBROSIS MANAGEMENT   Respiratory Inhalant
  (DNase)   **Oral/GI:** Sore throat, laryngitis.
  Pulmozyme   **S/Cond**: Caution $\bar{c}$ lactation.
  preservative free   **Pregnancy:** Category B.
    Other: <u>Chest pain</u>, <u>voice changes</u>, conjunctivitis, cough,
    mild & transient <u>rash</u>.

Doryx ANTIBIOTIC   See **Tetracyclines p 310**
  doxycycline

doxazosin ANTIHYPERTENSIVE, BPH TREATMENT
  Cardura   See **Alpha$_1$-Adrenergic Blockers p 28**

doxepin   ANTIDEPRESSANT, ANTIANXIETY   See **Tricyclic Antidepressants p 323**
   Sinequan previous brand name   Cream- ANTIPRURITIC

doxercalciferol   HYPERPARATHYROIDISM TREATMENT in renal failure   See **calcitriol p 69**
   Hectorol   Oral or Parenteral (IV)   Cap- fractionated TG of coconut oil,
               Metabolized to $1\alpha,25\text{-}(OH)_2D_2$ alcohol

doxorubicin   ANTINEOPLASTIC, Anthracycline Antibiotic   Parenteral only (IV)
   Adriamycin previous   (used to treat many cancers)
     brand name   **Doxil** for Kaposi's sarcoma, ovarian, multiple myeloma.
   Doxorubicin generic   **Diet:** Insure adequate fluid intake/hydration.
   Caelyx (Canada only)   **Nutr:** Anorexia, ↓ wt.
    94 mg sucrose/mL   **Oral/GI:** <u>Dry mouth</u>, oral candidiasis, dysphagia, <u>glossitis</u>, <u>stomatitis</u>,
   Doxil   <u>ESOPHAGITIS</u>, <u>ACUTE NAUSEA/VOMITING</u>, abdominal pain,
    sucrose   GI ulceration, diarrhea, constipation. Rare- pseudomembranous colitis.
               S/Cond: Avoid alcohol.[13] Not c̄ lactation. Do dental care cautiously.
               Caution c̄ ↓ hepatic func. Not c̄ severe ↓ hepatic func. Not c̄ ↓ cardiac func.
               Caution c̄ ANC < 1000 or platelets < 50,000 cells/mm³.
               Caution c̄ moderate palmar-plantar erythrodyesthesia.
               Not c̄ severe palmar-plantar erythrodyesthesia.
               Pregnancy: Category D.
               Other: <u>BONE MARROW SUPPRESSION</u>, <u>HAIR LOSS</u>, cardiotoxicity/<u>CHF</u>,
               <u>acute infusion reactions</u>, fever, chills, headache, chest pain,
               back pain, hypotension, tachycardia, infection, dyspnea, retinitis,
               dizziness, drowsiness, allergic reaction, rash,
               palmar-plantar erythrodyesthesia (skin eruptions), herpes simplex eruption.
               Rare- anaphylaxis, leukemia.
               Blood/Serum: ↓ <u>WHITE BLOOD CELLS</u>, ↓ <u>platelets</u>, <u>anemia</u>, ↑ <u>uric acid</u>,
               ↑ glucose, ↓ Ca, ↑ alk phos, ↑ AST, ↑ ALT, ↑ bil, ↑ PT/INR.
               Urinary: ↑ <u>uric acid</u>, <u>red color</u>, pro.
               Monitor: CBC c̄ diff, platelets, hepatic, renal & cardiac func, uric acid.
               Chest X-ray.

D

doxycycline   ANTIBIOTIC, Adjunct to periodontitis treatment (**Periostat**)
  Doryx, Vibramycin, Oracea, Periostat   See **Tetracyclines p 310**

Dramamine   ANTIVERTIGO, ANTIEMETIC, ANTINAUSEANT See **dimenhydrinate p 111**

dronabinol   APPETITE STIMULANT, ANTIEMETIC, marijuana derivative
  Marinol   **Drug:** As appetite stimulant- Take BID before lunch & dinner to ↑ appetite.
  Cap- sesame oil   As antiemetic- Take 1-3 hr before chemotherapy. **Nutr:** ↑ *APPETITE*, ↑ *WT*.
    Oral/GI: Dry mouth, <u>N/V</u>, <u>abdominal pain</u>, <u>diarrhea</u>.
    S/Cond: Avoid alcohol. Not c̄ lactation. 97% serum pro bound.
    May be habit forming c̄ LT use of high dose, but abuse potential is low.[7]
    Caution c̄ cardiac or psychiatric disease, geriatrics. Not for use in children.
    Pregnancy: Category C.
    Other: <u>EUPHORIA</u>, <u>drowsiness</u>, <u>dizziness</u>, <u>tachycardia</u>, palpitations,
    hypotension, ataxia, headache, weakness, blurred vision,
    hallucinations, mood changes, paranoid reaction,
    confusion, abnormal thinking, amnesia, anxiety, flushing.

dronedarone   ANTIARRHYTHMIC
  Multaq   **Drug:** Take twice daily c̄ food; morning meal & evening meal.
  Tab- lactose,   High fat meal ↑ bioavailablity from 4% to 15%.
  starch   **Diet:** Avoid grapefruit/related citrus, see p 390. Avoid SJW, see p 286.
    Oral/GI: Diarrhea, nausea, abdominal pain, vomiting, dyspepsia.
    S/Cond: Not c̄ lactation. Not c̄ hypokalemia or hypomagnesemia.
    Not c̄ NYHA Class IV heart failure or Class II or III c̄ decompensation.
    Not c̄ bradycardia (< 50 bpm). Not c̄ QT interval > 500 msec.
    Not c̄ sick sinus syndrome. > 98% serum pro bound.
    Not c̄ severe ↓ hepatic func. **Pregancy:** Category X.
    Other: ↑ QT interval. New or worsening CHF. Weakness, bradycardia,
    rashes, itching, eczema, dermatitis. **Blood/Serum:** ↑ SCr > 10%.
    Monitor: Baseline electrolytes, Mg, ECG. Signs of heart failure eg: edema,
    shortness of breath, rapid weight gain.

Droxia   PROPHYLAXIS OF SICKLE CELL CRISIS, Antimetabolite See **hydroxyurea p 168**

DTIC-Dome	ANTINEOPLASTIC, Alkylating Agent	See **dacarbazine p 99**

Duetact	ANTIHYPERGLYCEMIC, Type 2 Diabetes	See **sulfonylureas p 299**
Tab- lactose	Combination drug **glimeperide** & **pioglitazone** See **thiazolidinediones p 312**	

Duexis
Tab- lactose,   ANTIARTHRITIC, NSAID, STOMACH PROTECTION, Combination Drug
polyethylene glycol

(ibuprofen, famotidine)   See **ibuprofen p 170**
See listing for **Histamine H$_2$ Receptor Antagonists p 162**

Dulcolax	LAXATIVE, Stimulant	See **bisacodyl p 57**

Dulcolax	STOOL SOFTENER	See **docusate Na p 115**

Dulera
Inhaler- anhydrous alcohol   ANTIASTHMA, Long Acting Beta$_2$ Agonist & Coticosteroid
(fomoterol & mometasone)   See listing for **fluticasone p 144**
See listing for **salmeterol p 286**

duloxetine   ANTIDEPRESSANT, ANTIANXIETY, FIBROMYALGIA TREATMENT
  Cymbalta   ANALGESIC for Diabetic Peripheral Neuropathy, SNRI
  Cap (DR)   **Drug:** Take s̄ regard to food. Swallow cap whole, do not open, chew, crush.
  contains EC pellets   **Nutr:** ↓ appetite, ↓ wt, anorexia.
  sucrose, sugar spheres   **Oral/GI:** Dry mouth, nausea/vomiting, dyspepsia, gastritis, constipation, diarrhea.
  (sucrose & starch)   **S/Cond:** Avoid alcohol. Not c̄ lactation. > 90% serum pro bound.
  Not c̄ ↓ hepatic func, uncontrolled narrow angle glaucoma,
  dialysis or severe ↓ renal func. **Pregnancy:** Category C.
  Other: Insomnia, fatigue, drowsiness, dizziness, headache, tremor,
  rigors, syncope, orthostatic hypotension, ↑ sweating, blurred vision,
  anxiety, fever, rash, sexual dysfunction, suicidal thinking & behavior.
  Slightly ↑ BP. Rare- hepatotoxicity (may be fatal), SIADH.
  Blood/Serum: ↑ ALT, ↑ AST, ↑ CPK, ↑ alk phos, ↓ glucose, ↓ Na.
  Urinary: ↑ frequency, dysuria. **Monitor:** Baseline & periodic BP.

Duraclon	ANALGESIC	See **clonidine p 88**

Duragesic patch	ANALGESIC, Narcotic, Opioid	See **fentanyl p 139**

Duricef	ANTIBIOTIC	See **cefadroxil p 76**

dutasteride
  Avodart
  Cap

BPH TREATMENT, Androgen Hormone Inhibitor
    5 alpha-reductase inhibitor for treatment of prostate hyperplasia
      Drug: Swallow whole s̄ regard to food   See listing for **finasteride p 142**

Dyazide
  Cap- benzyl alcohol,
  lactose, starch

ANTIHYPERTENSIVE, DIURETIC
    Combination drug

See **triamterene p 322**
See **hydrochlorothiazide p 166**

Dynacin
  minocycline

ANTIBIOTIC

See **Tetracyclines p 310**

Dyrenium

DIURETIC, K Sparing

See **triamterene p 322**

echinocandins

ANTIFUNGAL (esophageal candidiasis, other fungal infections)
    Only **caspofungin** is indicated for aspergillosis   Parenteral only (IV infusion only)

Drug: caspofungin- Not c̄ diluents containing dextrose.[26]
anidulafungin- diluent contains 20% w/w dehydrated alcohol.
Oral/GI: N/V, dyspepsia, diarrhea.
S/Cond: Caution c̄ lacatation. **caspofungin** & **micafungin** 97->99% serum pro bound.
Not c̄ severe ↓ hepatic func. **caspofungin**- caution c̄ moderate ↓ hepatic func. **Pregnancy:** Category C.
Other: <u>Fever</u>, flushing, headache, rigors, headache, rash, edema, phlebitis at injection site.
Rare- severe hypersensitivity, hemolysis or hemolytic anemia, hepatic or renal dysfunction.
Blood/Serum: ↑ bil, ↑ alk phos, ↑ ALT, ↑ AST, ↑ GGT, ↓ K, ↓ P, ↓ Mg, anemia, ↓ WBC, ↓ neutrophils, ↑ eosinophils.
Urinary: ↑ pro, ↑ RBC.
Monitor: Baseline then periodic hepatic func, CBC c̄ diff, renal func.

anidulafungin   **Eraxis** 50 mg fructose, 250 mg mannitol/vial
caspofungin   **Cancidas** vial- sucrose, mannitol
micafungin   **Mycamine** 200 mg lactose/vial

Ecotrin Tab- starch
  enteric-coated aspirin

ANALGESIC, ANTIPYRETIC, ANTIARTHRITIC, NSAID   See **aspirin p 44**
    Drug: Swallow whole. Drug has very low Na content.

Edarbi/Edarbyclor
  azilsartan

ANTIHYPERTENSIVE   See **Angiotensin II Receptor Antagonists p 38**
    Edarbyclor also contains **chlorthalidone** see p 82

Edecrin ethacrynic acid	DIURETIC	See **Diuretics, Loop p 114**

S/Cond: May be used $\bar{c}$ sulfa allergy, unlike other loop diuretics.

Edluar sublingal form	SLEEP AID	See **zolpidem p 351**
E.E.S.	ANTIBIOTIC	See **erythromycin p 128**

efavirenz (EFV)
  Sustiva
  Cap- lactose,
   Na starch glycolate
  Tab- lactose

ANTIRETROVIRAL (HIV/AIDS), NNRTI
  Drug: Take HS on an empty stomach. Not $\bar{c}$ a high fat meal
  (test meal = 54 g fat). Food may ↑ adverse effects.
  Diet: Avoid SJW, see p 286. **Nutr:** Anorexia.
  Oral/GI: N/V, dyspepsia, abdominal pain, <u>diarrhea</u>, flatulence.
  S/Cond: Avoid alcohol. Not $\bar{c}$ lactation. > 99% serum pro bound.
  Caution $\bar{c}$ ↓ hepatic func, seizures[6] or geriatric.
  Pregnancy: Category D. Teratogenic in monkeys.
  Other: <u>RASH</u>, <u>dizziness</u>, headache, insomnia, fatigue, drowsiness,
  abnormal dreams, ↑ sweating, depression, impaired concentration,
  delusions, hallucinations, anxiety, agitation, hypesthesia.[13]
  Rare- SJS, arthritis, fat redistribution, pancreatitis, seizures.
  Blood/Serum: ↑ <u>CHOL</u>, ↑ <u>HDL</u>, ↑ <u>TRIGLYCERIDES</u>, ↑ AST, ↑ ALT, ↑ GGT,
  ↑ amylase, ↓ neutrophils. **Urinary:** Blood, renal calculus. False + cannabinoid test.
  Monitor: Chol, TG, possibly hepatic func.
  Note- CNS & GI effects generally ↓ after 2-4 wk, are more common in children.

Effexor/Effexor XR	ANTIDEPRESSANT, SNRI	See **venlafaxine p 331**
Effient	ACUTE CORONARY SYNDROME TREATMENT Platelet Aggregation Inhibitor	See **prasugrel p 262**
Elavil (generics only) amitriptyline	ANTIDEPRESSANT	See **Tricyclic Antidepressants p 323**
Eldepryl	ANTIPARKINSON, MAO-B Inhibitor	See **selegiline p 289**

Elestrin
  estradiol
	HORMONE REPLACEMENT THERAPY
	  topical gel
		See **Hormone Therapy p 165**

D/E

eletriptan	ANTIMIGRAINE, Serotonin 5-HT$_1$ Receptor Agonist	
Relpax		See **Antimigraine p 39**
Eligard	ANTINEOPLASTIC, Hormone	See **leuprolide p 190**
Elixophyllin	ANTIASTHMA, BRONCHODILATOR	See **theophylline p 311**
Ellence	ANTINEOPLASTIC, Anthracycline Antibiotic	See **epirubicin p 125**
Eloxatin	ANTINEOPLASTIC	See **oxaliplatin p 239**

eltrombopag
 Promacta
 Tab- mannitol,
 Na starch glycolate

IDIOPATHIC THROMBOCYTOPENIC PURPURA TREATMENT (ITP)
Thrombopoietin Receptor Agonist Stimulates bone marrow to
produce ↑ platelets $\geq$ 50X 10^9/L to ↓ bleeding risk.
Drug: Take drug on an empty stomach- 1 hr before or 2 hrs after a meal.
See **Diet:** below.
Diet: Take Ca, Fe, Mg, Zn, Se suppl, antacids c̄ Al, dairy products or
mineral fortified foods (eg OJ c̄ Ca) $\geq$ 4 hrs before or after drug.
Oral/GI: N/V, dyspepsia.
S/Cond: Not c̄ lactation. Caution c̄ geriatric.
Caution c̄ moderate to severe ↓ hepatic func. $\geq$ 99% serum pro bound.
Caution c̄ pt of east Asian ancestry- 70% ↑ drug levels.
Pregnancy: Category C.
Other: Menorrhagia, paresthesia, cataract, ecchymosis,
conjunctival hemorrhage, muscle pain. Rare- reticulin fiber deposition
in bone marrow, hematological malignancies.
Blood/Serum: ↑ ALT, ↑ AST, ↑ bil, thrombocytopenia,
↑ *PLATELETS*. ↓ RISK OF BLEEDING.
Monitor: ALT, AST bil prior to therapy; q 2 wk during adjustment period,
then q mo. CBC c̄ platelets & peripheral blood smears prior to therapy,
then q wk until stable platelet count, then q mo.

| **Emend** | ANTIEMETIC, ANTINAUSEANT | See **aprepitant p 40** |
| **Emsam** | ANTIDEPRESSANT, patch | See **selegiline p 289** |

emtricitabine
Emtriva
Cap
Soln- EDTA, xylitol,
propylene glycol

ANTIRETROVIRAL (HIV/AIDS), NRTI, fluorinated derivative of **lamivudine**
Drug: Take once a day s̄ regard to food. **Oral/GI:** N/V, <u>diarrhea</u>.
S/Cond: Avoid alcohol. Not c̄ lactation.
Caution c̄ ↓ renal func or geriatric.
Caution c̄ obesity- ↑ risk of lactic acidosis.[13] **Pregnancy:** Category B.
Other: <u>Headache</u>, cough, rhinitis, rash, asthenia, muscle pain, drowsiness,
hyperpigmentation of palms & soles. Rare- lactic acidosis, hepatomegaly
c̄ steatosis (can be fatal), fat redistribution.
Blood/Serum: ↑ TG, ↑ CPK, ↑ AST, ↑ ALT, ↑ amylase, ↓ neutrophils.
Monitor: Prior to use- Hepatitis B test. Possibly hepatic func.

Enablex
darifenacin

ANTIMUSCARINIC   See **Bladder Control Agents p 61**

enalapril/enalaprilat
Vasotec/Vasotec IV

ANTIHYPERTENSIVE   See **Angiotensin Converting Enzyme Inhibitors p 36**

Enbrel

ANTIARTHRITIC (Rheumatoid Arthritis)   See **etanercept p 130**

Endocet
Tab- cornstarch

ANALGESIC, Narcotic, Opioid   See **oxycodone p 241**
        Combination drug **Pregnancy:** Category C.   See **acetaminophen p 22**

enfuvirtide (T-20)
Fuzeon
preservative free
mannitol- 22.5 mg/mL

ANTIRETROVIRAL (HIV/AIDS), Fusion Inhibitor   Parenteral only (SC)
Affects membrane fusion dependent on glycoprotein 41
Nutr: ↓ appetite, ↓ wt.
Oral/GI: Taste change, N/V, constipation.
S/Cond: Not c̄ lactation. 92% serum pro bound.
Pregnancy: Category B.
Other: <u>INJECTION SITE REACTION</u>, ↓ BP, rash, insomnia, peripheral neuropathy,
anxiety, depression, pancreatitis, sinusitis, cough, weakness, muscle pain,
flu-like illness, fever, chills, lymph node tenderness/swelling,
allergic reaction, pneumonia. Rare- ↑ risk of bacterial pneumonia.
Blood/Serum: <u>Eosinophilia</u>, ↑ amylase, ↑ lipase, ↑ AST, ↑ ALT, ↑ TG,
↑ CPK, anemia.

See "Guide to the Use of This Book" inside front cover.

E

Enjuvia	HORMONE	See **Hormone Therapy p 165**

enoxaparin
Lovenox
prefilled syringes-
 preservative free
multi-dose-
 15 mg/ml benzyl alcohol

ANTICOAGULANT
 Low molecular weight **heparin**
 S/Cond: Not c̄ pork allergy- derived from porcine intestinal mucosa.
 Caution c̄ ↓ renal func GFR < 30- ↓ dose. **Pregnancy:** Category B.
 Monitor: CBC, platelet count, UA, fecal occult blood, possibly Anti-Factor Xa.
 Unlike **heparin**, APTT monitoring is not recommended.

See listing for **heparin p 161**
Parenteral only (SC)

entacapone
Comtan
Tab- mannitol,
 vegetable oil,
 sucrose

ANTIPARKINSON, COMT Inhibitor (Adjunct to **levodopa-carbidopa**)
 Drug: Take s̄ regard to food, but concomitantly c̄ **levodopa-carbidopa**.
 Diet: Take Fe suppl 1 hr before or 2 hr after drug.
 Nutr: Drug chelates c̄ Fe.
 Oral/GI: Dry mouth, taste changes, dyspepsia, N/V, gastritis,
 abdominal pain, diarrhea, constipation, flatulence.
 S/Cond: Avoid alcohol. Caution c̄ lactation. 98% serum pro bound.
 Caution c̄ ↓ hepatic func.
 Pregnancy: Category C.
 Other: Dyskinesia, hyperkinesias, anxiety, agitation, hypokinesia,
 drowsiness, dizziness, dyspnea, ↑ sweating, back pain, fatigue, weakness,
 mild leg paresthesia, hallucinations. Rare- hypotension, syncope.
 Blood/Serum: ↓ Fe, but no reports of ↓ ferritin or anemia. Rare- ↑ AST, ↑ ALT.
 Urinary: Brown orange color.

entecavir
Baraclude
Tab- lactose
Soln- maltitol

ANTIVIRAL, Hepatitis B Treatment
 Drug: Take once daily on empty stomach at least 2 hr apart from food.
 Food ↓ abs & drug levels.
 Oral/GI: Dyspepsia, diarrhea.
 S/Cond: Not c̄ lactation. Caution c̄ ↓ renal func.
 Pregnancy: Category C.
 Other: Headache, dizziness, fatigue. Acute exacerbation of hepatitis B
 after DC of drug. Rare- (can be fatal) lactic acidosis, hepatomegaly c̄ steatosis.
 Blood/Serum: ↑ AST, ↑ ALT, ↑ bil, ↑ amylase, ↑ lipase, ↑ glucose.

< 1%- ↓ alb, ↓ platelets.
Urinary: <u>Hematuria</u>, glucose.
Monitor: Baseline & periodic renal & hepatic func.
Hepatic func for several mo after DC of drug.

Entocort EC CROHN'S DISEASE TREATMENT, Corticosteroid See **budesonide p 64**

Enulose LAXATIVE, ANTIHYPERAMMONEMIC See **lactulose p 186**

epirubicin ANTINEOPLASTIC, Breast Cancer, Anthracycline Antibiotic
  Ellence Parenteral Only (IV)
  preservative free **Diet:** Insure adequate fluid intake/hydration.
  Pharmorubicin PFS **Nutr:** Anorexia, ↓ wt.
  Canada only **Oral/GI:** <u>STOMATITIS</u>, <u>ESOPHAGITIS</u>, <u>hyperpigmentation of the oral mucosa</u>,
  preservative free <u>NAUSEA/VOMITING</u>, GI ulceration/bleeding, <u>abdominal pain</u>, <u>DIARRHEA</u>.
  (also indicated for **S/Cond:** Avoid alcohol.[13] Not c̄ lactation. Do dental care cautiously,
  lung, Hodgkin's, see p 11 & 15. Caution c̄ ↓ hepatic func (not c̄ severe ↓ func).
  ovarian or gastric Caution c̄ severe ↓ renal func or c̄ severe ↓ cardiac func.
  cancer) Not c̄ ANC < 1500.
  Pregnancy: Category D.
  Other: <u>BONE MARROW SUPPRESSION</u>, <u>AMENORRHEA</u>, <u>HOT FLASHES</u>, <u>HAIR LOSS</u>,
  <u>cardiotoxicity/CHF</u>, <u>fever</u>, <u>conjunctivitis</u>, <u>rash</u>, ↓ LVEF, chills, infection,
  lethargy, photosensitivity, dark- soles, palms, nails. Rare- leukemia.
  Blood/Serum: ↓ <u>WHITE BLOOD CELLS</u>, ↓ <u>platelets</u>, <u>anemia</u>, ↑ AST, ↑ ALT,
  ↑ bil. Rare- ↑ uric acid.
  Urinary: Red color.
  Monitor: Cardiac func, especially LVEF. Baseline & during each cycle-
  CBC c̄ diff, platelets, hepatic func, crea, Ca, P, K, uric acid.

Epivir ANTIRETROVIRAL (HIV/AIDS), NRTI See **lamivudine p 187**

Epivir-HBV CHRONIC HEPATITIS B TREATMENT, NRTI See **lamivudine p 187**

eplerenone
Inspra
Tab- lactose

ANTIYPERTENSIVE, CHF TREATMENT post MI, Aldosterone Blocker
Drug: Take s̄ regard to food.
Diet: Avoid excessive K intake, K suppl, salt subs.
No significant interaction c̄ grapefruit/related citrus, see p 390.
↓ Na, ↓ cal may be recommended.
Avoid natural licorice, see p 374. SJW ↓ blood levels.
Oral/GI: Abdominal pain, diarrhea.
S/Cond: Not c̄ lactation. Caution c̄ diabetes, especially c̄ microalbuminemia.
Caution c̄ moderate ↓ renal func. Not severe ↓ renal func (crea clearance
≤ 30 mL/min c̄ CHF or ≤ 50 c̄ HTN). Not c̄ K blood level ≥ 5.5 prior
to use or 6 during use. **Pregnancy:** Category B.
Other: ↓ _BP_ possible hypotension, dizziness, fatigue, flu-like symptoms,
coughing. Rare- vaginal bleeding, gynecomastia.
Blood/Serum: ↑ <u>K</u> (more common c̄ ↓ renal func), ↓ <u>Na</u>, ↓ <u>Cl</u>, ↑ chol, ↑ TG,
↑ crea. Rare- ↑ uric acid, ↑ ALT, ↑ GGT.
Urinary: ↑ _WATER_, ↑ _Na_, ↑ _Cl_, ↓ _K_, alb.
Monitor: Baseline & periodic BP, electrolytes, renal func.

epoetin alfa
Aranesp
darbepoetin alfa
 long acting form
 2.5 mg albumin/mL
Epogen
 erythropoietin
Procrit
 erythropoietin
 all contain human
 albumin
 Multidose-
 1% benzyl alcohol

RECOMBINANT HUMAN ERYTHROPOIETIN, ANTIANEMIC
Stimulates RBC production   Parenteral only (IV or SC)
 For use in ESRD, chemotherapy or **zidovudine** induced anemia
Diet: May need Fe, Vit B_{12} or Fol suppl. ESRD- Diet compliance mandatory.
S/Cond: Caution c̄ lactation. Not c̄ Fe, Vit B_{12} or Fol def anemia, hemolysis,
uncontrolled HTN or GI bleeding.[26] Caution c̄ seizures or vascular disease.
Not c̄ Hb > 12- ↑ risk of CV complication.[1] If Hb ↑ > 1g/dL in 2 wk, ↓ dose.
Oral/GI: N/V, diarrhea. **Pregnancy:** Category C.
Other: ↑ <u>BLOOD PRESSURE</u>, <u>bone</u> or muscle <u>pain</u>, <u>fever</u>, <u>rash</u>,
<u>respiratory</u> <u>congestion</u>, headache, seizures, cough.
Blood/Serum: ↑ _RBC_, ↑ _HEMOGLOBIN_, ↑ _HEMATOCRIT_, ↓ Fe, ↓ ferritin,
↓ transferrin saturation, ↓ bleeding time. Rare- red cell aplasia/severe anemia.
Monitor: Baseline- Hb/HCT, BP, renal func, electrolytes, P.
Fe studies, Vit B_{12}, Fol (adequate levels essential).
During use- BP, CBC c̄ diff, platelets, Fe studies, renal func, uric acid, K, P.

| eprosartan | ANTIHYPERTENSIVE | See **Angiotensin II Receptor** |
| **Teveten/Teveten HCT*** | | **Antagonists p 38** |

also contains **hydrochlorothiazide, see **p 166***

| **Epzicom** | ANTIRETROVIRAL (HIV/AIDS), NRTI | See **abacavir p 19** |
| Tab- Na starch glycolate | Combination drug | See **lamivudine p 187** |

| **Equetro** | ANTIMANIC | See **carbamazepine p 72** |

| **Eraxis** | ANTIFUNGAL | See **echinocandins p 120** |
| anidulafungin | | |

| **Erbitux** | ANTINEOPLASTIC, Epidermal Growth Factor Inhibitor   See **cetuximab p 81** |

| **ergocalciferol** | VITAMIN | See **vitamin D p 340** |

erlotinib
Tarceva
Tab- lactose,
 Na starch glycolate

ANTINEOPLASTIC, Epidermal Growth Factor Inhibitor   Lung or Pancreatic Cancer
Drug: Take on empty stomach, 1 hr before or 2 hr after food.
Diet: Avoid SJW. Theoretical interaction c̄ grapefruit/related citrus, see p 390.
Nutr: <u>Anorexia</u>, ↓ <u>wt</u>.
Oral/GI: <u>Stomatitis</u>, <u>N/V</u>, dyspepsia, abdominal pain, <u>DIARRHEA</u>, flatulence. Rare- GI bleeding/perforation.
S/Cond: Not c̄ lactation. Caution c̄ ↓ hepatic func. 93% serum pro bound.
Pregnancy: Category D.
Other: <u>RASH</u>, <u>dry skin</u>, <u>itching</u>, <u>conjunctivitis</u>, <u>infection</u>, <u>fever</u>, <u>fatigue</u>, <u>dyspnea</u>, <u>depression</u>, <u>headache</u>, cough, edema, anxiety, neuropathy, bone/muscle pain, hair loss, DVT.
Rare- ocular disorders eg corneal perforation/ulcer, pulmonary toxicity, CVA, skin conditions eg SJS/TEN.
Blood/Serum: ↑ AST, ↑ ALT, ↑ bil.
Monitor: PT/INR, hepatic func.

ertapenem
  Invanz
  137 mg Na
  (6 mEq)/vial
  IM diluent-
  1% lidocaine

ANTIBIOTIC, Carbapenem   Parenteral only (IV or IM)

Drug: Not c̄ diluents containing dextrose.[26]
Oral/GI: Dyspepsia, <u>nausea</u>/V, regurgitation, diarrhea, <u>constipation</u>.
Rare- pseudomembranous colitis.
S/Cond: Caution c̄ lactation. 85-95% serum pro bound.
Caution c̄ severe ↓ renal func or geriatric. **Pregnancy:** Category B.
Other: Edema, chest pain, HTN or hypotension, tachycardia, headache,
altered mental status, fever, insomnia, dizziness, fatigue, anxiety, rash, vaginitis.
Rare- seizures, jaundice, allergic reaction, anaphylaxis.
Blood/Serum: ↑ <u>AST</u>, ↑ <u>ALT</u>, ↑ <u>platelets</u>, ↑ alk phos, eosinophilia,
↓ neutrophils, ↓ alb. < 1%- ↑ BUN, ↑ PTT, ↑ Na, ↑ bil, ↓ CO_2.
Monitor: Baseline & periodic CBC c̄ diff, platelets, renal & hepatic func.

erythromycin

ANTIBIOTIC, Macrolide   Oral or Parenteral (IV)
IV also used as Diabetic Gastroparesis Treatment.[26]

Drug: Optimal- Take ERYC, PCE or filmtab base or stearate forms c̄ full glass water on empty stomach
2 hr before or after meal- food ↓ abs.[3] Take estolate, ethylsuccinate & enteric-coated base forms c̄ food to
↓ GI distress. Swallow enteric-coated tab whole. Chew chewable tab well.
Diet: Caution c̄ grapefruit/related citrus,[3a] see p 390. Caution c̄ SJW,[12] see p 286. **Nutr:** Anorexia.
Oral/GI: Oral candidiasis,[13] ↑ gastric motility, <u>epigastric</u> <u>distress</u>, N/V, <u>ABDOMINAL</u> <u>CRAMPS</u>, diarrhea.
Rare- pseudomembranous colitis.
S/Cond: Avoid concurrent alcohol use- may ↓ abs of **erythromycin** &/or ↑ alcohol effects.[13]
Caution c̄ lactation. Estolate form is 96% serum pro bound.[6] Caution c̄ ↓ hepatic func or
severe ↓ renal func.[58] Estolate oral suspension- not c̄ ↓ hepatic func. **Pregnancy:** Category B.
Other: Cholestatic hepatitis (↑ c̄ estolate form), jaundice, allergic reaction, rash.
Rare- ↑ QT interval, arrhythmia, other ECG changes, pancreatitis, anaphylaxis, SJS, TEN.[7]
Blood/Serum: ↑ alk phos, ↑ bil, ↑ AST, ↑ ALT, eosinophilia. **Urinary:** False + catecholamines.
Monitor: Hepatic func c̄ high dose, LT use or estolate form.

E.E.S. (ethylsuccinate) Liquid & Granules- sucrose. Tab- cornstarch, sugar
EryPed (ethylsuccinate) Susp & drops- sucrose.
Ery-Tab (DR) (base) Tab
ERYC (base) Cap- lactose
erythromycin lactobionate- IV only- benzyl alcohol

Erythrocin Stearate (stearate) Tab- cornstarch
Erythromycin Base Filmtab
Erythromycin DR Cap
PCE (base)- lactose, vegetable oil wax,
propylene glycol, Na starch glycolate (333 mg Tab)

| erythropoietin | ANTIANEMIC | See **epoetin alfa p 126** |

escitalopram
  Lexapro
  Tab
  Soln- sorbitol, propylene glycol

ANTIDEPRESSANT, ANTIANXIETY, SSRI   See listing for **citalopram p 86**
s-isomer of **citalopram**

Eskalith   ANTIMANIC   See **lithium carbonate p 197**

esomeprazole
  Nexium/Nexium I.V.

ANTIULCER, ANTISECRETORY, ANTIGERD
s-isomer of **omeprazole**   See **Proton Pump Inhibitors p 268**

Estrace, Estraderm   HORMONE, Estradiol   See **Hormone Therapy p 165**
Estradiol Oral, Estrasorb, EstroGel, estropipate

estrogen

HORMONE (HT), ORAL CONTRACEPTIVE (OC)
  See **Hormone Therapy p 165** or See **Oral Contraceptives p 237**

Estrostep Fe   ORAL CONTRACEPTIVE, ANTI-ACNE   See **Oral Contraceptives p 237**

eszopiclone
  Lunesta
  Tab- lactose

SLEEP AID, Non-Benzodiazepine, 8 hr duration
  Drug: Take just at bedtime, not after high fat/heavy meal.
  Diet: High fat/heavy meal ↓ rate & extent of abs of drug, may ↓ effect.
  Theoretical interaction c̄ grapefruit/related citrus, see p 390. Avoid SJW.[9b]
  Oral/GI: UNPLEASANT/METALLIC TASTE, dry mouth, dyspepsia, N/V, diarrhea.
  S/Cond: Avoid alcohol. Caution lactation. Caution c̄ geriatric, depression,
  severe ↓ hepatic func or ↓ respiratory func.
  Pregnancy: Category C.
  Other: Headache, depression, anxiety, dizzinesss, abnormal dreams,
  hallucinations, confusion, nervousness, migraine, latent drowsiness, rash,
  itching, infection, edema. Rare- parasomnias c̄ amnesia (eg sleep walking).
  Blood/Serum: < 1%- ↑ chol, anemia

etanercept
Enbrel
Multi Use Vial
0.9% benzyl alcohol,
mannitol- 40 mg/vial,
sucrose- 10 mg/vial
Single Use Prefilled Syringe
sucrose- 10 mg/mL

ANTIARTHRITIC (Rheumatoid or Psoriatric Arthritis),
ANKYLOSING SPONDYLITIS or PLAQUE PSORIASIS TREATMENT
TNF Inhibitor   Parenteral only (SC)
Drug: Once or twice/wk injection.
Oral/GI: Mouth ulcer, dyspepsia, vomiting, abdominal pain.
Rare- GI bleeding c̄ high dose, gastroenteritis.
S/Cond: Not c̄ lactation. Caution c̄ CHF or demyelinating disorder.
Not c̄ active infection.
Pregnancy: Category B.
Other: INJECTION SITE REACTION, upper respiratory infection, other infection,
allergic reaction, headache, dizziness, cough, asthenia, rash, rhinitis,
pharyngitis, edema, fever. Rare- lupus-like syndrome, seizure, CVA, CHF,
multiple sclerosis, myelitis, optic neuritis, malignancies (eg lymphoma),
serious infection (can be fatal).
Blood/Serum: Aplastic anemia, + ANA. Rare- dyscrasias.
Monitor: For active TB prior to & during treatment.

ethacrynic acid
Edecrin

DIURETIC   See **Diuretics, Loop p 114**
S/Cond: May be used c̄ sulfa allergy, unlike other loop diuretics.

ethambutol
Myambutol
Tab- sucrose,
sorbitol

TUBERCULOSIS TREATMENT
Drug: May take c̄ food or milk to ↓ GI distress.
Nutr: Anorexia.
Oral/GI: Abdominal pain, N/V, GI distress.
S/Cond: Caution c̄ lactation. Caution c̄ ↓ renal func. Not c̄ optic neuritis.
Pregnancy: Category B.
Other: Optic neuritis, ↓ visual acuity, blurred vision, headache,
dizziness, confusion, joint pain, transient hepatic impairment.
Rare- acute gout, peripheral neuritis, dermatitis, anaphylaxis.
Blood/Serum: ↑ URIC ACID. Abnormal liver function tests, eosinophilia.
Urinary: ↓ uric acid.
Monitor: Uric acid, ophthalmologic exams.
Renal func, hepatic func & CBC c̄ LT use.[6]

etidronate
  Didronel
  Didrocal (Canada)
  90 day pack c̄ 14 day **Didronel**, then 76 day **Ca Carbonate** Tabs

PAGET'S DISEASE TREATMENT, ANTIBONE RESORPTION,
Also used to treat osteoporosis

See **Bisphosphonates, Oral p 59**

etodolac
  Lodine previous brand name
  Cap- lactose,
   Na starch glycolate
  Tab- lactose,
   Na starch glycolate
  Lodine XL (SR)
  previous brand name
  Tab- lactose

ANALGESIC, ANTIARTHRITIC, NSAID

Drug: Take c̄ food or milk to ↓ GI irritation. Swallow SR form whole.
Diet: Caution c̄ GI irritants eg K suppl (↑ risk of GI irritation).
Limit caffeine to ↓ GI effects.
Oral/GI: <u>Dyspepsia</u>, <u>N</u>/V, GI ulcer & bleeding (may be sudden & serious), <u>abdominal pain</u>, <u>diarrhea</u>, colitis, <u>flatulence</u>, constipation.
S/Cond: Avoid alcohol. Caution c̄ lactation. 99% serum pro bound.
Caution c̄ severe ↓ renal func or ↓ hepatic func. Not c̄ gastritis/ulcer.
Caution c̄ HTN, CHF or edema. Not c̄ aspirin allergy.
Pregnancy: Category C, but not recommended in pregnancy.
Category D in 3rd trimester due to ↑ risk to fetus & mother, including death.
Other: <u>Dizziness</u>, <u>weakness</u>, blurred vision, headache, nervousness, rash, tinnitus, pharyngitis, rhinitis, depression. Rare- jaundice, hepatitis, TEN, edema.
Risk of CV problems, eg HTN, CHF, MI, CVA.
Blood/Serum: Anemia, ↑ AST, ↑ ALT, ↓ <u>uric acid</u>, ↑ crea.
Rare- dyscrasias, ↑ bleeding time.
Urinary: False + bil, false + ketones (dipstick).
Monitor: Hepatic, renal func & Hb/HCT c̄ LT use.

etoposide
 VePesid (VP-16)
 Cap- sorbitol
 IV- 30 mg benzyl
  alcohol/mL,
  30.5% alcohol

ANTINEOPLASTIC, Mitotic Inhibitor (Testicular or Lung Cancer)
 Oral or Parenteral (IV)
  Diet: Insure adequate fluid intake/hydration. Avoid grapefruit/related citrus c̄ oral form- ↓ drug abs & serum levels, see p 390. **Nutr:** <u>Anorexia</u>.
  Oral/GI: <u>Stomatitis</u>, <u>taste changes</u>, dysphagia, nausea/vomiting, abdominal pain, constipation, <u>diarrhea</u>.
  S/Cond: Not c̄ lactation. Do dental care cautiously, see p 11 & 15. 97% serum pro bound. Caution c̄ ↓ hepatic or ↓ renal func or geriatric.
  Pregnancy: Category D.
  Other: <u>Bone marrow suppression</u>, <u>hair loss</u>, drowsiness, fatigue, peripheral neuropathy, ↑ infection, rash, anaphylaxis. Transient hypotension, confusion[6] c̄ IV. Rare- transient cortical blindness, optic neuritis.
  Blood/Serum: ↓ <u>platelets</u>, ↓ <u>white blood cells</u>, <u>anemia</u>. Transient ↑ bil, ↑ AST, ↑ ALT, ↑ alk phos.[6]
  Monitor: CBC c̄ diff & platelets prior to each dose. Baseline & periodic renal & hepatic func & during treatment.

etravirine
 Intelence
 Tab- lactose

ANTIRETROVIRAL, Second Generation   NNRTI
  Drug: Take twice daily after a meal to ↑ drug level. May disperse Tab in water, drink immediately, then rinse glass & drink rinse.
  Diet: Caution c̄ grapefruit/related citrus.[134] Not c̄ SJW. **Oral/GI:** Nausea.
  S/Cond: Not c̄ lactation. 99.9% serum pro bound. **Pregnancy:** Category B.
  Other: <u>Rash</u> (more common in women).[5] Peripheral neuropathy. Rare- SJS/TEN, hypersensitivity, hepatic failure.
  Blood/Serum: ↑ chol, ↑ LDL, ↑ TG, ↑ glucose, ↑ ALT.

EvaMist
 estradiol transdermal

HORMONE, Estradiol   See **Hormone Therapy p 165**

everolimus
 Zortess
 Tab- lactose

IMMUNOSUPPRESSANT (To prevent organ transplant rejection)
Adjunct to corticosteroids, some effects may be due to steroids, see p ___.
  Drug: Take consistently c̄ or s̄ food to ↓ absorption variability. High fat meal (44.5g fat) ↓ drug absorption. Take c̄ a glass of water.

Do not crush or chew tab.
Diet: Avoid grapefruit/related citrus, see p 390. Not c̄ SJW, see p 286.
Nutr: Anorexia, ↓ Fe, ↓ B$_{12}$
Oral/GI: N/V, <u>CONSTIPATION</u>, <u>DIARRHEA</u>, <u>abdominal pain</u>, <u>stomatitis/mouth ulceration</u>, dyspepsia, gingival hyperplasia, GERD, abdominal distention.
S/Cond: Not lacatation. Caution c̄ moderate ↓ hepatic func.
Not c̄ severe ↓ hepatic func. **Pregnancy:** Category C.
Other: <u>PERIPHERAL EDEMA</u>, <u>HYPERTENSION</u>, <u>FEVER</u>, <u>VIRAL INFECTIONS</u>, <u>POOR WOUND HEALING</u>, <u>FLUID COLLECTION</u>, <u>fatigue</u>, <u>back/extremity pain</u>, <u>headache</u>, <u>tremor</u>, <u>URTI</u>, <u>diabetes/hyperglycemia</u>, <u>insomnia</u>, <u>cough</u>, <u>rash</u>, <u>acne</u>, <u>night sweats</u>, <u>muscle/bone pain</u>, <u>osteopenia</u>, <u>osteoporosis</u>, <u>gout</u>, <u>dizziness</u>, <u>fainting</u>, <u>paresthesia</u>, <u>somnolence</u>, <u>agitation</u>, <u>anxiety</u>, <u>depression</u>, hydronephrosis, pulmonary edema, pleural effusion, hyperparathyroidism, osteonecrosis, angioedema, pancreatitis, renal artery/vein thromboses.
Blood/Serum: ↓ <u>HEMOGLOBIN</u>, ↓ <u>HEMATOCRIT</u>, ↑ or ↓ WBC, ↑ or ↓ platelets, ↑ <u>crea</u>, ↑ <u>BUN</u>, ↑ <u>chol</u>, ↑ TG, ↑ or ↓ <u>glucose</u>, ↑ or ↓ <u>P</u>, ↓ Ca, ↓ Na, ↑ uric acid, ↑ or ↓ <u>K</u>, ↓ <u>Mg</u>, ↑ AST, ↑ ALT, ↓ testosterone, ↑ FSH.
Urinary: <u>INFECTION</u>, <u>hematuria</u>, <u>dysuria</u>, <u>pro</u>, bladder spasm, urgency, frequency, pyuria, retention.
Monitor: Baseline & periodic- lipid panel, TG, serum glucose, BP, electrolytes, Mg, P, renal func, hepatic func, CBC c̄ diff, platelets, drug level.

Exalgo	ANALGESIC, ANTITUSSIVE, Narcotic, Opioid See listing for **morphine p 221**	
Evista	OSTEOPOROSIS TREATMENT & PREVENTION, SERM	See **raloxifene p 274**

Excedrin Migraine
  Combination drug
  Tab- mineral oil
	ANTIMIGRAINE, ANALGESIC
	  250 mg **acetaminophen**,
	  250 mg **aspirin**, 65 mg **caffeine**
		See **acetaminophen p 22**
		See **aspirin p 44**
		See **caffeine p 67**

Exelon	ANTIALZHEIMER'S	See **rivastigmine p 283**
exemestane **Aromasin**	ANTINEOPLASTIC	See **aromatase inhibitors p 42**

E

exenatide
  Byetta prefilled pen
  Buffered Soln-
  mannitol, 2.2 mg
  metacresol/mL

ANTIHYPERGLYCEMIC, Incretin Mimetic protein   Parenteral Only (SC)
  Adjunct to **metformin** &/or **sulfonylurea** for Type 2 diabetes only
  Drug: Use SC twice a day within 1 hr before AM and evening meals.
  Diet: Prescribed diabetic diet. ↓ cal if wt loss needed.
  Nutr: ↓ appetite. <u>MILD</u> <u>WEIGHT</u> <u>LOSS</u>.
  Oral/GI: ↓ *GASTRIC EMPTYING*. Dyspepsia, <u>NAUSEA</u>, <u>vomiting</u>, GERD, <u>diarrhea</u>.
  S/Cond: Caution c̄ lactation. <u>NOT</u> for Type 1 diabetes. Caution c̄ moderate
  ↓ renal func. Not c̄ severe ↓ renal func or severe GI disease.
  Pregnancy: Category C.
  Other: Dizziness, headache, jittery feeling, asthenia, ↑ perspiration.
  Production of anti-**exenatide** antibodies (may affect glycemic response
  to drug). Rare- acute pancreatitis, acute renal failure or insufficiency.
  Blood/Serum: ↓ *FASTING* & *POSTPRANDIAL GLUCOSE*. ↓ *HbA1$_C$,*
  ↑ *INSULIN* (in response to hyperglycemia), ↓ *POSTPRANDIAL GLUCAGON*.
  <u>Hypoglycemia</u> (↑ risk c̄ **sulfonylurea**).
  Urinary: ↓ *GLUCOSE*. **Monitor:** Serum glucose, HbA1$_C$. Renal func. Body wt.

Exforge/Exforge HCT*

ANTIHYPERTENSIVE   See **amlodipine p 32**
  Combination drug **amlodipine** & **valsartan**
                 See **Angiotensin II Receptor Antagonists p 38**
                 * See also **hydrochlorothiazide p 166**

Ex-Lax Regular & Max   LAXATIVE, Stimulant   See **senna p 290**

Ex-Lax Ultra   LAXATIVE, Stimulant   See **bisacodyl p 57**

Extavia   MULTIPLE SCLEROSIS TREATMENT   See **interferon beta 1-b p 178**

ezetimibe
  Zetia
  Tab- lactose

ANTIHYPERLIPIDEMIC, Cholesterol Absorption Inhibitor
  To treat ↑ Chol or Homozygous Sitosterolemia
  Often prescribed c̄ HMG-CoA Reductase Inhibitors (Statins)
  Drug: Take s̄ regard to food.
  Diet: Adjunct to ↓ fat, ↓ chol diet.

Oral/GI: Diarrhea.
S/Cond: Not c̄ lactation. Not c̄ moderate to severe ↓ hepatic func.
Pregnancy: Category C.
Other: Headache, dizziness, URTI, sinusitis, pharyngitis, chest pain, muscle/joint pain.
Blood/Serum: ↓ _CHOL_, ↓ _LDL_, ↑ _HDL_, ↓ _TG_, ↓ APO B, ↓ _SITOSTEROL_, ↓ _CAMPESTEROL_.
Monitor: Chol, lipid profile.

ezogabine
  Potiga
  Tab- polyethylene
  glycol

ANTIEPILEPTIC, Adunctive Treatment of Partial Onset Seizures in Adults
  Drug: Take s̄ regard to food. Swallow tab whole (do not break, crush chew or dissolve).
  Nutr: ↑ appetite, ↑ wt.
  Oral/GI: <u>N</u>, constipation, dyspepsia, dry mouth, dysphagia.
  S/Cond: Avoid alcohol. Not c̄ lactation. Caution c̄ geriatrics. Caution c̄ moderate - severe ↓ renal or ↓ hepatic func. Not c̄ hypokalemia or hypomagnesemia.
  Pregnancy: Category C.
  Other: <u>DIZZINESS</u>, <u>SOMNOLENCE</u>, <u>confusion</u>, <u>fatigue</u>, <u>weakness</u>, <u>diplopia</u>, <u>blurred vision</u>, <u>memory impairment</u>, <u>tremor</u>, <u>vertigo</u>, <u>abnormal coordination</u>, <u>attention disturbance</u>, ↑ QT interval rash, dyspnea, gait disturbance, dysarthria, balance disorder, hypokenesia, myoclonus, paresthesia, sweating, hallucinations, amnesia, dysphasia/aphasia, anxiety, disorientation, psychosis, encephalopathy, coma, syncope, nystagmus, suicidal thinking and behavior.
  Blood/Serum: ↑ AST, ↑ ALT, ↓ WBC, ↓ neutrophils, ↓ platelets.
  Urinary: Retention, hesitation, dysuria, hematuria, abnormal color.
  Monitor: Urinary symptoms especially in at risk pts (eg BPH). S/S of emergence or worsening of depression, mood changes, suicidal thinking or behavior.

Factive

ANTIBIOTIC, Fluoroquinolone   See **gemifloxacin p 156**

E/F

famciclovir	ANTIVIRAL (Herpes Zoster-Shingles, Herpes Simplex-Genital Herpes, Recurrent Herpes Labialis-Cold Sores)

famciclovir
Famvir
Tab- lactose,
 Na starch glycolate

ANTIVIRAL (Herpes Zoster-Shingles, Herpes Simplex-Genital Herpes, Recurrent Herpes Labialis-Cold Sores)
Drug: Take s̄ regard to food.
Oral/GI: N/V, dyspepsia, diarrhea.
S/Cond: Not c̄ lactation. Caution c̄ ↓ renal func or severe ↓ hepatic func.
Pregnancy: Category B.
Other: <u>Headache</u>, paresthesia, drowsiness, fatigue, itching, joint pain.
Blood/Serum: ↑ ALT, ↑ AST, ↑ bil, ↓ neutrophils.

famotidine
Pepcid/Pepcid AC/Pepcid IV

ANTIULCER, ANTIGERD, ANTISECRETORY   Oral or Parenteral (IV)
See **Histamine H$_2$ Receptor Antagonists p 162**

Famvir   ANTIVIRAL   See **famciclovir above**

Fanapt   ANTIPSYCHOTIC (Second Generation)   See **iloperidone p 171**

Fareston
 toremifene
ANTINEOPLASTIC (Breast Cancer), Estrogen Antagonist
Tab- lactose, Na starch glycolate   See listing for **tamoxifen p 302**

Faslodex   ANTINEOPLASTIC, Estrogen Receptor Blocker   See **fulvestrant p 152**

FazaClo   ANTIPSYCHOTIC (Second Generation)   See **clozapine p 90**

febuxostat
Uloric
Tab- lactose

ANTIGOUT, Xanthine Oxidase Inhibitor
For the chronic management of hyperuricemia in patients c̄ gout
Drug: Take s̄ regard to food or antacids. **Oral/GI:** Nausea.
S/Cond: Caution c̄ lactation. Caution c̄ severe ↓ renal func
or severe ↓ hepatic func. > 99% serum pro bound. **Pregnancy:** Category C.
Other: Arthralgia, rash, gout flare, < 1%- cardiovascular death,
non-fatal MI, non fatal CVA.
Blood/Serum: ↓ <u>*URIC ACID*</u>, ↑ ALT, ↑ AST, < 1%- anemia, neutropenia,
thrombocytopenia, ITP.
Urinary: ↓ <u>*URIC ACID*</u>.
Monitor: LFTs at 2 & 4 mo after initiation, then periodically.
Serum uric acid as early as 2 wk after initiation. S/S of cardiovascular events.

| **Feldene** | ANTIARTHRITIC, NSAID | See listing for **ibuprofen p 170** |
| piroxicam | Cap- lactose, starch | |

felodipine
Plendil (SR)
previous brand name
Tab- lactose

ANTIHYPERTENSIVE, Ca Channel Blocker (dihydropyridine derivative)
Drug: High fat/high CHO meal ↑ peak blood level 60%.
Take regularly s̄ food or c̄ a light, low fat meal.[10] Swallow whole.
Do not crush or chew.
Diet: ↓ Na, ↓ cal may be recommended. Caution c̄ grapefruit/related citrus or Seville orange juice,[80] see p 390. Avoid natural licorice, see p 374. Avoid peppermint oil- may ↑ drug effect.[9b] Caution c̄ lime juice- may ↑ drug effect.[9b] Caution c̄ red wine- may cause dose dumping.[135]
Oral/GI: Dry mouth, dyspepsia, N/V, abdominal pain, constipation, diarrhea, flatulence. Rare- mild gingival hyperplasia.
S/Cond: Avoid alcohol.[9b] Not c̄ lactation. 99% serum pro bound. Caution c̄ ↓ hepatic func, geriatric.
Pregnancy: Category C.
Other: ↓ _BP_ c̄ possible hypotension, <u>peripheral edema</u>, <u>headache</u>, <u>flushing</u>, dizziness, URTI, cough, paresthesia, rash, weakness, tachycardia.
Monitor: BP.

| **Femara** | ANTINEOPLASTIC | See **Aromatase Inhibitors p 42** |
| letrozole | | |

| **Femcon Fe** | ORAL CONTRACEPTIVE | See **Oral Contraceptives p 237** |

| **Femhrt** | HORMONE | See **Hormone Therapy p 165** |

| **Femiron** | HEMATINIC, ANTIANEMIC | See **ferrous salts p 140** |

| **Femring** | HORMONE, **Estradiol** | See **Hormone Therapy p 165** |

| **Femtrace** | HORMONE, **Estradiol** | See **Hormone Therapy p 165** |

fenofibrate
  TriCor
  Tab- sucrose, lactose,
    soy lecithin,
    xanthan gum
  Triglide
  Tab- lactose, mannitol,
    egg lecithin
  Lofibra
  Cap- lactose, starch
  Tab- lactose, xanthan gum,
    Na starch glycolate
  Antara
  Cap- sugar sheres,
    simethicone

ANTIHYPERLIPIDEMIC, Fibrate (to treat ↑ chol &/or ↑ triglycerides)
Also used as adjunct to gout treatment
Drug: Lofibra, **Tricor** or **Antara**- Take c̄ meals to ↑ abs & to ↓ GI distress.
Triglide PI states take s̄ regard to food, but food ↑ abs 55%.
Diet: Adjunct to ↓ LF, ↓ chol (↓ cal if needed).
Oral/GI: N/V, constipation, flatulence.
S/Cond: Avoid alcohol. Not c̄ lactation. 99% serum pro bound.
Tricor- caution c̄ soy allergy. **Triglide**- caution c̄ egg allergy.
Caution c̄ geriatric. Not c̄ ↓ hepatic func or severe ↓ renal func.
Not c̄ gallbladder disease.
Pregnancy: Category C.
Other: Headache, myopathy, fatigue, flu-like syndrome, dizziness,
rhinitis, rash, itching, infections. Rare- pancreatitis, hepatitis,
photosensitivity, gall stones, allergic reaction, SJS, TEN.
Blood/Serum: ↓ _TRIGLYCERIDES_, ↓ _VLDL_, ↓ _chol_, ↓ _LDL_, ↓ _apoB_, ↑ _HDL_,
↑ _apoAl_, ↑ _apoAll_, ↓ URIC ACID, ↓ fibrinogen, ↑ AST, ↑ ALT, ↑ CPK,
anemia, ↓ WBC, ↑ BUN, ↑ crea. **Urinary:** ↑ URIC ACID.
Monitor: Lipid panel baseline & periodically.
CBC periodically for the first 12 mo.[13] Hepatic func.
Possibly CPK if S/S of myopathy.

fentanyl   ANALGESIC, Narcotic, Opioid

Duragesic transdermal patch   **Drug:** Do not chew or crush buccal tab. Suck lozenge.
alcohol- < 0.2 mL   Allow to dissolve in mouth. After 30 minutes, swallow rest of tab c̄ water.
released during use   Apply film to inside of cheek- do not eat food until film dissolves.
Fentora Buccal Tab   May drink liquid after 5 minutes. Place SL tab under tongue.
mannitol, Na starch glycolate   May use water to moisten mucosa in pts c̄ dry mouth. Do not chew,
Actiq/Fentyl OTFC   suck or swllow SL tab. Allow tab to dissolve completely before eating or
lozenge on a handle   drinking. Prime nasal spray before use. Inserrt tip of sprayer 1/2 inch into
confectioners sugar   one nostril to spray as directed.
food starch = 2g total sugar   **Nutr:** Anorexia.
Onsolis   **Oral/GI:** <u>Dry</u> <u>mouth</u>, <u>dyspepsia</u>, <u>N/V</u>, hiccups,
Buccal Soluble Film   <u>abdominal</u> <u>pain</u>, <u>constipation</u>, flatulence, <u>diarrhea</u>.
Abstral- SL   **S/Cond:** Avoid alcohol. Not c̄ lactation. May be habit forming c̄ LT use.
Tab- mannitol   Caution c̄ ↓ hepatic func, ↓ renal func or ↓ pulmonary func.
Lazanda- Nasal Spray   Heat ↑ fentanyl abs from patch- e.g. heating pads, hot tubs, sunbathing,
mannitol, pectin, sucrose   high fever.[1]
    Patch, buccal tab, film or **Actiq** are not for children- may be fatal.
    Pregnancy: Category C.
    Other: <u>Sedation</u>, <u>respiratory</u> <u>depression</u>, <u>drowsiness</u>, <u>confusion</u>,
    <u>weakness</u>, <u>dizziness</u>, <u>anxiety</u>, <u>mental</u> <u>depression</u>, <u>hallucinations</u>,
    <u>headache</u>, <u>sweating</u>, <u>dyspnea</u>, amnesia, ↑ or ↓ BP, ataxia, edema, rash,
    migraine, dehydration, ↑ cough, pharyngitis, back pain, chest pain,
    chills, fever, infection, pain.
    Blood/Serum: ↑ amylase, ↑ lipase.
    Urinary: <u>Retention</u>.

Fentora   ANALGESIC, Narcotic, Opioid   See **fentanyl above**
Buccal Tab

ferrous salts (oral) HEMATINIC, ANTIANEMIC, Mineral Supplement, Iron (Fe)

Drug: Take c̄ 8 oz water or juice on empty stomach. May take c̄ food to ↓ GI distress, but food ↓ abs 50%.[6]
Drink liquid form c̄ straw to ↓ dental stains. Take 1 hr before or 2 after bran, high phytate foods, see p 382, fiber suppl, tea, coffee, caffeine, red grape juice/wine, soy, dairy products or egg.[13, 47e]

Diet: 200 mg Vit C/ 30 mg Fe will ↑ Fe abs.[6] Meat/fish/poultry ↑ abs.[47e]
Take carbonate antacids,[9b] Ca, P, Zn or Cu suppl separately by ≥ 2 hr.
High dose Vit E (> 10 IU/kg body wt) ↓ hematologic response to Fe in children c̄ Fe def anemia.[6]
Vit A def ↓ Fe mobilization from stores.[47e]

Nutr: <u>Anorexia</u>. High dose Fe ↓ Zn abs- may need Zn suppl.[13] **RDA** (mg/day)- Infant 7-12 mo = **11**.
Children 1-3 yr = **7**. 4-8 = **10**. 9-13 = **8**. Males 14-18 = **11**. 19-70+ = **8**. Females 14-18 = **15**. 19-50 = **18**.
51+ = **8**. Lactation = **9-10**. Vegetarian- Female 14-18 = **26**. 19-50 = **33**. Males 19-70+ = **14**.

Oral/GI: <u>DENTAL STAINS</u> c̄ liquid forms, <u>NAUSEA</u>/V, <u>DYSPEPSIA</u>, <u>bloating</u>, <u>CONSTIPATION</u>, <u>diarrhea</u>, <u>DARK STOOLS</u>. False + guaiac test for occult fecal blood.

S/Cond: Limit alcohol. 90% serum pro bound. Achlorhydria or malabsorption ↓ Fe abs.

Feosol Elixir precipitates TF. Caution c̄ alcoholism/cirrhosis, ↓ hepatic func.[47e] Not c̄ peptic ulcer, enteritis, colitis, hemochromatosis, thalassemia or non Fe def anemia eg hemolytic anemia.

Pregnancy: RDA = 27 mg/day. Category A.

Other: UL (mg/day) Children = **40**. Adults = **45**. 60-250 mg elemental Fe/kg body wt in one dose can be fatal.[6] As low as 20 mg/kg may be toxic in some individuals.[47]
Iron overload (hemosiderosis) & toxicity may result from LT use of high dose (not reported c̄ Fe bisglycinate).[118]

Blood/Serum: ↑ <u>Hb</u>, ↑ <u>HCT</u>, ↑ <u>ferritin</u>, ↑ <u>Fe</u>, ↑ <u>% transferrin saturation</u>. ↓ <u>TIBC</u>. False ↓ Ca.[13]

Urinary: Dark color. **Monitor:** Hb/HCT, ferritin, Fe, TIBC, transferrin.

ferrous fumarate	**ferrous gluconate**	**ferrous sulfate-** generics	**iron polysaccharide**
33% elemental Fe	12% elemental Fe	20% elemental Fe	**Niferex** Elixir =
Femiron	**Fergon**	**ferrous sulfate exsiccated**	100 mg Fe/5mL
Tab = 20 mg Fe	Tab = 27 mg Fe	30% elemental Fe	10% alcohol, sorbitol
Ferro-Sequels (SR)	Tab- cornstarch,	**Feosol** Tab = 65 mg Fe,	**Niferex 150** Cap = 150 mg Fe,
Tab = 50 mg Fe	sucrose	lactose, sorbitol	Vit C 50 mg, succinic acid
(+ 100 mg docusate Na)	**carbonyl Fe**	**Slow Fe** Tab (SR) =	50 mg
Tab- lactose	**Feosol** Caplet	50 mg Fe	
	Caplet = 45 mg Fe	**ferrous sulfate elixir**	
	lactose, sorbitol	5 ml- 44 mg Fe, sucrose, corn syrup, alcohol 5%, saccharin Na	
		(Total CHO = 2g, Na 1mg)	
		ferrous bisglycinate (chelate c̄ glycine) also called **Ferrochel**	
		20% elemental Fe	

ferrous salts (Parenteral IV or IM)   HEMATINIC, ANTIANEMIC, Mineral Supplement, Iron (Fe)
    Fe Deficiency Treatment[a]   Fe supplementation c̄ **erythropoietin** use in Renal Dialysis[b]
Nutr: See **ferrous salts** (oral) above for **RDA** & **UL** for iron. Parenteral Fe ↓ abs of concomitant oral Fe.
Oral/GI: <u>Taste loss</u>, <u>N/V</u>, abdominal pain, <u>diarrhea</u>, constipation.
S/Cond: Caution c̄ lactation. **ferumoxytol**- not c̄ lactation. Not c̄ Fe def anemia eg hemolytic anemia.
Pregnancy: Category B. Category C- **Fe dextran** & **ferumoxytol**.
Other: Hypotension (↑ IN DIALYSIS PTS), <u>chest pain</u>, <u>edema</u>, <u>dizziness</u>, <u>headache</u>, <u>HTN</u>, fever, muscle pain/<u>cramp</u>, back pain, flushing, cough, dyspnea, rash, itching. Very rare- anaphylactic reaction (may be fatal).
Blood/Serum: Fe dextran- false ↑ bil, false ↓ Ca, unreliable Fe & ferritin.
Urinary: Dark color.
Monitor: Hb/HCT, ferritin, Fe, TIBC, transferrin.

iron dextran (IV, IM)	**iron sucrose** (IV)	**Na ferric gluconate complex** (IV)
InFeD[a]	**Venofer**[b]	**Ferrlecit**[b]
Single Dose Vial =	Single Dose Vial =	Single Dose Vial =
2 mL = 100 mg Fe,	5 mL = 100 mg Fe,	5 mL = 62.5 mg Fe,
0.9% NaCl	30% sucrose (1.5 g)	20% sucrose (0.98 g), benzyl alcohol 45 mg

iron oxide Feraheme (**ferumoxytol**[b]) Single dose vial- 17 mL = 510 mg Fe, 748 mg mannitol

fesoterodine   ANTIMUSCARINIC   See **Bladder Control Agents p 61**
    Toviaz (SR)   Tab- lactose

fexofenadine   ANTIHISTAMINE
    Allegra   **Drug:** Take s̄ regard to food, but not c̄ apple, orange or grapefruit juice.[76]
    Tab- starch   Dissolve ODT on tongue c̄ or s̄ liquid, swallow saliva.
    Susp- propylene glycol,   **Diet:** Fruit juice (apple, orange or grapefruit) ↓ drug bioavailability > 70%.[76]
    xanthan gum, sucrose,   **S/Cond:** Caution c̄ alcohol.[7] Caution c̄ lactation. Caution c̄ ↓ renal func.
    xylitol   Caution c̄ SJW,[9b] see p 286.
    ODT- aspartame, mannitol   **Pregnancy:** Category C.
    5.3 mg phenylalanine   **Other:** Menstrual pain, cold or flu, headache, drowsiness, dizziness,
    Na starch glycolate   back pain, cough.

FiberCon	LAXATIVE, Bulk Forming	See **calcium polycarbophil p 71**

fidaxomicin
Dificid
Tab-
pre-gelatinized starch,
Na starch glycolate,
ethylene glycol,
lecithin (soy)

ANTIBIOTIC, Macrolide, To treat C. difficile associated diarrhea in adults
    Drug: Take s̄ regard to food.
    Oral/GI: <u>N/V</u>, <u>abdominal</u> <u>pain</u>, GI hemorrhage, abdominal distension,
    abdominal tenderness, dyspepsia, dysphagia, flatulence,
    intestinal obstruction, megacolon.
    S/Cond: Caution c̄ lactation, Not for systemic infections- poorly absorbed.
    Only for infection proven or strongly suspect to be caused by C. difficile.
    Pregnancy: Category B.
    Other: Skin drug eruption, rash, pruritis, metabolic acidosis.
    Blood/Serum: ↓ Hb, ↓ HCT, ↓ neutrophils, ↓ platelets, ↑ alk phos,
    ↑ AST, ↑ ALT, ↓ bicarb, ↑ glucose.

filgrastim (G-CSF)
Neupogen
single dose vials or
prefilled syringes
sorbitol = 50 mg/mL,
preservative free

COLONY STIMULATING FACTOR (↑ production & activity of neutrophils)
    Given > 24 hr before or after chemotherapy   Parenteral only (IV or SC)
    S/Cond: Caution c̄ lactation. Not c̄ allergy to E. coli derived pro.
    Caution c̄ sickle cell patients- ↑ risk of crisis.
    Pregnancy: Category C.
    Other: <u>BONE</u> <u>PAIN</u>, <u>SPLENOMEGALY</u>, <u>nosebleed</u>, fever. Transient ↓ BP.
    Rare- ARDS (IV), allergic reaction (↑ c̄ IV within 30 min of use).
    Blood/Serum: ↑ <u>NEUTROPHILS</u>, ↑ <u>WBC</u>.
    Transient- ↑ <u>URIC</u> <u>ACID</u>, ↑ <u>LDH</u>, ↑ <u>ALK</u> <u>PHOS</u>, ↓ platelets.
    Urinary: Hematuria, pro.
    Monitor: CBC c̄ diff & platelets baseline, then daily to 2-3 X/wk.

finasteride
Propecia
Tab- lactose, starch,
Na starch glycolate,
docusate Na
Proscar
Tab- lactose, starch,
Na starch glcolate,

BPH TREATMENT (**Proscar**), Androgen Hormone Inhibitor
MALE PATTERN BALDNESS TREATMENT (**Propecia**)
    5 alpha-reductase inhibitor for treatment of prostate hyperplasia
    Drug: Take s̄ regard to meals.
    S/Cond: 90% serum pro bound. Caution c̄ ↓ hepatic func.[6]
    Not for women or children.
    Pregnancy: Category X.
    Pregnant women should <u>NOT</u> handle crushed or broken tab.

docusate Na

Blood/Serum: ↓ PSA.
Urinary: BPH patients- ↑ _FLOW_, ↓ _RESIDUAL URINE_, ↓ _FREQUENCY_, ↓ _NOCTURIA_, ↑ _EASE OF STARTING MICTURITION_.
Monitor: Digital rectal exams for prostate cancer.
Note- No nutritionally-related effects reported.

Firmagon   ANTINEOPLASTIC, (Advanced Prostate Cancer)   See **degarelix p 103**

fingolimod   TREATMENT OF RELAPSING FORMS OF MULTIPLE SCLEROSIS,
  Gilenya   TO REDUCE THE FREQUENCY OF CLINICAL EXACERBATIONS,
  Cap- mannitol,   TO DELAY THE ACCUMULATION OF PHYSICAL DISABILITIES,
  gelatin   Sphingosine 1-phosphate receptor modulator
Drug: Take cap s̄ regard to food.
Nutr: ↓ wt.
Oral/GI: Gastroenteritis, diarrhea.
S/Cond: Avoid alcohol. Not c̄ lacatation. Caution c̄ ↓ renal func or severe ↓ hepatic func. Caution c̄ uveitis or diabetes mellitus- ↑ risk of macular edema.
Pregnancy: Category C.
Other: Back pain, influenza viral infection, herpes viral infection, bronchitis, fungal infection, ↓ HR (after first dose) bradycardia, HTN, headache, dizziness, paresthesia, migraine, weakness, alopecia, eczema, pruritis, cough, dyspnea, depression, blurred vision,eye pain, lymphoma. < 1%- macular edema.
Blood/Serum: ↑ AST, ↑ ALT ↑ GGT, ↑ TG, ↓ LYMPHOCYTES (effect persists up to 2 mos after treatment cessation), lymphopenia, ↓ leukocytes.
Monitor: Baseline CBC, LFTs and ophthalmic evaluation. ECG in pts taking antiarrhythmics, or pts c̄ cardiac risk factors, slow /irregular beat prior to first dose. Varicella zoster vaccine in pts who test varicella antibody negative before initiating **fingolimod** therapy.
S/S of bradycardia for 6 hrs after first dose. S/S of infection.
Ophthalmic evaluation q 3-4 mos. Respiratory func if clinically indicated. CBC and LFT during therapy if clinically indicated.

F

Fioricet	ANALGESIC, SEDATIVE, Barbiturate, Combination drug	
Tab- starch	50 mg **butalbital**, 40 mg **caffeine**, 325 mg **acetaminophen**	
Fiorinal		
Cap- starch	50 mg **butalbital**, 40 mg **caffeine**, 325 mg **aspirin**	
may contain benzyl alcohol		
	See **butalbital p 66**, **caffeine p 67**, **acetaminophen p 22** or **aspirin p 44**	
fish oil	ANTIHYPERLIPIDEMIC to reduce triglyceride levels	
	Also used as Anticoagulant & to Prevent Cardiac Disease	
		See **Omega-3 Fatty Acids p 234**
Fisol	ANTIHYPERLIPIDEMIC	See **Omega-3 Fatty Acids p 234**
5-ASA	ANTI-INFLAMMATORY (in ulcerative colitis & Crohn's) See **mesalamine p 209**	
5-FU	ANTINEOPLASTIC, Antimetabolite	See **fluorouracil p 147**
Flagyl	ANTIBIOTIC	See **metronidazole p 216**
Flector	ANALGESIC, NSAID, Patch	See **diclofenac sodium p 107**
Fleet Stimulant Laxative	LAXATIVE, Stimulant	See **bisacodyl p 57**
Flexeril	SKELETAL MUSCLE RELAXANT	See **cyclobenzaprine p 95**
Flomax	BPH TREATMENT	
tamsulosin		See **Alpha₁ Adrenergic Blockers p 28**
Flonase	ANTIALLERGIC RHINITIS	See listing for
fluticasone	Corticosteroid, Nasal	**beclomethasone p 51**
Florinef	CORTICOSTEROID, Mineralocorticoid	See **fludrocortisone p 146**
(previous brand name)		
Flovent HFA/Flovent Diskus	ANTIASTHMA (maintenance therapy)	Aerosol or Rotadisk
fluticasone	Corticosteroid, Inhalant	See listing for **beclomethasone p 51**
Aerosol (inhalation aerosol)- soy lecithin		
Disk- lactose		

fluconazole
  Diflucan
  Susp- sucrose
  Tab
  IV- 9 mg NaCl
  <u>or</u> 56 mg dextrose/mL

ANTIFUNGAL, ANTICRYPTOCOCCAL MENINGITIS, ANTICANDIDIASIS

Oral or Parenteral (IV)

Drug: Take s̄ regard to food. Take c̄ food if GI distress occurs.
Oral/GI: Taste changes, dry mouth, dyspepsia, N/V, abdominal pain, diarrhea.
S/Cond: Not c̄ lactation. Caution c̄ diabetics on sulfonylurea- hypoglycemia.
Caution c̄ ↓ renal func or pre-existing hepatic disease.
Pregnancy: Category C.
Other: <u>Headache</u>, rash, tremor, ↑ sweating, dizziness,
hepatotoxicity (can be fatal). Rare- ↑ QT interval.[26]
Blood/Serum: ↑ <u>AST</u>, ↑ <u>ALT</u>, ↑ <u>alk phos</u>, ↑ <u>bil</u>, ↑ <u>GGT</u>.
Rare- ↑ TG, ↓ K.
Monitor: Baseline & periodic hepatic func.

fludarabine
  Fludara
  Single dose vial-
   50 mg mannitol
  Oforta
  Tab- lactose

ANTINEOPLASTIC , Antimetabolite (Leukemia)   Oral, Parenteral (IV)

Nutr: <u>ANOREXIA</u>.
Oral/GI: <u>Stomatitis</u>, dysphagia, <u>NAUSEA/VOMITING</u>, <u>bleeding diarrhea</u>,
constipation.
S/Cond: Not c̄ lactation. Caution c̄ geriatric or ↓ renal func.
Pregnancy: Category D.
Other: <u>BONE MARROW SUPPRESSION</u>, <u>FEVER</u>, <u>INFECTION</u>, <u>PNEUMONIA</u>, <u>WEAKNESS</u>,
<u>COUGH</u>, <u>PAIN</u>, <u>asthenia</u>, <u>dyspnea</u>, <u>severe</u> <u>neurotoxicity</u> (may be fatal),
<u>paresthesia</u>, <u>chills</u>, <u>edema</u>, <u>visual changes</u>, <u>hearing loss</u>, <u>rash</u>,
<u>muscle pain</u>, hair loss, dehydration, headache, DVT, phlebitis.
Blood/Serum: <u>ANEMIA</u>, ↓ <u>PLATELETS</u>, ↓ <u>NEUTROPHILS</u>, ↑ glucose.
Urinary: Dysuria, Pro, blood, infection.
Monitor: Baseline & periodic CBC, platelets.

fludrocortisone
Florinef
(previous brand name)
Tab- lactose
Generic brands only

CORTICOSTEROID, Mineralocorticoid
ADRENOCORTICAL INSUFFICIENCY TREATMENT IN ADDISON'S
DISEASE (Partial replacement therapy)
TO TREAT SALT-LOSING ADRENOGENITAL SYNDROME
Also used to manage orthostatic hypotension
At usual doses, adverse reactions are caused by ↑ Na & ↑ water retention
as compared to glucocorticoids.
LT high dose may cause glucocorticoid effects. See also **corticosteroids p 94**
Diet: ↓ Na (except ↑ Na if used to manage hypotension), ↑ Ca, ↑ Vit D.
May need ↑ K (or suppl). Ca-Vit D suppl recommended c̄ LT use.
S/Cond: Avoid alcohol. Caution c̄ lactation. Highly pro bound.
Hypoalbuminemia (< 3 g/dL)- may ↑ drug effects. Caution c̄ ↓ renal func.
Not c̄ systemic fungal infection or TB.
Pregnancy: Category C. **Other:** <u>EDEMA</u>, ↑ <u>BLOOD</u> <u>PRESSURE</u>, dizziness,
headache, cardiac enlargement, CHF, hypokalemia.
Blood/Serum: ↑ <u>Na</u>, ↓ K. **Urinary:** ↓ <u>Na</u>, ↑ <u>K</u>, ↑ <u>Ca</u>. **Monitor:** Electrolytes, BP.

fluoride (F)
Sodium Fluoride
2.2 mg = 1 mg F
Luride
Pediaflor
Drops - sorbitol,
< 0.5% alcohol

DENTAL CARIES PROPHYLACTIC, MINERAL SUPPLEMENT
Drug: Take separately by ≥ 2 hr from dairy products, Ca, Fe or Mg suppl.[7]
Tab- dissolve in mouth, chew or swallow whole or add to water or juice.
Drops- Take undiluted or mix with fluids or non dairy food.
Nutr: AI (mg/day) Children 0-6 mo = **0.01**. 7-12 mo = **0.5**. 1-3 yr = **0.7**.
4-8 = **1**. 9-13 = **2**. 14-18 = **3**. Males 19+ = **4**. Females 19+ = **3**.
Lactation = 3.
UL (mg/day) Children 0-6 mo = **0.7**. 7-12 mo = **0.9**. 1-3 yr = **1.3**.
4-8 = **2.2**. Children > 8 & Adults = **10**. **Lactation = 10**.
Ca, Fe or Mg ions ↓ abs. High conc of dietary Ca forms insoluble
complexes c̄ F.[73] Caution- swallowed F in toothpaste or rinse is 100%
abs- may contribute to dental fluorosis.[47b]
Oral/GI: Dental fluorosis, gastric distress. GI bleeding, N/V c̄ LT high dose. [6]
S/Cond: Do not use in areas c̄ > 0.3 ppm F in water.[7]
≥ 1 mg not recommended for children < 6 years old.
Pregnancy: Consult physician. **AI = 3** mg/day. **UL = 10** mg/day.

Other: Headache, eczema, rash.
↑ osteoblast activity & BMD, but may ↓ bone strength & elasticity.[93]
<u>In children</u>- 0.1 mg F/kg body wt daily causes dental fluorosis.
<u>In adults</u>- 20 to 80 mg F/day leads to chronic toxicity & skeletal fluorosis after > 10 years of use.[47]
Acute dose of 10-20 mg NaF causes ↑ salivation & GI upset.
Estimated adult lethal dose of NaF is 5-10 g (70 to 140 mg/kg); 500 mg for children.[6]

fluorouracil
(5-FU)
Fluorouracil

ANTINEOPLASTIC, Antimetabolite   Parenteral (IV)
(colorectal, breast, stomach or pancreatic cancer)
Used c̄ **leucovorin** to ↑ effect of **fluorouracil**, see p 190
Diet: Bland diet may ↓ GI distress.
Oral Pyr may treat palmar-plantar erythrodyesthesia.[13]
Nutr: <u>ANOREXIA</u>, ↓ <u>wt</u>. May ↑ Thi requirement.
Oral/GI: <u>Bitter/sour taste</u>, STOMATITIS, <u>esophagitis</u>, <u>dyspepsia</u>, severe <u>NAUSEA/VOMITING</u>, <u>enteritis</u>, GI ulceration & bleeding, <u>DIARRHEA</u>.
Rare- pseudomembranous colitis.
S/Cond: Not c̄ lactation. Do dental care cautiously, see p 11 & 15.
Caution c̄ ↓ hepatic func or ↓ renal func.
Contraindicated c̄ poor nutritional status.
Caution c̄ obesity, edema, ascites- base dose on LBM.[7]
Pregnancy: Category D.
Other: <u>BONE MARROW SUPPRESSION</u>, <u>WEAKNESS</u>, <u>RASH</u>, <u>HAIR LOSS</u>, <u>fatigue</u>, <u>dermatitis</u>, ataxia, photosensitivity. Rare- hand-foot syndrome, acute cerebellar syndrome (balance dysfunction).
Blood/Serum: ↓ <u>WHITE BLOOD CELLS</u>, ↓ <u>platelets</u>, <u>anemia</u>, ↓ alb, ↑ alk phos, ↑ AST, ↑ ALT, ↑ bil, ↑ LDH, ↓ T_3, ↓ T_4.
Monitor: WBC c̄ diff & platelets before each dose.
CBC, hepatic func. Oral exams.
DC if S/S of toxicity or severe Oral-GI effects.

fluoxetine
  Prozac
  Cap (Pulvule)- starch
  Prozac Weekly (DR)
  Cap- sucrose,
   sugar spheres (sugar & starch)
  generic liquid-
   0.23% alcohol,
   sucrose

  Sarafem
  Cap- starch
  Tab

ANTIDEPRESSANT, TREATMENT OF OCD, BULIMIA NERVOSA, PANIC DISORDER,   SSRI

Sarafem- PMDD TREATMENT (premenstrual dysphoric disorder)
Drug: Take in AM s̄ regard to meals.
Diet: Avoid tryptophan suppl- will ↑ drug side effects.[3]
Avoid SJW, see p 286.
Nutr: <u>Anorexia</u>, ↓ wt. ↑ appetite, ↑ wt. May ↓ abs of leucine.[77]
Oral/GI: <u>Dry mouth</u>, taste changes, <u>dyspepsia</u>, <u>N</u>/V, <u>diarrhea</u>, constipation.
Rare- upper GI bleeding.[68]
S/Cond: Avoid alcohol. Not c̄ lactation. Caution c̄ diabetes-
hypoglycemia. Caution c̄ geriatric[84]- ↑ incidence of <u>ANOREXIA</u>.[21]
94.5% serum pro bound. Caution c̄ ↓ hepatic func. Caution c̄ seizures.
Caution c̄ bipolar disorder.
Pregnancy: Category C.
Other: <u>Tremor</u>, <u>headache</u>, <u>drowsiness</u>, <u>dizziness</u>, <u>insomnia</u>, <u>asthenia</u>,
<u>anxiety</u>, <u>sweating</u>, <u>flu-like</u> <u>syndrome</u>, <u>yawning</u>, <u>pharyngitis</u>, sinusitis,
headache, chills, visual disturbances, photosensitivity, rash,
sexual dysfunction, HTN, ear pain, tinnitus, amnesia, confusion,
palpitation, chest pain, hemmorhage.
Rare- SIADH,[10] akathisia, EPS, hepatitis, seizures, galactorrhea.[21]
Rare- serotonin syndrome, suicidal thinking & behavior
Blood/Serum: ↑ or ↓ glucose, ↓ Na. < 1%- ↑ AST, ↑ ALT, ↑ prolactin.[21]
Urinary: ↑ frequency. < 1%- ↑ alb. **Monitor:** Wt.

fluphenazine
  Prolixin

ANTIPSYCHOTIC   See **Phenothiazines p 254**

flurazepam
  Dalmane

SLEEP AID   See **Benzodiazepines p 54**

fluticasone
  Flonase (spray)
  Flovent /Flovent Diskus

ANTIALLERGIC RHINITIS (**Flonase**, **Vermyst**)   See listing for **beclomethasone p 51**
ANTIASTHMA (**Flovent**)   Corticosteroid
Nasal Spray- dextrose, 0.25% phenylethyl alcohol

Veramyst (spray)
Aerosol- soy lecithin (inhalation aerosol)   Diskus- lactose
S/Cond: Caution c̄ severe ↓ hepatic func.
Other: Cataracts, ↑ intraocular pressure.[9a]

fluvastatin
Lescol/Lescol XL
ANTIHYPERLIPIDEMIC   See **HMG-CoA Reductase Inhibitors p 164**
To ↓ chol or TG

fluvoxamine
Luvox
(previous brand name)
Tab- mannitol,
potato starch,
cornstarch

Generic Brands Only

Luvox CR
Cap- sugar spheres
(gluten free)

OCD or SOCIAL ANXIETY DISORDER TREATMENT,
Also used to treat depression, SSRI
Drug: Take HS s̄ regard to food. Do not crush or chew CR Cap.
Diet: Avoid tryptophan suppl- ↑ drug effects.[3] Limit caffeine,
melatonin- drug ↓ metabolism & ↑ levels (≥ 5X caffeine[21]; ≥ 20X melatonin[93]).
Caution c̄ grapefruit/related citrus,[109] see p 390. Avoid SJW, see p 286.
Nutr: <u>Anorexia</u>. ↑ or ↓ wt. ↑ thirst.
Oral/GI: Dry mouth, taste changes, tooth disorder, dysphagia, <u>NAUSEA</u>/V,
<u>dyspepsia</u>, <u>diarrhea</u>, <u>constipation</u>, flatulence. Rare- upper GI bleeding.[68a]
S/Cond: Avoid alcohol. Not c̄ lactation.
Caution c̄ ↓ hepatic func or seizures. Caution c̄ geriatric.
Caution c̄ bipolar disorder. Caution c̄ CYP2D6 slow metabolizer.
Pregnancy: Category C.
Other: <u>Asthenia</u>, <u>drowsiness</u>, <u>insomnia</u>, <u>nervousness</u>, <u>dizziness</u>,
headache, tremor, chills, flu syndrome, edema, ↑ cough, palpitations,
tachycardia, agitation, anxiety, depression, amnesia, HTN or hypotension,
yawning, dyspnea, blurred vision, sweating, flushing, sexual dysfunction.
Rare- SIADH, akathisia, EPS, hepatitis, seizures, galactorrhea,
serotonin syndrome, NMS-type reactions, suicidal thinking & behavior.
Blood/Serum: ↑ AST, ↑ ALT. < 1%- dyscrasias, ↑ chol, ↓ Na.
Urinary: ↑ frequency, retention.

Focalin/Focalin XR
dexmethylphenidate
ANTI-ADHD, Stimulant   See listing for **methylphenidate p 214**
Focalin Tab- starch, lactose, Na starch glycolate
Focalin XR Cap- sugar spheres (sucrose & starch)

folic acid
(folate)
generic Parenteral-
1.5% benzyl alcohol
Folgard Tab
Fol 800 µg
Vit B$_{12}$ 115 µg
Pyr 10 mg
Folgard RX 2.2 Tab
Fol 2.2 mg
Vit B$_{12}$ 1 mg
Pyr 25 mg
Folgard OS
Fol 1.1 mg
Vit B$_{12}$ 250 µg
Pyr 12.5 mg
Ca 500 mg as Ca Carbonate
Mg 100 mg as Mg Oxide
Vit D-3 300 IU, Boron 1.5 mg

B COMPLEX VITAMIN, ANTIANEMIC   Oral or Parenteral (IM, IV or SC)
Also used to treat depression[93]
Drug: Usual therapeutic dose- 1 mg daily for megaloblastic/macrocytic anemia.
Nutr: AI (µg/day) Infants 0-6 mo = **65**. 7-12 mo = **80**.
RDA (µg/day) Children 1-3 yr = **150**. 4-8 = **200**. 9-13 = **300**.
14-18 & Adult = **400**. Lactation = **500**.
UL (µg/day) Children 1-3 yr = **300**. 4-8 = **400**. 9-13 = **600**.
14-18 = **800**. Adult = **1000**. Lactation = **800-1000**.
S/Cond: Not c̄ untreated pernicious anemia.
Fol metabolism inhibited by def of Vit B$_{12}$[26], Vit C or Fe.
↑ need in alcoholism, hemodialysis,[13] celiac disease, chronic diarrhea,
tropical sprue, HIV. HIV- ↓ abs of Fol.
Pregnancy: Category A. **RDA** = **600** µg/day. **UL** = 800-1000 µg/day.
400 µg minimum before conception & in early pregnancy is
recommended to prevent neural tube defects in infants.
Other: Rare- allergic reaction.
Blood/Serum: ↓ Vit B$_{12}$ c̄ LT high dose, ↓ HOMOCYSTEINE. ↑ RBC, ↑ WBC,
↑ platelets, ↑ Hb, ↑ HCT, ↓ MCH, ↓ MCV when used to treat anemia.
Monitor: CBC. Vit B$_{12}$ c̄ LT high dose.

folinic acid

CHEMOTHERAPY RESCUE OR ADJUNCT See **leucovorin p 190**

formoterol
Foradil
Perforomist

ANTIASTHMA (not for acute symptoms), COPD TREATMENT
Beta-2 Agonist Inhalation Aerosol Cap- lactose
Inhalation aerosol- preservative free See listing for **salmeterol p 286**

Fortamet

ANTIHYPERGLYCEMIC AGENT, Biguanide See **metformin p 210**

Fortaz

ANTIBIOTIC, **ceftazidime** See **cephalosporins p 80**

Forteo

OSTEOPOROSIS TREATMENT See **teriparatide p 308**
Human Parathyroid Hormone

Fortesta

MALE HORMONE REPLACEMENT, Androgen See **testosterone p 308**

Fortical	OSTEOPOROSIS TREATMENT	See **calcitonin p 68**

Fosamax
  alendronate   OSTEOPOROSIS TREATMENT, PAGET'S DISEASE TREATMENT
                                          See **Bisphosphonates, Oral p 59**

Fosamax plus D   OSTEOPOROSIS TREATMENT   See **Bisphosphonates, Oral p 59**
  alendronate & **cholecalciferal (Vit D-3)**   Combination drug,   See **Vitamin D p 340**
  Tab- lactose, gelatin, sucrose, modified food starch, 2800 IU Vit D   once a week dosing

fosamprenavir   ANTIRETROVIRAL (HIV/AIDS), Protease Inhibitor
  Lexiva   pro-drug of **amprenavir**, taken c̄ **ritonavir**
  Tab   **Drug:** Adults- take s̄ regard to food. High fat meal does not affect drug.
  Susp- propylene glycol,   Children should take susp c̄ food to ↓ GI upset.
    sucralose   **Diet:** Avoid SJW. Caution c̄ garlic- may ↓ drug level.[1]
                       Oral/GI: <u>Nausea</u>/vomiting, abdominal pain, GI upset, diarrhea.
                       S/Cond: Avoid alcohol. Not c̄ lactation. 90% serum pro bound.
                       Caution c̄ ↓ hepatic func, diabetes, geriatric or sulfonamide allergy.
                       Not c̄ hemophilia. **Pregnancy:** Category C.
                       Other: <u>Rash</u>, paresthesia, headache, diabetes, depressive or mood
                       disorders, fatigue, neuropathy. May ↑ risk of lipodystrophy.
                       Rare- diabetes, jaundice, nephrolithiasis, angioedema,[5] SJS, MI.
                       Blood/Serum: ↑ lipase, ↑ glucose, ↑ Hb A1$_c$, ↑ <u>triglycerides</u>, ↑ chol.
                       Rare- hemolytic anemia, ↑ ALT, ↑ AST.
                       Monitor: Baseline & periodic lipid panel & hepatic func.

fosaprepitant   **Emend** for injection   ANTIEMETIC, ANTINAUSEANT
  Prodrug of **aprepitant**   See **aprepitant p 40**

fosinopril   ANTIHYPERTENSIVE, CHF TREATMENT
  Monopril   See **Angiotensin Converting Enzyme Inhibitors p 36**

fosphenytoin   ANTIEPILEPTIC   See listing for **phenytoin p 256**
  Cerebyx   Water soluble prodrug   Parenteral only (IV or IM)
                       Pregnancy: Category D.

Fosrenol	PHOSPHATE BINDER (for use in ESRD)	See **lanthanum p 188**
Fragmin	ANTICOAGULANT, low molecular weight **heparin**	See **dalteparin p 101**

frovatriptan
  Frova
ANTIMIGRAINE, Serotonin 5-HT$_1$ Receptor Agonist
See **Antimigraine p 39**

fulvestrant
  Faslodex
  alcohol,
  benzyl alcohol,
  castor oil
ANTINEOPLASTIC, Estrogen Receptor Blocker (Breast Cancer) Parenteral (IM)
  Drug: Once a month use.
  Oral/GI: <u>NAUSEA</u>, <u>vomiting</u>, <u>abdominal pain</u>, <u>constipation</u>, <u>diarrhea</u>.
  S/Cond: Not c̄ lactation. Not studied in moderate to severe ↓ hepatic func.
  99% serum pro bound, largely to lipoproteins. **Pregnancy:** Category D.
  Other: <u>ASTHENIA</u>, <u>headache</u>, <u>back</u>, <u>chest</u>, <u>pelvic</u> and/or <u>bone pain</u>,
  <u>hot flushes</u>, <u>rash</u>, <u>sweating</u>, <u>flu syndrome</u>, <u>fever</u>, <u>pharyngitis</u>, <u>edema</u>,
  <u>cough</u>, <u>dyspnea</u>, <u>dizziness</u>, <u>insomnia</u>, <u>paresthesia</u>, <u>depression</u>, <u>anxiety</u>.
  Blood/Serum: <u>Anemia</u>. < 1%- ↓ WBC. **Urinary:** <u>UTI</u>.

Fungizone	ANTIBIOTIC	See **amphotericin B p 34**
Furadantin	ANTIBIOTIC	See **nitrofurantoin p 230**
furosemide **Lasix**	DIURETIC, ANTIHYPERTENSIVE	See **Diuretics, Loop p 114**
Fuzeon	ANTIRETROVIRAL (HIV/AIDS), Fusion Inhibitor	See **enfuvirtide p 123**

gabapentin
  Neurontin[a]
  Cap- lactose,
   cornstarch
  Tab- cornstarch
  Soln- xylitol, glycerin
  Generic Tab- lactose
gabapentin encarbil
  Horizant[b]
  Tab (ER)
ANTIEPILEPTIC, POSTHERPETIC NEURALGIA TREATMENT[a]
TREATMENT OF MODERATE TO SEVERE RESTLESS LEG SYNDROME IN ADULTS[b]
  Also used as a mood stabilizer to treat Bipolar Disorder.[21][a]
  Also used to treat Neuropathy, Hot Flashes, Migraine[a]
  Drug: Take s̄ regard to food.[a] Swallow ER tab whole. Do not cut, crush,
  split or chew. Take extended release tab around 5:00 PM c̄ food[b]
  Do not cut, chew or crush extended release tab.[b] Take Mg suppl
  separately by 2 hr.
  Nutr: ↑ <u>WT</u>, ↑ <u>APPETITE</u>,[21] anorexia.[a] ↑ wt, ↑ appetite.[b]
  Oral/GI: Dental abnormalities, gingivitis, dry mouth or throat, dyspepsia,

Galise[b]
Tab- ER
  300 mg tab- polyethylene
    glycol, soy lecithin,
  600 mg tab
    polyethylene glycol

N/V, flatulence, diarrhea, constipation. **S/Cond:** Caution c̄ alcohol. Not c̄ lactation. Caution c̄ ↓ renal func. Not with severe ↓ renal func.[b]
Pregnancy: Category C.
Other: <u>Drowsiness</u>, <u>dizziness</u>, <u>fatigue</u>, <u>ataxia</u>, <u>edema</u>, abnormal gait, twitching, tremor, visual changes, asthenia, face edema, HTN, fever, pharyngitis, bronchitis, infection, joint pain.[a] <u>Somnolence/sedation</u>, <u>dizziness</u>, headache, vertigo, irritability, disorientation, lethargy, blurred vision.[b] Neuropsychiatric problems (↑ in children 3-12 yr)- emotional lability, hostility, hyperkinesia, thought disorders, amnesia, anxiety, depression, confusion. Rare- suicidal thinking & behavior. Rare- drug rash c̄ eosinophilia and systemic symptoms (DRESS).
Blood/Serum: < 1%- ↓ WBC, dyscrasias, ↑ glucose.
Urinary: False + pro c̄ Ames N-Multistix SG dipstick.
Monitor: Emergence or worsening of depression, mood changes, suicidal thoughts or behavior.

Gabitril

ANTIEPILEPTIC

See **tiagabine p 313**

galantamine
  formerly **Reminyl**
  (still Canadian name)
  Razadyne
  Tab- lactose,
   propylene glycol
  Soln- saccharin
  Razadyne ER (SR)
  Cap- sugar spheres
   (sucrose & starch)

ANTIALZHEIMER'S, Acetylcholinesterase Inhibitor
  Also used to treat vascular & mixed dementia, cognitive problems in schizophrenia[21]
  Drug: Take tab or soln BID preferably c̄ breakfast & evening meal. Take **ER** Cap once a day c̄ breakfast.
  Diet: Insure adequate fluid intake/hydration to ↓ N/V. **Nutr:** <u>Anorexia</u>, ↓ <u>wt</u>.
  Oral/GI: <u>N/V</u>, dyspepsia, abdominal pain, flatulence, <u>diarrhea</u>.
  S/Cond: Not intended for lactating mothers. Caution c̄ moderate ↓ hepatic func or ↓ renal func. Not c̄ severe ↓ hepatic func or ↓ renal func. Caution c̄ peptic ulcer, cardiac disease, asthma, COPD or seizures.
  Pregnancy: Category B. **Other:** Dizziness, syncope, bradycardia, headache, fatigue, drowsiness, tremor, depression, insomnia, rhinitis, chest pain, fever, asthenia, dehydration.
  Blood/Serum: Anemia, ↓ K. < 1%- ↑ glucose, ↑ alk phos, ↓ platelets.
  Urinary: UTI, hematuria, incontinence.

ganciclovir
Cytovene
Cap
Cytovene IV-
46 mg (2 mEq)
Na/500 mg

ANTIVIRAL, ANTI-CMV, Nucleoside Analog   Oral or Parenteral (IV)
Intravitreal Implant for CMV Retinitis only
Drug: Take oral form c̄ food (test diet was 602 cal, 46.5% fat)
to ↑ bioavailability. **Diet**: Insure adequate fluid intake/hydration.
Nutr: Anorexia, ↓ wt.
Oral/GI: Dry mouth, N/V, GI hemorrhage, abdominal pain, flatulence, <u>diarrhea</u>.
S/Cond: Not c̄ lactation. Do dental care cautiously- ↑ bleeding or
infection, ↓ healing. Caution c̄ ↓ renal func or geriatric.
Not c̄ ANC < 500 or platelets < 25,000.
Pregnancy: Category C.
Other: <u>FEVER</u>, <u>neuropathy</u>, <u>weakness</u>, chills, paresthesia, headache,
sweating, sepsis, confusion,[5] rash.
Rare- SIADH, anaphylaxis, SJS, pancreatitis, seizures.[5]
Blood/Serum: ↓ <u>WHITE BLOOD CELLS</u>, <u>ANEMIA</u>, ↓ <u>platelets</u>, ↑ <u>crea</u>, ↑ BUN,
↑ AST, ↑ ALT, ↑ alk phos, ↑ bil. < 1%- ↓ glucose, ↓ K.
Monitor: Baseline & frequent CBC c̄ diff, platelets. Renal & hepatic func.
Ophthalmologic exams when used for CMV retinitis.

Garamycin
previous brand name

ANTIBIOTIC

See **gentamicin p 156**

GasAid Maximum Strength

ANTIFLATULENT

See **simethicone p 292**

Gelusil
Chew Tab- mannitol,
sorbitol, sugar

ANTACID, ANTIFLATULENT
Sodium Free, contains simethicone

See **aluminum hydroxide &
magnesium hydroxide p 29**

Gelnique
oxybutynin

ANTIMUSCARINIC
Topical Gel

See **Bladder Control Agents p 61**

gemcitabine
Gemzar
Pwd for Inj- mannitol

ANTINEOPLASTIC, Antimetabolite (Breast, Ovarian, Lung, Pancreatic Cancer)
Parenteral only (IV)
Diet: ↑ fluid intake/hydration essential.
Nutr: <u>Anorexia</u>, ↓ <u>wt</u>.

Oral/GI: <u>Stomatitis</u>, <u>nausea/vomiting</u>, <u>diarrhea</u>, <u>constipation</u>.
S/Cond: Not c̄ lactation. Do dental care cautiously, see p 11 & 15.
Caution c̄ ↓ hepatic func or ↓ renal func.[7]
Pregnancy: Category D.
Other: <u>BONE MARROW SUPPRESSION</u>, <u>PAIN</u>, <u>FEVER</u>, <u>RASH</u>, <u>DYSPNEA</u>, <u>EDEMA</u>,
<u>HAIR LOSS</u>, <u>infection</u>, <u>fatigue</u>, <u>hemorrhage</u>, <u>paresthesia</u>, <u>bruising</u>,
<u>flu syndrome</u>, <u>hypotension</u>, headache, muscle/joint pain.
Rare- pulmonary toxicity or nephrotoxicity.
Blood/Serum: ↓ <u>WBC</u>, ↓ <u>PLATELETS</u>, <u>ANEMIA</u>, ↑ <u>ALK PHOS</u>, ↑ <u>AST</u>, ↑ <u>ALT</u>,
↑ <u>bil</u>, ↑ <u>GGT</u>,[26] ↑ <u>BUN</u>, ↑ <u>crea</u>, ↑ <u>glucose</u>, ↓ <u>Ca</u>, ↓ <u>Mg</u>.
Urinary: <u>PRO</u>. <u>HEMATURIA</u>.
Monitor: Baseline CBC c̄ diff, renal & hepatic func.
CBC c̄ diff, platelets before each dose. Periodic renal & hepatic func.

gemfibrozil
  Lopid
   Tab- starch
   Cap (Canada only)
    cornstarch

ANTIHYPERLIPIDEMIC, Fibrate   To treat ↑ TG, ↓ CHD Risk
                   (Types IIb, IV & V hyperlipidemia)
Drug: Take 1/2 hr before breakfast & supper.
Diet: ↓ fat, low sucrose, cal controlled.
Oral/GI: <u>Taste changes</u>, <u>dyspepsia</u>, <u>abdominal pain</u>, N/V, diarrhea,
constipation, flatulence. Rare- acute appendicitis.
S/Cond: Avoid alcohol to ↓ TG. Not c̄ lactation.
Caution c̄ diabetes- possible ↑ glucose.[6] 95% serum pro bound.
Caution c̄ ↓ renal func. Not c̄ ↓ hepatic func,
severe ↓ renal func or gallbladder disease.
Pregnancy: Category C.
Other: Headache, dizziness, drowsiness, blurred vision, fatigue, rash,
gallstones, cholestatic jaundice, paresthesia, muscle/joint pain,
angioedema. Rare- myopathy, rhabdomyolysis.
Blood/Serum: ↓ <u>_TG_</u>. Slightly ↓ <u>_CHOL_</u>, ↑ <u>_HDL_</u>, ↓ <u>_VLDL_</u>, ↓ <u>_LDL_</u>.
↑ AST, ↑ ALT, ↑ alk phos, ↑ bil, ↑ LDH, ↑ CPK.
Slightly ↑ glucose, ↓ K, ↓ Hb/HCT, ↓ WBC.
Monitor: CBC for first 12 mo, hepatic func, lipid profile q 3-6 mo.[6]

gemifloxacin
Factive
Tab

ANTIBIOTIC, Fluoroquinolone
Drug: Swallow whole $\bar{s}$ regard to food, $\bar{c}$ 4-8 oz fluid.
Diet: Insure liberal fluid intake/hydration. Milk/dairy product does not affect drug. Take tab at least 2 hr before or 3 hr after antacids, Mg, Fe or Zn suppl, MVI $\bar{c}$ minerals.[3]
Nutr: Minor interaction if taken $\bar{c}$ Ca suppl, not clinically significant.
Oral/GI: Taste changes, N/V, abdominal pain, diarrhea.
Rare- pseudomembranous colitis.
S/Cond: Not $\bar{c}$ lactation. Caution $\bar{c}$ ↓ renal func or seizures.
Pregnancy: Category C. **Other:** <u>Rash</u> (↑ $\bar{c}$ use > 7 days & in young female), headache, dizziness. Rare- CNS toxicity, allergic reaction, photosensitivity, SJS, TEN, anaphylaxis, tendonitis/tendon rupture, ↑ QT interval.
Blood/Serum: ↑ AST, ↑ ALT. < 1%- ↑ glucose, dyscrasias, ↑ bil, ↑ CPK.
Monitor: Renal func.

Gemzar

ANTINEOPLASTIC, Nucleoside Analog   See **gemcitabine p 154**

gentamicin
Garamycin
previous brand name
3.2 mg
Na bisulfite/mL

ANTIBIOTIC, Aminoglycoside   Parenteral (IM or IV) or Intrathecal
Diet: Insure adequate fluid intake/hydration. **Nutr:** Anorexia, ↓ wt.
Oral/GI: Stomatitis, ↑ salivation, N/V. Rare- pseudomembranous colitis.
S/Cond: Dose based on IBW. In obesity, dose based on IBW + 0.4(TBW-IBW).[12]
Not $\bar{c}$ lactation. Caution $\bar{c}$ ↓ renal func, neuromuscular disorder, geriatric, pediatric, dehydration or hypocalcemia.[6]
Pregnancy: Category D.[7]
Other: <u>Nephrotoxicity</u>, <u>ototoxicity</u>, <u>neurotoxicity</u> (dizziness, ataxia, headache, lethargy, confusion, depression). Rare- peripheral neuropathy, ↑ or ↓ BP, edema, rash, respiratory depression/paralysis, acute organic brain syndrome.
Blood/Serum: ↑ <u>BUN</u>, ↑ <u>crea</u>, ↑ <u>N</u>, ↓ Mg, ↑ AST, ↑ ALT, ↑ LDH, ↑ bil, ↑ alk phos, ↓ K, ↓ Na, ↓ Ca. Rare- anemia, dyscrasias.
Urinary: Pro, oliguria.
Monitor: Renal func, electrolytes, Ca, Mg, urinalysis.
Hearing tests.[7] Possibly drug level.

Geodon	ANTIPSYCHOTIC (Second Generation)	See **ziprasidone HCl p 350**
Gilenya	TREATMENT OF RELAPSING FORMS OF MULTIPLE SCLEROSIS, Sphingosine 1-phosphate receptor modulator	See **fingolimod p 143**
Gleevec/Glivec	ANTINEOPLASTIC (Leukemia)	See **imatinib p 172**
Gliadel Wafer	ANTINEOPLASTIC, Alkylating Agent	See **carmustine p 74**
glimepiride **Amaryl**	ORAL HYPOGLYCEMIC	See **sulfonylureas p 299**
glipizide **Glucotrol/Glucotrol XL**	ORAL HYPOGLYCEMIC	See **sulfonylureas p 299**
Glucophage/ **Glucophage XR**	ANTIHYPERGLYCEMIC AGENT, Biguanide See **metformin p 210**	

glucosamine
Many Generic forms
Tab or liquid
Dona
Pwd-
crystalline sulfate form
150 mg (6.53 mEq) Na/pkt,
aspartame, sorbitol,
10 cal

NATURAL PRODUCT (Not FDA approved)
    ANTIARTHRITIC (Osteoarthritis)   Oral or Parenteral (not in US)
    Drug: Often taken in combination $\bar{c}$ **chondroitin**, see p 83.
    Dissolve pwd in a glass of water or juice.
    Oral/GI: Nausea, dyspepsia, diarrhea, constipation.
    S/Cond: Caution $\bar{c}$ diabetes- may theoretically ↑ insulin resistance,
but has not caused insulin resistance in human studies.[4]
    Caution $\bar{c}$ shellfish allergy. Not $\bar{c}$ peptic ulcer.[4]
    Pregnancy: Not studied. Avoid use. **Other:** Drowsiness, headache, rash.
    Blood/Serum: Possibly ↑ glucose in diabetics, ↑ insulin.

Glucotrol/Glucotrol XL glipizide	ORAL HYPOGLYCEMIC	See **sulfonylureas p 299**
Glucovance Tab	ANTIHYPERGLYCEMIC AGENT (**metformin**) & ORAL HYPOGLYCEMIC (**glyburide**) **Pregnancy:** Category B. See **metformin p 210** & See **sulfonylureas p 299**	

Glumetza   ANTIHYPERGLYCEMIC AGENT, Biguanide   See **metformin p 210**

glyburide   ORAL HYPOGLYCEMIC   See **sulfonylureas p 299**
  DiaBeta
  Glynase PresTab

Glycolax   LAXATIVE, Osmotic   See **polyethylene glycol p 259**

Glyset   ANTIDIABETIC AGENT for TYPE 2 diabetes   See **miglitol p 217**

golimumab   ANTIARTHRITIC (Rheumatoid c̄ **methotrexate**; Psoriatic Arthritis c̄ or s̄
  Simponi   **methotrexate**), ANKYLOSING SPONDYLITIS TREATMENT
  L-histidine 0.44 mg,   TNF Inhibitor   Parenteral (SC)
  sorbitol 20.5 mg
         Oral/GI: Oral herpes.
         S/Cond: Not c̄ lactation. Caution c̄ CHF, immune or demyelinating
         disorder, cytopenias. Caution c̄ geriatric- ↑ infection risk.
         Pregnancy: Category B.
         Other: Injection site reaction, URTI, nasopharyngitis, HTN, bronchitis,
         dizziness, sinusitis, influenza, rhinitis, paresthesia, fever, reactivation of
         HBV, opportunistic infections.
         Rare- malignancies (eg lymphoma), serious infection (can be fatal).
         Blood/Serum: ↑ ALT, ↑ AST, sepsis.
         Monitor: For active TB prior to & during treatment.
         For S/S of fungal, viral, bacterial infections.

goserelin   ENDOMETRIOSIS TREATMENT, ANTINEOPLASTIC, Hormone Implant
  Zoladex   (Prostate or Breast Cancer)   See listing for **leuprolide p 190**

granisetron   ANTIEMETIC, ANTINAUSEANT   Oral or Parenteral (IV)
  Kytril   (Post Operative - IV only or c̄ Chemotherapy/Radiation- IV or oral)
  Tab- lactose,   serotonin 5HT$_3$ receptor antagonist
  Na starch glycolate   **Oral/GI:** Taste disorder, dyspepsia, abdominal pain, <u>constipation</u>, diarrhea.
  IV- Single dose vial-   **S/Cond:** Caution c̄ lactation.
  preservative free   **Pregnancy:** Category B.

Multi-dose vial- benzyl alcohol 10 mg/mL	**Other:** <u>Headache</u>, <u>asthenia</u>, <u>dizziness</u>, drowsiness, <u>insomnia</u>, <u>fever</u>, anxiety, transient ↓ or ↑ BP, allergic reaction.
Sancuso- patch	**Blood/Serum:** Transient ↑ AST, ↑ ALT.

guaifenesin   EXPECTORANT

Robitussin Chest Congestion syrup- corn syrup, glucose, saccharin Na, propylene glycol	**Drug:** Take c̄ 8 oz water. Swallow SR forms whole- do not break, crush or chew. Put granules on tongue & swallow- do not chew.
	Oral/GI: N/V, GI distress, diarrhea.
	S/Cond: Not c̄ lactation. Not c̄ persistent cough.
	Syrup precipitates tube feedings.[8] **Pregnancy:** Category C.
	Other: Headache, dizziness, rash. **Urinary:** False + VMA.

Mucinex (SR) Tab- Na starch glycolate
Mucinex Liquid- dextrose, propylene glycol, saccharin Na, sucralose, xanthan gum.   3 mg Na/5 mL
mini-melt grape granules- aspartame (phenylalanine 0.6 mg/pkt), Mg stearate (6 mg Mg), sorbitol. 2 mg Na/pkt
mini-melt bubble gum granules- aspartame (phenylalanine 1.0 mg/pkt), Mg stearate (10 mg Mg), sorbitol.
   3 mg Na/pkt

guanfacine   ANTIHYPERTENSIVE   Also as ADHD, tics[17] Treatment

Tenex Tab- lactose	**Drug:** Take HS s̄ regard to food.
	Diet: for HTN- ↓ Na, ↓ cal may be recommended.
	Avoid natural licorice, see p 374. Caution c̄ SJW, see p 286.
Studies done in adults	Caution c̄ grapefruit/related citrus, see p 390.
	Insure adequate fluid intake/hydration.
	Oral/GI: <u>D</u><u>RY</u> <u>MOUTH</u>, taste changes, dysphagia, nausea, <u>constipation</u>.
	S/Cond: Caution c̄ alcohol. Caution c̄ lactation.
	Caution c̄ severe ↓ renal func or severe ↓ hepatic func.
	Caution c̄ CV disease, recent MI, severe CHF.
	↑ risk of dental problems, see p 11 & 15.
	Pregnancy: Category B.
	Other: ↓ *BP* c̄ possible hypotension, sedation, <u>drowsiness</u>, <u>fatigue</u>, dizziness, headache, insomnia, asthenia, depression, bradycardia, palpitations.
	Monitor: BP prior to use & periodically

G

guanfacine
Intuniv
SR Tab- lactose

**Studies done
in children/adolescents**

ADHD TREATMENT for children ≥ 6 yr old.
 Drug: Take once daily. Swallow whole c̄ water, milk or other liquid.
Do not break, crush or chew tab. Do not take c̄ high fat meal- will
↑ exposure to drug.
 Diet: Insure adequate fluid intake/hydration. Caution c̄ SJW, see p 286.
Caution c̄ grapefruit/related citrus, see p 390. **Nutr:** ↑ <u>weight</u>, ↑ appetite.
 Oral/GI: Dyspepsia, nausea, <u>vomiting</u>, dry mouth, constipation,
abdominal pain.
 S/Cond: Avoid alcohol. Caution c̄ lactation. Caution c̄ moderate to
severe ↑ renal func. Caution c̄ CV disease.
 ↑ risk of dental problems, see p 11 & 15.
 Pregnancy: Category B.
 Other: <u>SOMNOLENCE</u>, <u>headache</u>, <u>fatigue</u>, lethargy, dizziness, irritability,
insomnia, hypotension, bradycardia, syncope.
 Blood/Serum: ↑ ALT. **Urinary:** ↑ frequency, enuresis
 Monitor: BP, HR prior to use & peridically.

Halcion
 triazolam

SLEEP AID   See **Benzodiazepines p 54**

haloperidol
 Haldol
 (previous brand name)
 Tab- cornstarch
 Haldol Decanoate
 Injection long acting
 sesame oil,
 1.2% benzyl alcohol
 Generic **haloperidol**
 Conc- lactic acid
 Haldol Lactate
 Injection rapid acting
 (also used IV)

ANTIPSYCHOTIC, TOURETTE'S TREATMENT, Butyrophenone
 To Treat HYPERACTIVITY or BEHAVIORAL PROBLEMS IN CHILDREN
          Oral or Parenteral (IM)
 Drug: Take c̄ food or milk to ↓ GI distress.
Do not mix conc c̄ coffee or tea- drug may precipitate.[13] Dilute conc
c̄ ≥ 60 ml milk, pudding, carbonated drinks,[23] acidic beverage or water.[13]
 Nutr: ↑ <u>appetite</u>, ↑ wt, ↓ wt, anorexia.
 Oral/GI: <u>DRY MOUTH</u>, ↑ salivation, dyspepsia, N/V, <u>constipation</u>, diarrhea.
 S/Cond: Avoid alcohol. Not c̄ lactation. ↑ risk of dental problems, see p 11 & 15.
92% serum pro bound. Caution c̄ HTN, ↓ hepatic func, cardiac disease or
seizures.[17] Caution c̄ geriatric. Not c̄ Parkinson's disease.[17]
 Pregnancy: Category C.
 Other: <u>EXTRAPYRAMIDAL SYMPTOMS (EPS)</u>, <u>DROWSINESS</u>, <u>restlessness</u>, <u>blurred</u>

<u>vision</u>, galactorrhea, gynecomastia, amenorrhea, HTN or hypotension,
dizziness, syncope, headache, photosensitivity, ↑ heat/cold sensitivity,
tachycardia, seizures, arrhythmias, rash, wheezing, dyspnea, ↑ salivation.
<u>Tardive dyskinesia</u> c̄ LT use. Rare- NMS, ↑ QT interval,
torsades de pointes (↑ risk c̄ IV use), jaundice.
↑ mortality in geriatrics c̄ dementia related psychosis.
Blood/Serum: ↑ <u>prolactin</u>, ↑ or ↓ WBC, anemia, ↑ or ↓ glucose, ↓ Na.
Urinary: Retention, hesitancy.
Monitor: Possibly CBC c̄ diff, hepatic function c̄ LT use.[13]

HCTZ ANTIHYPERTENSIVE, DIURETIC, Thiazide

See **hydrochlorothiazide p 166**

Hectorol HYPERPARATHYROIDISM TREATMENT in renal dialysis
doxercalciferol metabolized to $1,25\text{-}(OH)_2D_2$
Cap- fractionated TG of coconut oil, alcohol See listing for **calcitriol p 68**

heparin ANTICOAGULANT Parenteral only (IV or SC)
Heparin **Oral/GI:** N/V, <u>abdominal pain</u>, <u>GI bleeding</u>, <u>constipation</u>, <u>black tarry stools</u>.
< 10 mg benzyl **S/Cond:** Caution c̄ diabetes & ESRD- hyperkalemia.[7]
alcohol/mL, Do dental care cautiously- ↑ bleeding.
7 mg Na/2 mL vial Caution c̄ ↓ hepatic or severe ↓ renal func. Caution c̄ geriatric.
Pregnancy: Category C.
Other: <u>BLEEDING</u>, <u>hemorrhage</u>, <u>dizziness</u>, <u>headache</u>, <u>bruising</u>,
hypersensitivity reaction c̄ chills, fever, hives,
skin & subcutaneous necrosis. Osteoporosis, bone & muscle pain,
hair loss c̄ LT use (> 6 mo).[13]
Blood/Serum: ↓ <u>PLATELETS</u> (may be delayed 7-12 days)[7], ↑ <u>AST</u>, ↑ <u>ALT</u>,
↑ <u>PT/INR</u>, ↑ K, ↓ TG, ↑ FFA, ↓ chol, ↓ T_4.
Urinary: Hematuria.[26]
Monitor: Baseline & periodic APTT, platelet count, CBC.
Fecal occult blood, K.

Hepsera CHRONIC HEPATITIS B TREATMENT, NRTI See **adefovir p 24**

Heptovir (Canada)	ANTIRETROVIRAL (HIV/AIDS), NRTI	See **lamivudine p 187**
Herceptin	ANTINEOPLASTIC, Monoclonal Antibody	See **trastuzumab p 320**
Hexadrol dexamethasone	CORTICOSTEROID IV- Na bisulfite, benzyl alcohol	See **corticosteroids p 94**

Histamine H_2 Receptor Antagonists

ANTIULCER including H. pylori, ANTIGERD, ANTISECRETORY   Oral or Parenteral (IM or IV)

Drug: Take c̄ a glass of water s̄ regard to meals, HS if once a day. Dissolve **Zantac Efferdose** tab in 6-8 oz water- do not swallow whole, dissolve on tongue or chew.

Mix **Pepcid** susp pwd c̄ water as directed just before use.

Diet: Bland diet may be recommended. Take drug at least 2 hr before or after Fe suppl.[3]

Take Mg suppl or Al/Mg antacids separately by at least 2 hr. Limit caffeine/xanthine, see p 379.

Nutr: ↓ Fe[3] & Vit B_{12} abs.[74] Mg or Al/Mg antacids ↓ drug abs.

Oral/GI: ↓ *GASTRIC ACID SECRETIONS*, ↑ *GASTRIC pH*, N/V, diarrhea, constipation.

S/Cond: Avoid alcohol. Not c̄ lactation. Caution c̄ ↓ hepatic func or ↓ renal func, COPD, asthma. Avoid or limit smoking. Liquid **cimetidine** precipitates tube feeding.[8]

Pregnancy: Category B.

Other: Drowsiness, dizziness, headache (severe c̄ IV), confusion, hallucinations, rash, bruising. Rare- hepatitis, jaundice, pneumonia.[44] **Cimetidine**- gynecomastia c̄ use > 1 mo.

Cimetidine & **ranitidine**- rare- pancreatitis.

Blood/Serum: ↑ AST, ↑ ALT, ↑ alk phos. ↓ Fe, [9b]↓ Vit B_{12} c̄ LT use.[11]

Cimetidine- ↑ prolactin after IV bolus.

Rare- ↓ WBC, other dyscrasias. **Cimetidine** & **ranitidine** only- ↑ crea.

Urinary: Ranitidine only- false + pro c̄ Multistix. **Nizatidine**- false + urobilinogen test.

Monitor: Hepatic func, Vit B_{12} c̄ LT use.

cimetidine
Tagamet
Tab- Na starch glycolate
Generic Soln-
 2.8% alcohol,
 sorbitol,
 saccharin
Tagamet HB (OTC)
Tab- Na starch glycolate,
 cornstarch
Generic Parenteral
 may contain
 benzyl alcohol

famotidine
Pepcid
Tab- cornstarch
Susp pwd- sucrose, xanthan gum
Pepcid AC (OTC)
Tab- cornstarch
GelCap- benzyl alcohol,
 castor oil, cornstarch,
 propylene glycol
Maximum Strength Pepcid AC
Tab- starch
Pepcid Preservative free IV

nizatidine
 (oral only)
Axid
Cap- starch
Soln- glycerin,
 saccharin Na,
 sucrose
Axid AR (OTC)
Tab- starch,
 cornstarch,
 propylene glycol

ranitidine
Zantac Tab
Syrup- 7.5% alcohol,
 saccharin Na, sorbitol
Efferdose 25 Tab
 aspartame = 2.81 mg
 phenylalanine
 31 mg (1.33 mEq) Na
Zantac 75 or 150 (OTC)
Tab Na & sugar free

HMG-CoA Reductase Inhibitors (statins)   ANTIHYPERLIPIDEMIC (to ↓ total & LDL chol [a] or TG [b])
TO PREVENT [c] OR ↓ RISK [d] OF CARDIOVASCULAR EVENTS, TO SLOW PROGRESSION OF ATHEROSCLEROSIS[e]
Drug: atorvastatin or **rosuvastatin**- take s̄ regard to food or time of day. **lovastatin**- take c̄ meals to ↑ abs.
Take single dose c̄ last meal of the day.
fluvastatin, **pitavastatin**, **pravastatin** or **simvastatin**- Take s̄ regard to food. Take single dose HS. Swallow SR form whole.
Diet: ↓ fat, ↓ chol (↓ cal if needed). **atorvastatin**- caution c̄ grapefruit/related citrus, **lovastatin** or
simvastatin- avoid grapefruit/related citrus, see p 390 & avoid **SJW**, see p 286. **fluvastatin**, **pitavastatin**,
pravastatin or **rosuvastatin**- no or minor interaction c̄ grapefruit/related citrus. Not c̄ high dose niacin-
possible myopathy. Separate fiber, pectin or oat bran from drug by several hr- ↓ abs reported c̄ **lovastatin**.[33]
Avoid red yeast- contains **lovastatin**.[4]
Oral/GI: Nausea, dyspepsia, abdominal pain, constipation, diarrhea, flatulence.
S/Cond: Avoid substantial alcohol. Not c̄ lactation. **rosuvastatin** only- ↓ starting dose for Asian pts.
95-99% serum pro bound, except **pravastatin** (50%), **rosuvastatin** (88%). Not c̄ active hepatic disease or ↑ ALT/AST.
Caution c̄ ↓ renal func c̄ **lovastatin**, **pitavastatin**, **pravastatin**, **simvastatin** or **rosuvastatin**.[1]
Pregnancy: Category X.
Other: Myopathy, back pain, weakness, headache, rash, dizziness, chest pain, insomnia, bronchitis,
↓ <u>risk</u> of <u>fracture</u> due to ↓ bone resorption.[79, 79a] Edema (**atorvastatin** only).
Rare- rhabdomyolysis, neuropathy c̄ LT use.[1]
Blood/Serum: ↓ <u>*CHOL*</u>, ↓ <u>*TRIGLYCERIDES*</u>, ↓ <u>*LDL*</u>, ↓ <u>*VLDL*</u>, ↓ <u>*apoB*</u>, ↑ <u>*HDL*</u>, ↓ <u>*CRP*</u>, ↑ ALT, ↑ AST, ↑ alk phos.
Transient ↑ CPK. ↓ Coenzyme Q10.[54] Rare- dyscrasias, ↑ myoglobin. **Urinary:** Alb, hematuria.
Monitor: Baseline hepatic func, then at 6 (**lovastatin** only) & 12 wks after first use or after ↑ dose, then
periodically (eg semi-annually). Chol, lipid panel. Possibly Coenzyme Q10, CPK.

atorvastatin	**Lipitor** [a b d]	Tab- lactose, 13.6 mg Ca/10 mg **atorvastatin**	
fluvastatin	**Lescol** [a c e]	Cap- cornstarch, benzyl alcohol	**Lescol XL** [a c] (SR) Tab
lovastatin	**Mevacor** [a c d e]	Tab- lactose, starch	
	Altoprev [a c d] (SR)Tab- confectioner's sugar (contains cornstarch), propylene glycol		
pitavastatin	**Livalo** [a b]	Tab- lactose	
pravastatin	**Pravachol** [a b c d]	Tab-lactose	
rosuvastatin	**Crestor** [a b e]	Tab- lactose	
simvastatin	**Zocor** [a c d]	Tab- lactose, starch	

Horizant   TREATMENT OF MODERATE TO SEVERE RESTLESS LEG SYNDROME IN ADULTS
See **gabapentin** p 152

Hormone Therapy (HT)   Estrogen or Estrogen plus Progesterone
              MENOPAUSAL SYMPTOM TREATMENT, OSTEOPOROSIS PREVENTION

Drug: Take $\bar{c}$ food at same time each day to prevent nausea.[13]

Diet: ↑ food high in Ca, Vit D, Mg, Fol, Pyr. May need Ca/Vit D suppl. Vit C suppl > 1 g/day ↑ estrogen serum levels- possible toxicity.[9b] Caution $\bar{c}$ grapefruit/related citrus, see p 390.[136]
Limit caffeine- estrogen ↓ caffeine metabolism.[93]

Nutr: ↑ or ↓ wt, appetite changes, ↓ Ca bone loss. ↑ Ca abs.

Oral/GI: N/V, bloating, cramps, diarrhea.

S/Cond: Limit alcohol. Not $\bar{c}$ lactation. Caution $\bar{c}$ diabetes- may affect glucose tolerance.
Caution $\bar{c}$ ↓ hepatic func, ↓ renal func, cardiac disease, asthma, migraine, hormone dependent malignancy.
For ST use only $\bar{c}$ lowest effective dose. Do not use to ↓ risk of cardiac events.[42]

Pregnancy: Category X.

Other: ↓ *BONE RESORPTION*, edema, ↑ or ↓ BP, breast tenderness, vaginitis/BLEEDING, dizziness, headache, migraine, rash, jaundice, visual disturbances, gallbladder disease, thromboembolism, involuntary movements, paresthesia, back pain, nervousness, depression, hair loss. **Drospirenone**- less edema, ↓ BP. Rare- but significant ↑ risk of gallbladder disease, MI, CVA, endometrial or breast cancer, dementia.

Blood/Serum: ↑ TG, ↑ HDL, ↓ LDL, ↓ Fol, ↓ Mg, ↑ Ca, ↑ or ↓ glucose, ↑ T_4, ↑ T_3, ↓ Pyr, ↑ platelets, ↑ corticosteroids. Rare- abnormal thyroid func tests. **Drospirenone**- ↑ K.

Urinary: ↑ incontinence.[1]

Monitor: BP, hepatic func, lipid panel, TSH, bone density (if used to prevent osteoporosis).

Estrogen Therapy

Alora- transdermal patch
Cenestin- Tab- lactose, starch
Climara- Transdermal patch
Divigel- Topical gel
Elestrin- Topical gel
Enjuvia- Tab- lactose
Estrace- Tab- lactose, cornstarch, tartrazine in 2 mg Tab
Estraderm- transdermal patch
Estradiol Oral- Tab
Estrasorb Topical- soybean oil, alcohol

Estring- vaginal insert
Estrogel Topical- alcohol
Estropipate Tab
Evamist- Transdermal Spray
Femring- Vaginal Ring
Femtrace Tab- lactose
Menostar- transdermal patch
Ogen- Tab- lactose, cornstarch
Premarin- Tab- lactose, sucrose
Vivelle or Vivelle DOT- transdermal patch

Estrogen & Progesterone Therapy

Activella- Tab- lactose, cornstarch
Angeliq - estradiol & **drospirenone** Tab- lactose, cornstarch
Climara Pro- transdermal patch
Combipatch- transdermal patch
Femhrt- Tab- lactose, cornstarch
Premphase- Tabs- lactose, sucrose (2 Tabs) **(Premarin** Tab- days 1-14 & **Premarin + medroxyprogesterone acetate**- Tab- days 15-28)
Prempro- Tab-lactose, sucrose (single Tab)

| **Humalog**
insulin lispro | ANTIDIABETIC, HYPOGLYCEMIC | See **insulin p 175** |

| **Humira** | ANTIARTHRITIC (Rheumatoid Arthritis) | See **adalimumab p 24** |

| **Humulin** | ANTIDIABETIC, HYPOGLYCEMIC | See **insulin p 175** |

hydralazine
Apresoline (Canada)
10 mg Tab- cornstarch,
 mannitol
25 & 50 mg Tabs-
 cornstarch, gelatin,
 lactose, sucrose

ANTIHYPERTENSIVE, CHF Treatment, Vasodilator Oral or Parenteral (IM or IV)
Drug: Take oral form consistently $\bar{c}$ or $\bar{s}$ food. Food ↑ bioavailability.
Diet: ↓ Na, ↓ cal may be recommended. Avoid natural licorice, see p 374.
Pyr suppl (100-200 mg) may correct drug-induced peripheral neuropathy.[13]
Nutr: <u>Anorexia</u>, ↓ or ↑ wt, ↑ thirst.
Interferes $\bar{c}$ Pyr metabolism- possible Pyr def.
Oral/GI: Dry mouth,[26] unpleasant taste,[26] <u>N/V</u>, GI distress,
<u>diarrhea</u>, constipation.
S/Cond: Limit alcohol. Caution $\bar{c}$ lactation.
May cause lupus-like syndrome. 90% serum pro bound.[26]
Caution $\bar{c}$ severe ↓ renal func or geriatric. Not $\bar{c}$ CAD.[7]
Caution $\bar{c}$ pulmonary HTN. Caution $\bar{c}$ slow acetylators- ↑ drug effects.
Pregnancy: Category C. Drug of choice in eclampsia.[26]
Other: ↓ <u>*BP*</u> $\bar{c}$ possible hypotension, <u>edema</u>, <u>headache</u>, <u>tachycardia</u>,
<u>palpitations</u>, <u>angina</u>, dizziness, tremor, rash, dyspnea.
Rare- hepatotoxicity, peripheral neuropathy, lupus-like syndrome.
Blood/Serum: Dyscrasias, + <u>ANA</u>, + Coombs' test.[13]
Urinary: ↑ Pyr, difficult urination.
Monitor: BP, ANA. CBC $\bar{c}$ LT use.[6]

| **Hydrea** | ANTINEOPLASTIC, Antimetabolite | See **hydroxyurea p 168** |

hydrochlorothiazide
 (HCTZ)
Microzide
Cap- lactose,
 cornstarch,
 12.5 mg HCTZ

ANTIHYPERTENSIVE, DIURETIC, Thiazide (K-depleting)
Drug: Take in AM $\bar{c}$ food or milk.
Diet: May need ↓ Na, ↓ cal, ↑ K, ↑ Mg (or K or Mg suppl).
Discontinue Na restriction if hyponatremia occurs.
Avoid natural licorice, see p 374.
Caution $\bar{c}$ Ca &/or Vit D suppl[3]- risk of hypercalcemia.

Nutr: Anorexia, ↑ thirst.
Oral/GI: Dry mouth, N/V, GI irritation, diarrhea, constipation.
S/Cond: Limit alcohol. Not c̄ lactation. Caution c̄ diabetes- ↑ glucose.
Caution c̄ ↓ hepatic func[13] or severe ↓ renal func. Not c̄ anuria.[10]
Caution c̄ geriatric. Not c̄ sulfonamide allergy.
Pregnancy: Category B. Should be used only if clearly needed.
Other: ↓ _BLOOD PRESSURE_ c̄ possible hypotension, dizziness, weakness,
photosensitivity. Rare- gout, pancreatitis, jaundice, hyponatremia.
Blood/Serum: ↓ SODIUM, ↓ CHLORIDE, ↓ POTASSIUM, ↓ Mg, ↓ Zn,
↑ GLUCOSE,[18] ↑ Ca, dyscrasias, ↑ uric acid, ↑ bil, ↑ chol, ↑ LDL, ↑ VLDL,
↑ TG, ↑ BUN, ↑ crea. DC HCTZ before tests of parathyroid func.[10]
Urinary: ↑ _WATER_, ↑ SODIUM, ↑ CHLORIDE, ↑ POTASSIUM, ↑ Mg, ↑ Zn, ↓ Ca,
glucose, ↓ uric acid, ↑ bicarb.
Monitor: Electrolytes, Mg, Ca, renal func, uric acid, BP, glucose.

hydrocodone	ANALGESIC, ANTITUSSIVE, Narcotic, Opioid	See listing for **codeine p 91**
hydrocortisone	CORTICOSTEROID	See **corticosteroids p 94**
hydromorphone	ANALGESIC, ANTITUSSIVE, Narcotic, Opioid	See listing for **morphine p 221**

hydromorphone
Dilaudid
Tab- lactose, Liquid- sucrose
8 mg Tab & Oral liquid- Na bisulfite
Exalgo
Tab ER- lactose,   **Drug:** Do not crush, cut or chew ER tab.
polyethylene glycol

Oral, Parenteral (IM or SC) or
Suppository

hydroxycobalamin	B-COMPLEX VITAMIN, ANTIANEMIC	See **vitamin B₁₂ p 338**

hydroxychloroquine
  Plaquenil
  Tab- starch

ANTIMALARIAL, ANTIARTHRITIC (rheumatoid), LUPUS TREATMENT
  Drug: Take c̄ meals or milk to ↓ GI distress.
  May crush & mix c̄ 1 tsp jam, jelly or jello.
  Nutr: Anorexia, ↓ wt.
  Oral/GI: Blue-black mouth, N/V, abdominal cramps, diarrhea.
  S/Cond: Caution c̄ lactation. Caution c̄ obesity- dose by IBW.
  Caution c̄ G6PD def- risk of hemolytic anemia.
  Not for LT use in children. Caution c̄ ↓ hepatic func or ↓ renal func.[13]
  Pregnancy: Category C.[23] Not recommended c̄ pregnancy except to treat
  malaria or hepatic amebiasis.[13]
  Other: Headache, itching (↑ in BLACK PATIENTS),[6] dizziness, visual changes,
  corneal deposits, fatigue, muscle weakness/myopathy, ataxia,
  emotional or psychological changes, rash, blue-black skin & nails,
  photosensitivity, hair loss/bleaching. Rare- SJS, seizures, retinopathy.
  Blood/Serum: Dyscrasias.
  Monitor: CBC, platelets, ophthalmologic exams. Muscle strength c̄ LT use.[6]

hydroxyurea
  Droxia[b]
  Cap- lactose
  Hydrea[a]
  Cap- lactose
  Hydroxyurea[a]
  Cap- lactose

ANTINEOPLASTIC,[a] PROPHYLAXIS OF SICKLE CELL CRISIS[b]
  Antimetabolite (Ovarian or Squamous Cell Cancer, Melanoma, Leukemia)
  Also used to treat Psoriasis, Thrombocythemia or as Antiretroviral c̄ **didanosine**
  Drug: ↑ fluids recommended. If patient cannot swallow,
  may mix contents of cap c̄ water & drink immediately.
  Pwd must not touch skin or mucous membranes.
  Nutr: Anorexia.
  Oral/GI: Stomatitis, N/V, diarrhea, constipation.
  S/Cond: Not c̄ lactation. Not c̄ severe bone marrow suppression.
  Correct anemia before use. Caution c̄ geriatrics.
  Caution c̄ ↓ renal func. Do dental care cautiously, see p 11 & 15.
  Caution c̄ obesity- dose based on actual wt or IBW, whichever is less.
  Pregnancy: Category D.
  Other: Bone marrow suppression, drowsiness, hair loss, blackening of nails,
  rash, blisters, fever/chills. Rare- neurological disturbances,
  acute pulmonary reaction, renal impairment, gangrene.

Blood/Serum: ↓ <u>WBC</u>, <u>anemia</u>, ↓ platelets, ↑ BUN, ↑ crea, ↑ uric acid.
Rare- ↑ hepatic enzymes. **Urinary:** Rare- dysuria.
Monitor: Baseline & periodic CBC c̄ diff & platelets (q 2wk).
Renal & hepatic func.

hydroxyzine   ANTIHISTAMINE, ANTIANXIETY, ANTINAUSEANT (IM)
  Atarax (brand name in Canada)   Oral or Parenteral (IM)
  Tabs- lactose,   **Drug:** May crush tab or open cap & mix c̄ food or fluid.
   sucrose, gelatin   **Oral/GI:** <u>Dry</u> <u>mouth</u>, bitter taste, nausea.
  Syrup- 0.5% alcohol,   **S/Cond:** Avoid alcohol. Not c̄ lactation.
   sucrose, peppermint oil   ↑ risk of dental problems, see p 11 & 15.
  Cap- soybean oil, lecithin   Caution c̄ ↓ renal func.[58] Caution c̄ geriatric.[84] Caution c̄ asthma or COPD.
  Parenteral- 0.9% benzyl alcohol **Pregnancy:** Category C. Contraindicated in first trimester.
  Vistaril   **Other:** <u>DROWSINESS</u>, ataxia, dizziness, headache, weakness, wheezing,
  Cap- sucrose, starch   flushing, agitation. Rare- tremor, seizures, dyspnea.
  Oral Susp- sorbitol

hyoscyamine   ANTISPASMODIC, ANTICHOLINERGIC   Oral or Parenteral (SC, IM, IV)
  Levbid (SR) generic   See listing for **Bladder Control Agents p 61**
  Tab- lactose   Also used in IBS, colitis, peptic ulcer, Parkinsons, rhinitis.
  Levsin generic   Drops or Elixir also used as infant colic treatment.
  Tab- sugar, starch,   **Diet:** Antacids, Ca or Mg suppl may ↓ drug abs.
   lactose   Take drug before meals, antacids or suppl after meals.
  Elixir- 20% alcohol,   **Pregnancy:** Category C.
   sorbitol, sucrose
  Drops- 5% alcohol, sorbitol, sucrose
  Parenteral 10 mL Vial- 1.5% benzyl alcohol, 0.1% Na metabilsulfite[7]
  Levsin/SL generic sublingual/chew Tab- mannitol, lactose, starch

Hytrin   ANTIHYPERTENSIVE, BPH TREATMENT
  terazosin   See **Alpha₁ Adrenergic Blockers p 28**

Hyzaar   ANTIHYPERTENSIVE, DIURETIC   See **Angiotensin II Receptor Antagonists p 38**
  Tab- lactose, starch   Combination drug **losartan** & **hydrochlorthiazide** See **hydrochlorothiazide p 166**

H

ibandronate **Boniva/Boniva Injection**	OSTEOPOROSIS TREATMENT	See **Bisphosphonates, Oral p 59** See **Bisphosphonates, Parenteral p 60**

ibuprofen*

  Advil Tab
  Advil LiquiGels Cap
  Caldolor (IV)
  Pwd
  Children's Advil &
  Pediatric Drops
  Motrin Tab,
  Susp
  Infants' Oral drops

ANTIARTHRITIC, ANALGESIC, NSAID   Oral & Parenteral (IV)

Drug: Take c̄ food or milk to ↓ GI irritation.
Diet: Caution c̄ GI irritants eg K suppl (↑ risk of GI irritation).[13]
Limit caffeine to ↓ GI effects. Avoid or limit natural products which
affect coagulation (eg garlic, ginkgo, ginseng, ginger or horse chestnut).
Nutr: ↓ appetite.
Oral/GI: N/V, dyspepsia, abdominal pain, bloating, constipation, diarrhea,
colitis, flatulence, GI ulcers & bleeding (may be sudden & serious).
S/Cond: Avoid alcohol. Not detected in breast milk. ≥ 99% serum pro bound.
Hypoalbuminemia (< 3 g/dL)- may ↑ drug effects.
Not c̄ aspirin allergy. Caution c̄ HTN, CHF or edema. Caution c̄ geriatric.
Caution c̄ ↓ hepatic func or ↓ renal func. Not c̄ gastritis/ulcer.
Pregnancy: Category C, not recommended in pregnancy.
Category D in 3rd trimester due to ↑ risk to fetus & mother, including death.
Other: Dizziness, rash, edema, headache, tinnitus, depression,
nervousness, hypertension or hypotension.
Rare- SJS, acute renal failure, ↓ CrCl, aseptic meningitis.
Risk of CV problems, eg HTN, CHF, MI, CVA.
Blood/Serum: ↑ AST, ↑ ALT, ↑ alk phos, ↓ Hb (≥ 20% c̄ LT high dose),
↓ HCT, ↑ K, ↑ BUN, ↑ crea, ↓ CrCl, ↓ alb, ↓ glucose,
↓ platelet aggregation. Rare- dyscrasias, ↑ PT/INR.
Monitor: CBC, hepatic & renal func c̄ LT use.

*Check label for alcohol, aspartame, cornstarch, saccharin, sorbitol, starch, sucrose, sulfites or tartrazine

idarubicin HCl
  Idamycin PFS
  Preservative Free
	ANTINEOPLASTIC, Anthracycline Antibiotic (Leukemia) Parenteral only (IV)
	Analog of **daunorubicin**
		See listing for **doxorubicin p 117**

iloperidone
   Fanapt
    Tab- lactose

ANTIPSYCHOTIC (Second Generation)
   Drug: Take s̄ regard to food.
   Diet: Not c̄ SJW, see p 286.
   Insure adequate fluid intake/hydration.
   Nutr: ↑ <u>weight</u>. ↓ weight.
   Oral/GI: <u>Dry</u> <u>mouth</u>, nausea, diarrhea, abdominal discomfort.
   S/Cond: Not c̄ alcohol. Not c̄ lactation. Not c̄ ↓ hepatic func.
   Not c̄ dementia related psychosis. 95% serum pro bound.
   Caution c̄ Hx of seizures. Caution c̄ CYP2D6 poor metabolizers.
   Caution c̄ CV or cerebrovascular disease.
   Pregnancy: Category C.
   Other: ↑ <u>QT</u> INTERVAL, <u>dizziness</u>, <u>drowsiness</u>, <u>tachycardia</u>, <u>nasal congestion</u>, <u>orthostatic</u> <u>hypotension</u>, tremor, palpitations, dyspnea, fatigue, lethargy, joint/muscle pain, muscle spasms, URTI, restlessness, aggression, delusion, erectile dysfunction.
   Rare- gynecomastia, galactorrhea.
   ↑ mortality in geriatrics c̄ dementia-related psychosis.
   Blood/Serum: ↑ <u>prolactin</u>, ↓ WBC. < 1%- ↓ K.
   Urinary: Incontinence.
   Monitor: Prior to use- ECG, Mg, K. Possibly CYP2D6 genetic testing.
   Baseline FBS, HbA1$_c$ & lipids then at 12 wk, then at least annually.

imatinib
Gleevec/Glivec
Tab
Cap (Canada)

ANTINEOPLASTIC (Leukemia, GI Stromal Tumor, Systemic Mastocytosis)
Protein-Tyrosine Kinase Inhibitor
Drug: Take c̄ food & a large glass of water to ↓ GI irritation.
Diet: Avoid SJW, see p 286.
Nutr: <u>Anorexia</u>, ↑ <u>wt</u> (due to edema).
Oral/GI: <u>Taste changes</u>, stomatitis, <u>NAUSEA/VOMITING</u>, <u>dyspepsia</u>, reflux, <u>ABDOMINAL</u> <u>PAIN</u>, <u>DIARRHEA</u>, <u>constipation</u>, <u>hemorrhage</u>, <u>FLATULENCE</u>.
S/Cond: Avoid alcohol. Not c̄ lactation. Caution c̄ ↓ hepatic func. Not c̄ severe ↓ hepatic func or fluid retention.[7] Do dental care cautiously- ↑ risk of bleeding/infections. 95% serum pro bound.
Pregnancy: Category D. **Other:** <u>HEMORRHAGE (ANY)</u>, <u>EDEMA</u>, <u>FEVER</u>, <u>MUSCULOSKELETAL</u> <u>PAIN</u>, <u>RASH</u>, <u>MUSCLE</u> <u>CRAMPS</u>, <u>HEADACHE</u>, <u>FATIGUE</u>, <u>COUGH</u>, <u>itching</u>, <u>dizziness</u>, <u>dyspnea</u>, <u>nasopharyngitis</u>, <u>pneumonia</u>, <u>night</u> <u>sweats</u>, <u>insomnia</u>, <u>petechiae</u>, <u>weakness</u>, <u>nosebleed</u>, hepatotoxicity, CHF, paresthesia, blurred vision. Rare-SJS.
Blood/Serum: ↑ <u>alk phos</u>, ↑ <u>bil</u>, ↑ <u>AST</u>, ↑ <u>ALT</u>, ↓ <u>K</u>, ↓ <u>WBC</u>, ↓ <u>PLATELETS</u>, <u>ANEMIA</u>.
Monitor: Weight. CBC weekly for 1st mo, biweekly for 2nd mo, then q 2-3 mo. Hepatic func q mo.

Imdur previous brand name ANTIANGINA, Vasodilator   See **isosorbide mononitrate p 180**

imipenem & cilastatin
Primaxin
IV- 250- 19 mg
(0.8 mEq) Na
IV- 500- 38 mg
(1.6 mEq) Na
IM- 500- 32 mg
(1.4 mEq) Na
IM- 750- 48 mg
(2.1 mEq) Na

ANTIBIOTIC, Carbapenem   Parenteral only (IM or IV)
Oral/GI: (↑ c̄ IV)- N/V, cramps, diarrhea. Rare- pseudomembranous colitis.
S/Cond: Caution c̄ lactation. Caution c̄ seizures, ↓ renal func or wt < 70 kg.
Pregnancy: Category C.
Other: IV- CNS toxicity including seizures, tinnitus, <u>thrombophlebitis</u>.[6]
Rare- allergic reaction, anaphylaxis, hypotension, SJS, TEN.
Blood/Serum: ↑ <u>alk phos</u>, ↑ <u>AST</u>, ↑ <u>ALT</u>, ↑ BUN, ↑ crea, ↑ K, ↑ Cl, ↓ Na, eosinophilia, ↑ PT/INR, false + Coombs' test.[6] Rare- dyscrasias, anemia, ↑ bil, ↑ LDH. **Urinary:** Pro, RBC, WBC, ↑ frequency.
Rare- discoloration. **Monitor:** CBC c̄ diff, hepatic & renal func.

imipramine
Tofranil/Tofranil PM

ANTIDEPRESSANT, ANTIENURESIS   See **Tricyclic Antidepressants p 323**

| **Imitrex** | ANTIMIGRAINE, Serotonin 5-HT$_1$ Receptor Agonist | |
| sumatriptan | | See **Antimigraine p 39** |

| **Imodium** | ANTIDIARRHEAL | See **loperamide p 198** |

| **Imuran** | IMMUNOSUPPRESSANT | See **azathioprine p 48** |

Incivek   TREATMENT FOR CHRONIC HEPATITIS C See **telaprevir p 304**

indacaterol   COPD TREATMENT, Beta2 Agonist, (Not for rapidly deteriorating COPD or asthma)
  Arcapta Neohaler- lactose   Pwd for inhalation, long acting   See listing for **salmeterol p 286**

indapamide   ANTIHYPERTENSIVE, DIURETIC, (K-depleting)
  Lozol   **Blood/Serum:** Does **not** cause ↑ chol.
  Tab- lactose, starch, cornstarch   See listing for **hydrochlorothiazide p 166**

Inder al   ANTIHYPERTENSIVE, Beta-Blocker   See **propranolol p 267**

indinavir (IDV)   ANTIRETROVIRAL (HIV/AIDS), Protease Inhibitor
  Crixivan   Generally given c̄ **ritonavir** to boost **indinavir** serum levels
  Cap- lactose   **Drug:** Take 1 hr before or 2 hr after a high fat meal if administered s̄ **ritonavir**. Light, fat free meal does not affect drug level. Take s̄ regard to meals if administered c̄ **ritonavir**. Separate from high dose (1 g) Vit C. [119]
              Diet: Adequate hydration essential to prevent kidney stones. Drink at least 1500 mL fluids daily. Caution c̄ grapefruit/related citrus, see p 390. Avoid SJW, see p 286. **Nutr:** Concomitant high dose (1 g) Vit C ↓ drug level.[119]
              Oral/GI: Taste changes, <u>nausea</u>, vomiting, regurgitation, <u>abdominal pain</u>, diarrhea. **S/Cond:** Not c̄ lactation. Caution c̄ diabetes- ↑ glucose. Caution c̄ ↓ hepatic func due to cirrhosis. **Pregnancy:** Category C.
              Other: <u>Headache</u>, <u>kidney stones</u> (↑ incidence in children), back or flank pain, dizziness, asthenia, blurred vision. Rare- hepatotoxicity, diabetes. ↑ risk of lipodystrophy. **Blood/Serum:** ↑ <u>bil</u>, ↑ AST, ↑ ALT, ↑ amylase, dyscrasias, ↑ glucose, ↑ TG, ↑ chol. **Urinary:** Hematuria, crystalluria, ↑ WBC. **Monitor:** Urinalysis q 3-4 mo. Baseline lipid panel & glucose. Possibly hepatic func.

Indomethacin
  generic Cap
Indomethacin CR
  generic Cap
Indocin
  Susp- 1% alcohol,
  sorbitol
Indocin SR
  Cap- lactose, lecithin,
  propylene glycol

ANTIARTHRITIC, ACUTE GOUT TREATMENT, NSAID
    Drug: Take c̄ food or milk to ↓ GI irritation. Swallow SR Cap whole.
    Diet: Caution c̄ GI irritants eg K suppl (↑ risk of GI irritation).[13]
    Limit caffeine to ↓ GI effects. Avoid or limit natural products which
    affect coagulation (eg garlic, ginger, ginkgo, ginseng or horse chestnut).
    Nutr: ↓ appetite. **Oral/GI:** <u>N/V</u>, <u>dyspepsia</u>, <u>abdominal pain</u>, constipation,
    diarrhea, colitis,[13] GI ulcers & bleeding (may be sudden & serious).
    S/Cond: Avoid alcohol. Not c̄ lactation. 99% serum pro bound.
    Not c̄ aspirin allergy. Caution c̄ seizures, Parkinsons, geriatric,[84] HTN,
    CHF or edema. Caution c̄ ↓ hepatic func or ↓ renal func. Not c̄ gastritis/ulcer.
    Pregnancy: Category C, but not recommemed in pregnancy.
    Category D in 3rd trimester due to ↑ risk to fetus & mother, including death.
    Other: <u>Headache</u>, <u>dizziness</u>, <u>edema</u>, anxiety, drowsiness, depression, fatigue,
    tinnitus. Rare- nephrotoxicity. Risk of CV problems, eg HTN, CHF, MI, CVA.
    Blood/Serum: ↑ <u>AST</u>, ↑ <u>ALT</u>, ↑ alk phos.[7] ↓ <u>platelet</u> <u>aggregation</u>.
    <1%- ↑ K, ↑ BUN, ↑ crea, ↑ or ↓ glucose, dyscrasias.
    Urinary: < 1%- glucose, pro. **Monitor:** CBC, hepatic & renal func c̄ LT use.

InFeD
  Iron dextran

HEMATINIC, ANTIANEMIC, Mineral Supplement, Iron
See **Ferrous Salts Parenteral p 141**

Infergen
  interferon alfacon-1

To Treat CHRONIC HEPATITIS C   See listing for **interferon alfa p 177**

infliximab
  Remicade
  500 mg sucrose/vial

ANTIARTHRITIC (Rheumatoid Arthritis), CROHN'S DISEASE TREATMENT,
    ULCERATIVE COLITIS OR ANKYLOSING SPONDYLITIS TREATMENT,
    TNF inhibitor   Parenteral only (IV)
See listing for **etanercept p 130**
    As antiarthritic, used in combination c̄ **methotrexate**
    Monitor: For active TB prior to & during treatment.
    Hepatic func- baseline & periodically.[1]

INH (previous brand name)   TUBERCULOSIS TREATMENT   See **isoniazid p 180**

InnoPran XL   ANTIHYPERTENSIVE, Non-selective Beta-Blocker See **propranolol p 267**

Inspra   ANTIHYPERTENSIVE, Aldosterone Blocker See **eplerenone p 126**

insulin   ANTIDIABETIC, HYPOGLYCEMIC   Parenteral only [(SC or IV- **Regular** only)]
Drug: Timing of injection or pump bolus in relation to food varies $\bar{c}$ insulin form. See PI.
Diet: Diabetic meal plan to balance carbohydrate $\bar{c}$ insulin.
Nutr: ↑ <u>wt</u>. No ↑ wt in Type 1 diabetes $\bar{c}$ **insulin detemir**.
S/Cond: Use alcohol $\bar{c}$ caution and under advice from a physician. Alcohol ↑ hypoglycemic effect of insulin.
Caution $\bar{c}$ lactation. **Insulin detemir** is 98% serum pro bound- caution $\bar{c}$ severe hypoalbuminemia.
Exercise, stress, illness, pregnancy, heavy smoking[99] or large wt gain ↑ insulin needs.
Caution $\bar{c}$ ↓ hepatic func or ↓ renal func, hyperthyroidism or hypothyroidism.[13]
Pregnancy: See pregnancy categories below.
Other: <u>HYPOGLYCEMIA</u>. Transient edema, vision changes. Rare- allergic reaction.
Blood/Serum: ↓ <u>GLUCOSE</u>, ↓ <u>Hb A1</u>_C. ↓ K, ↓ Mg, ↓ P,[13] ↑ T$_4$.[7]
Urinary: ↓ <u>GLUCOSE</u>. **Monitor:** Serum glucose, Hb A1$_C$. Urine ketones.
human insulins:
Regular	**Humulin R/Novolin R** bolus, short acting **Pregnancy:** B	
NPH	**Humulin N/Novolin N** basal, intermediate acting (contains protamine* & Zn) **Pregnancy:** B	
Mixtures	**Humulin 70/30** or **Novolin 70/30** = 70% NPH + 30% Regular **Pregnancy:** B	
	Humulin 50/50 = 50% NPH + 50% Regular **Pregnancy:** B	

human insulin analogs:
insulin aspart	**Novolog** bolus. May mix $\bar{c}$ NPH only for SC use. **Pregnancy:** C	
Novolog 70/30	= 30% insulin aspart + 70% insulin aspart protamine*, mannitol 36.4 mg/mL **Pregnancy:** B	
insulin detemir	**Levemir** basal, once or twice daily. Do not mix $\bar{c}$ any other insulin. **Pregnancy:** C	
insulin glulisine	**Apidra** bolus. May mix $\bar{c}$ NPH only. **Pregnancy:** C	
insulin glargine	**Lantus** basal, once daily. Do not mix $\bar{c}$ any other insulin. **Pregnancy:** C	
insulin lispro	**Humalog** bolus. May mix $\bar{c}$ NPH only. **Pregnancy:** B	
	Humalog 75/25 Pregnancy: B	
	= 25% insulin lispro + 75% insulin lispro protamine*.	

*Note: Addition of protamine slows abs & prolongs action of insulin.
Recombinant DNA (rDNA) products (analogs) are created by changes in amino acid(s) on the A &/or B chain of the human insulin molecule. Pharmacokinetics are affected as compared to human insulin.
For pharmacokinetics of insulins see next page

I

INSULIN	TRADE NAME	ONSET	PEAK	DURATION	ANALOG
Rapid Acting Bolus Insulin					
Insulin Aspart	Novolog	10-20 minutes	40-50 min	3-5 hr	Yes
Insulin Lispro	Humalog	15-30 minutes	2.4 hr (0.5-2.5 hr)	3-6.5 hr	Yes
Insulin Glulisine	Apidra	10-15 minutes	1-1.5 min	3-5 hr	Yes
Short Acting Bolus Insulin					
Human Regular	Humulin R Novolin R	0.5-1 hr	1-5 hr (4-4.5 hr)	6-10 hr	No
Intermediate Acting Basal Insulin					
Insulin NPH	Humulin N Novolin N	1-2 hr	6-14 hr	16-24+ hr*	No
Long Acting Basal Insulin					
Insulin Glargine	Lantus	1.1 hr	no peak	20-24+ hr	Yes
Insulin Detemir	Levemir	0.8-2 hr*	no peak	12-24 hr*	Yes
Premixed Insulin (mixture of short acting and intermediate acting)					
Biphasic Lispro	Humalog 75/25	<30 minutes 0.25-0.5 hr	2.6 hr (1-6.5 hr)	10-16 hr up to 24	Yes
Biphasic Lispro	Humalog 50/50	0.25-0.5 hr	2.3 hr (0.8-4.8 hr)	~24 hr	Yes
Biphasic Aspart	Novolog 70/30	<30 minutes	1-4 hr	15-18 up to 24 hr	Yes
Biphasic Human	Humulin 70/30	0.5-1 hr	4.4 hr (1.5-16 hr)	10-16 hr up to 24	No
Biphasic Human	Humulin 50/50	0.5-1 hr	3.3 hr (2-5.5 hr)	10-16 hr up to 24	No
Biphasic Human	Novolin 70/30	30 minutes	2-12 hr	10-16 hr~24 hr	No

* Dose dependent

References 1 (21(8)- detail document 210803), 7, 10, Manufacturer's information,
Triplitt, C, How to titrate and intensify insulin treatment in type 2 diabetes. US Pharm. 2007; 32(10):10-16

Intelence	ANTIRETROVIRAL, NNRTI	See **etravirine p 132**

Intermezzo	SLEEP AID, Non Benzodiazepine	See **zolpidem p 351**

interferon
alfa-2b
Intron-A
alfa-2a
Roferon-A (SC only)

ANTINEOPLASTIC (**Intron**) (**Roferon-A**- Hairy Cell Leukemia)
(Kaposi's Sarcoma, Leukemia, Malignant Melanoma, Follicular Lymphoma)
Parenteral only (IV, SC, IM, intralesional)
CHRONIC HEPATITIS B (**Intron**) or C (**Intron**, **Roferon-A**) TREATMENT
Diet: Insure adequate fluid intake/hydration.
Nutr: <u>ANOREXIA</u>, ↓ <u>WEIGHT</u>, ↑ <u>THIRST</u>.
Oral/GI: <u>DRY</u> <u>MOUTH</u>, <u>TASTE</u> <u>CHANGES</u>, <u>gingivitis</u>, stomatitis, dysphagia,
↑ saliva, <u>NAUSEA/VOMITING</u>, <u>dyspepsia</u>, gastritis, <u>ABDOMINAL</u> <u>PAIN</u>, <u>DIARRHEA</u>,
flatulence, <u>constipation</u>. Rare- GI hemorrhage.
S/Cond: Avoid alcohol. Not c̄ lactation. ↑ risk of dental problems.
Caution c̄ diabetes. Caution c̄ cardiac or pulmonary disease,
severe ↓ renal func or severe ↓ hepatic func,
seizures or bone marrow suppression.[10]
Pregnancy: Category C.
Other: <u>FLU-LIKE</u> <u>SYMPTOMS</u>, <u>FEVER/CHILLS</u>, <u>HEADACHE</u>, <u>FATIGUE</u>,
<u>MUSCLE/JOINT</u> <u>PAIN</u>, <u>COUGH</u>, <u>BONE</u> <u>MARROW</u> <u>SUPPRESSION</u>, <u>DIZZINESS</u>, <u>HAIR</u> <u>LOSS</u>,
<u>DEPRESSION</u> c̄ suicidal thinking & behavior, <u>anxiety</u>, <u>irritability</u>, <u>amnesia</u>,
<u>rash</u>, dyspnea, <u>pharyngitis</u>, <u>sinusitis</u>, <u>night</u> <u>sweats</u>, <u>insomnia</u>,
<u>chest</u> <u>pain</u>, <u>edema</u>, psychosis, confusion, visual changes,
peripheral neuropathy, HTN, hypotension, flushing, paresthesia.
Rare- pancreatitis, allergic reaction, nephrotoxicity.[6]
Blood/Serum: ↓ <u>WHITE</u> <u>BLOOD</u> <u>CELLS</u>, ↓ <u>PLATELETS</u>, ↑ <u>AST</u>, ↑ <u>ALT</u>,
↑ <u>alk</u> <u>phos</u>, ↑ <u>LDH</u>, ↑ <u>BIL</u>, <u>ANEMIA</u>, ↑ BUN, ↑ crea, ↑ fasting glucose,
↑ P, ↓ Ca, ↑ uric acid, ↑ or ↓ TSH, ↑ TG. **Urinary:** <u>PRO</u>.
Monitor: Baseline & during use- CBC c̄ diff, platelets,
electrolytes, hepatic func, TSH. BP. Possibly TG.[6] Baseline chest x-ray.

interferon alfacon-1 **Infergen**	CHRONIC HEPATITIS C TREATMENT	See listing for **interferon alfa above**

Parenteral only (SC), synthetic **interferon**, preservative free

interferon beta-1a
  Avonex (IM)
  pwd- 16.5 mg albumin human/vial
  prefilled syringe-
   albumin free
  Rebif (SC)
  prefilled syringes-
   albumin human,
   mannitol

interferon beta-1b
  Betaseron (SC)
  pwd- 15 mg mannitol,
  15 mg albumin
   human/vial
  Extavia (SC)
  pwd- 15 mg mannitol

MULTIPLE SCLEROSIS TREATMENT   Parenteral only (IM or SC)
Nutr: Anorexia. ↑ or ↓ wt.
Oral/GI: Dry mouth, <u>N</u>/V, dyspepsia, abdominal pain, <u>diarrhea</u>, <u>constipation</u>.
S/Cond: Not c̄ lactation. Caution c̄ cardiac disease or seizures.
Pregnancy: Category C.
Other: <u>FLU-LIKE SYMPTOMS</u>, <u>muscle ache</u>, <u>fever/chills</u>, <u>weakness</u>,
  <u>headache</u>, <u>infection</u>, chest pain, syncope, dyspnea, flushing, dizziness,
  insomnia, muscle spasm, seizures, ataxia, depression c̄ suicidal thinking
  & behavior, speech disorder, sinusitis, ovarian cyst, vaginitis, ↓ hearing,
  abnormal vision, dry eyes, rash, photosensitivity, thyroid disorder.
  Rare- severe hepatotoxicity (may be fatal).
Blood/Serum: beta-1a- <u>Anemia</u>, eosinophilia, ↑ AST.
beta-1b - ↓ <u>WBC</u>, ↑ <u>AST</u>, ↑ <u>ALT</u>, ↑ bil, ↓ <u>glucose</u>,[7] ↑ glucose, dyscrasias.
Monitor: Baseline & during use- CBC c̄ diff, platelets, blood chemistry
  including hepatic func at 1, 3 & 6 mo, then periodically.
  Possibly thyroid func.

Intron A   ANTINEOPLASTIC   See **interferon alfa 2b p 177**

Intuniv (SR)   ADHD TREATMENT for children ≥ 6 yr old.   See **guanfacine p 160**

Invanz   ANTIBIOTIC, Carbapenem   See **ertapenem p 128**

Invega   ANTIPSYCHOTIC, Second Generation   See listing for **risperidone p 280**
  Tab SR- propylene glycol   **paliperidone**- metabolite of **risperidone** ↑ QT interval
  3 mg Tab- lactose   **Drug:** IM starting dose, then 1/2 dose one wk later, then dose q mo.
Invega Sustenna (SR) Parenteral only (SC)

Invirase   ANTIRETROVIRAL (HIV/AIDS), Protease Inhibitor
                                              See **saquinavir p 288**

ipratropium bromide   BRONCHODILATOR, Anticholinergic   Oral Inhalant- COPD, chronic
  Atrovent HFA   bronchitis, emphysema. Nasal Spray- relief of rhinorrhea due to allergies, cold
  Inhaler-   **Oral/GI:** <u>Dry mouth/throat</u>, metallic/bitter taste, nausea, dyspepsia.

dehydrated alcohol **Atrovent** Nasal Spray	**S/Cond:** Caution c̄ lactation. Caution c̄ ↓ hepatic func or ↓ renal func. **Pregnancy:** Category B. **Other:** <u>Cough</u>, <u>headache</u>, <u>dyspnea</u>, dizziness, blurred vision, palpitations, back or chest pain, nervousness. **Urinary:** Retention, <u>UTI</u>.
irbesartan **Avapro/Avalide**	ANTIHYPERTENSIVE See **Angiotensin II Receptor Antagonists p 38** **Avalide** also contains **hydrochlorothiazide**, see **p 166**
irinotecan **Camptosar** IV- sorbitol, lactic acid	ANTINEOPLASTIC, Topoisomerase I Inhibitor (Colorectal Cancer) Parenteral only (IV) **Diet:** Insure adequate hydration/fluid intake. Avoid SJW, see p 286. Avoid caffeine, high fiber, high fat foods if diarrhea occurs.[13] **Nutr:** <u>ANOREXIA</u>, ↓ <u>WEIGHT</u>, dehydration. **Oral/GI:** <u>Stomatitis</u>, ↑ salivation, <u>NAUSEA/VOMITING</u>, <u>ABDOMINAL CRAMPS</u>, <u>CONSTIPATION</u>, <u>EARLY</u> & <u>LATE</u> <u>SEVERE</u> <u>DIARRHEA</u>, <u>flatulence</u>, colitis. **S/Cond:** Avoid alcohol. Not c̄ lactation. Metabolite SN-38 is 95% pro bound. Do dental care cautiously, see p 11 & 15. Caution c̄ ↓ hepatic func or ↓ pulmonary[26] func or geriatric. Caution c̄ ↓ renal func. Not c̄ dialysis. Not c̄ bil > 2 mg/dL.[26] **Pregnancy:** Category D. **Other:** <u>ASTHENIA</u>, <u>HAIR</u> <u>LOSS</u>, <u>FEVER</u>, <u>PAIN</u>, <u>DYSPNFA</u>, <u>headache</u>, chills, <u>edema</u>, <u>cough</u>, <u>rash</u>, <u>insomnia</u>, <u>rhinitis</u>, <u>flushing</u>, <u>sweating</u>, bone marrow suppression, infection. Dizziness, orthostatic hypotension due to dehydration. **Blood/Serum:** ↓ <u>WHITE</u> <u>BLOOD</u> <u>CELLS</u>, ↓ <u>NEUTROPHILS</u>, ↓ <u>eosinophils</u>, ↑ <u>alk phos</u>, ↑ <u>bil</u>, ↑ <u>AST</u>, <u>anemia</u>, ↑ glucose, ↓ platelets. Electrolyte imbalance due to diarrhea. **Monitor:** Before each dose- WBC c̄ diff, Hb, platelets.
iron	MINERAL SUPPLEMENT See **ferrous salts p 140 & 141**
Isentress	ANTIRETROVIRAL (HIV/AIDS) Integrase Inhibitor See **raltegravir p 274**
ISMO	ANTIANGINA, VASODILATOR See **isosorbide mononitrate p 180**

I

isocarboxazid	ANTIDEPRESSANT, MAOI	See listing for
Marplan	Tab- lactose, cornstarch	**phenelzine p 252**

isoniazid
  INH (oral)
  (previous brand name)
  Tab
  Syrup- sorbitol
  Nydrazid
  (previous brand name)
  (Parenteral)

TUBERCULOSIS TREATMENT, ANTIMYCOBACTERIUM   Oral or Parenteral (IM)

Drug: Food significantly ↓ abs. Take 1 hr before meals. May take c̄ food if drug causes GI distress.

Diet: <u>Pyr suppl</u> (25-50 mg daily) to prevent peripheral neuropathy. MAOI-like activity. Avoid high tyramine or histamine foods, see p 383. Caution c̄ **melatonin**- ↑ drug level.[4]

Nutr: Anorexia. Inhibits conversion of tryptophan to niacin. May cause Pyr def or pellagra (niacin def).[7] ↑ risk in slow acetylators.

Oral/GI: Dry mouth, N/V, epigastric distress, constipation, diarrhea.

S/Cond: Avoid alcohol- ↑ risk of hepatitis. Caution c̄ lactation. Caution c̄ ↓ hepatic func or severe ↓ renal func. Not c̄ acute hepatic disease. Caution c̄ malnourished patients- ↑ risk of Pyr &/or niacin def.

Pregnancy: Category C.

Other: <u>PERIPHERAL</u> <u>NEUROPATHY</u>, hepatitis (can be fatal or delayed- risk ↑ postpartum, in minority women & in geriatric), fatigue, weakness, fever, skin eruptions, vasculitis, joint pain. Rare neurotoxic effects- very uncommon c̄ usual dose- toxic encephalopathy, optic neuritis & atrophy, memory impairment, toxic psychosis, seizures. SLE-like syndrome.

Blood/Serum: ↑ <u>AST</u>, ↑ <u>ALT</u>, ↑ <u>bil</u>, ↑ glucose, ↓ Ca, ↓ P, ↓ Vit D, dyscrasias.

Urinary: False + glucose ($CuSO_4$), ↑ Pyr, ↑ bil.

Monitor: Hepatic func, bil, possibly eye exams.

Isoptin SR	ANTIARRHYTHMIC, Ca Channel Blocker See **verapamil p 332**

isosorbide dinitrate
  Isordil (previous brand name)
  Titradose Tab- lactose
  Dilatrate SR Cap-
  lactose, starch, sucrose
  Generic brand
  Sublingual Tab- lactose,

ANTIANGINA, Vasodilator

Drug: Take on empty stomach c̄ 8 oz water to ↑ rate of abs.[13] Swallow SR tab whole c̄ half glass of water. Do not crush or chew sublingual tab. Do not take sublingual form HS due to ↑ risk of aspiration. Chew chew tab well, hold in mouth 1-2 minutes.[13]

Oral/GI: Dry mouth, epigastric distress.

S/Cond: Avoid alcohol- risk of severe hypotension.[7]

starch   Caution c̄ lactation. Caution c̄ dry mouth- sublingual or chewable form may not be fully absorbed.[13]

isosorbide mononitrate
  Imdur previous brand name
  Tab (SR)
  ISMO Tab-
  lactose, Na starch glycolate

Pregnancy: Category C, except **Imdur**- Category B.[10]
Other: HEADACHE, flushing, dizziness, orthostatic hypotension, weakness, tachycardia, restlessness.
Blood/Serum: ↑ AST, ↑ ALT, ↑ uric acid, ↓ K.
Rare-↑ methemoglobin c̄ very high dose.
Monitor: BP, heart rate. Possibly K, methemoglobin.

isotretinoin
  Accutane
  previous brand name
  Cap- vegetable oil,
  soybean oil flakes,
  soybean oil

ANTIACNE, Retinoid (Only for severe recalcitrant, nodular acne)
Drug: Take c̄ high fat meals or milk to ↑ abs & swallow c̄ full glass liquid to ↓ GI irritation. Dosage based on body wt.
Diet: Do not take suppl c̄ Vit A or beta carotene. Do not take MVI.
Nutr: Anorexia, ↑ thirst.
Oral/GI: DRY MOUTH, CHEILITIS (LIP INFLAMMATION), esophagitis, N/V, stomach upset, abdominal pain. Rare- IBS, bleeding.
S/Cond: Limit alcohol. Not c̄ lactation. Do dental care cautiously, see p 11 & 15. Caution c̄ diabetes, obesity, osteoporosis/osteomalacia or hyperlipidemia. 99.9% serum pro bound. Caution c̄ soy allergy.
Pregnancy: Category X- absolutely contraindicated.
Other: CONJUNCTIVITIS, DRY NOSE/NOSE BLEEDS, BACK PAIN, headache, muscle/bone pain, ↓ bone density, photosensitivity, visual changes, dry eyes, rash, dry skin, fatigue, edema, hepatotoxicity, slow skin healing. Psychosis &/or severe depression c̄ suicidal thinking & behavior (but large study found no ↑ risk).[48] Rare- acute pancreatitis, pseudotumor cerebri, allergic reaction, ototoxicity, tinnitus, palpitation, tachycardia, ↓ night vision, aggressive/violent behavior, rhabdomyolysis, hyperostosis, tendon/ligament calcification, seizures, syncope.
Blood/Serum: ↑ TRIGLYCERIDES, ↑ chol, ↓ HDL, ↑ LDL, ↑ VLDL, ↑ LDH, ↑ AST, ↑ GGT, ↑ ALT, ↑ alk phos, ↓ Hb/HCT, ↓ RBC, ↓ WBC, ↓ or ↑ platelets, ↑ CPK, ↑ glucose, ↑ uric acid. **Urinary:** WBC, RBC, pro.
Monitor: Lipids & hepatic func baseline & weekly or biweekly until response established. CBC, glucose in diabetes, vision, psychological status.[21]

itraconazole
  Sporanox
  Cap- sucrose,
   starch
  Soln- sorbitol,
   saccharin Na,
   propylene glycol
  Ampule- propylene glycol

ANTIFUNGAL, ANTICANDIDIASIS (Soln for oral or esophageal candidiasis only)
Oral & Parenteral (IV infusion only)

Drug: Take cap c̄ full meal to ↑ abs. Take liquid on empty stomach to ↑ abs.
Diet: (oral forms) Take Ca or Mg suppl or antacid ≥ 2 hr after drug.
240 cc cola ↑ AUC & C_{max} of cap form in achlorhydria or AIDS patients.[7]
Caution c̄ grapefruit/related citrus- ↑ drug levels, see p 390. Do not
co-administer with OJ- significantly ↓ drug levels. Avoid SJW, see p 286.
Nutr: Anorexia. ↑ appetite. **Oral/GI:** Dyspepsia, gastritis, <u>N/V</u>,
abdominal pain, diarrhea, constipation, flatulence.
S/Cond: Not c̄ lactation. 99.8% serum pro bound.
Caution c̄ diabetic on sulfonylurea- ↑ effect of oral hypoglycemics.[9a]
Caution c̄ achlorhydria (must take in acidic liquid, eg cola).[13]
Caution c̄ ↓ hepatic func or severe ↓ renal func. Not c̄ CHF.
Pregnancy: Category C.
Other: <u>Rash</u>, <u>headache</u>, <u>rhinitis</u>, <u>URTI</u>, <u>sinusitis</u>, edema, fatigue, asthenia,
drowsiness, fever, headache, dizziness, abnormal dreaming, ↑ sweating,
cough, dyspnea, HTN, muscle pain, tremor.
Rare- hepatotoxicity, anaphylaxis, SJS, hair loss.
Blood/Serum: ↑ AST, ↑ ALT, ↑ alk phos, ↑ bil, ↓ K, ↑ TG. **Urinary:** Pro, UTI.
Monitor: Baseline & periodic hepatic func, K.

ixabepilone
  Ixempra
  Single use vials
   pwd & diluent
  diluent-
   52.8% polyoxyethylated
    castor oil,
   39.8% dehydrated alcohol

ANTINEOPLASTIC, Epothilone class of Antimicrotubule Agent (Breast Cancer)
Parenteral only (IV)

Drug: Insure adequate fluid intake/hydration.
Diet: Not c̄ SJW, see p 286. Avoid grapefruit/related citrus, see p 390.
Nutr: <u>ANOREXIA</u>, ↓ <u>weight</u>, dehydration.
Oral/GI: <u>STOMATITIS</u>, <u>taste changes</u>, gastritis, dysphagia, <u>GERD</u>,
<u>NAUSEA/VOMITING</u>, <u>abdominal pain</u>, hemorrhage, <u>DIARRHEA</u>, <u>constipation</u>.
S/Cond: Avoid alcohol. Not c̄ lactation.
Caution c̄ ↓ hepatic func or cardiac disease. Not c̄ severe ↓ hepatic func.
Pregnancy: Category D.
Other: <u>PERIPHERAL NEUROPATHY</u>, <u>BONE MARROW SUPPRESSION</u>, <u>ASTHENIA</u>,
<u>MUSCLE/JOINT/BONE PAIN</u>, <u>HAIR LOSS</u>, flushing, headache, <u>nail changes</u>,
<u>hand-foot syndrome</u>, <u>URTI</u>, edema, <u>chest pain</u>, <u>fever</u>, insomnia,

<u>dizziness</u>, <u>dyspnea</u>, skin changes, itching, cough, ↑ tearing.
Blood/Serum: ↓ <u>WHITE BLOOD CELLS</u>, ↓ <u>NEUTROPHILS</u>, <u>anemia</u>, ↓ <u>platelets</u>,
↑ AST, ↑ ALT, ↑ alk phos, ↑ GGT, ↓ K, ↓ Na. **Urinary:** UTI.
Monitor: Baseline & before each dose- CBC c̄ diff, platelets, hepatic func.

Jalyn Cap- gelatin, glycerin	BPH TREATMENT, Combination Drug (**dutasteride**, **tamsulosin**) Take cap 30 min after the same meal each day. Swallow whole. Do not open, chew or crush. Contact of cap contents c̄ oropharyngeal mucosa may cause irritation. See listing for **finasteride p 142** See **alpha₁ adrenergic blockers p 28**
Janumet Tab	ANTIDIABETIC AGENT Combination drug See **sitagliptin p 293** See **metformin p 210**
Januvia	ANTIDIABETIC AGENT See **sitagliptin p 293**
Kadian	ANALGESIC, Narcotic, Opioid See **morphine p 221**
Kaletra	ANTIRETROVIRAL (HIV/AIDS), Protease Inhibitor Also contains a small amount of **ritonavir** to ↓ drug metabolism Combination drug See **lopinavir/ ritonavir p 199**
Kaopectate	ANTIDIARRHEAL See **bismuth subsalicylate p 58**
Kaopectate Stool Softener	STOOL SOFTENER, LAXATIVE See **docusate calcium p 115**
Kapidex **dexlansoprazole** (DR) Cap- sugar spheres, sucrose	ANTIGERD, ANTISECRETORY *R*-enantiomer of **lansoprazole** Dual Action Release See **Proton Pump Inhibitors p 268**
Kariva	ORAL CONTRACEPTIVE See **Oral Contraceptives p 237**
Kayexalate	ANTIHYPERKALEMIA See **sodium polystyrene sulfonate p 294**
KCl/K-Dur	ELECTROLYTE, potassium supplement See **potassium chloride p 260**
Keflex	ANTIBIOTIC, Cephalosporin See **cephalexin p 79**

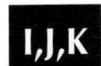

Kenalog	CORTICOSTEROID, **triamcinolone**	See **corticosteroids p 94**
Kepivance	ORAL MUCOSITIS TREATMENT	See **palifermin p 242**
Keppra	ANTIEPILEPTIC	See **levetiracetam p 191**

ketoconazole
  Nizoral
  Tab- lactose,
  cornstarch

ANTIFUNGAL, ANTICANDIDIASIS
  Drug: Take c̄ food to ↑ abs. Acidic pH < 5.0 needed to dissolve.
  Diet: Take Ca or Mg suppl or antacid ≥ 2 hr after drug.
  Must take c̄ acidic liquid- cola ↑ abs 65%.[6] Avoid SJW, see p 286.
  Oral/GI: N/V, abdominal pain, diarrhea.
  S/Cond: Avoid alcohol- possible disulfiram-like reaction.
  Not c̄ lactation. Caution c̄ achlorhydria (must take in acidic liquid).[13]
  84-99% serum pro bound.[6] Caution c̄ ↓ hepatic func.[13]
  Caution c̄ diabetic on sulfonylurea- ↑ effect of oral hypoglycemics.[9a]
  Caution c̄ med metabolized by CYP3A4,
  ketoconazole is a very potent CYP3A4 inhibitor. **Pregnancy:** Category C.
  Other: Headache, dizziness, drowsiness, itching.
  Rare- hepatotoxicity (can be fatal), anaphylaxis.
  Adrenal insufficiency c̄ high dose.
  Blood/Serum: ↑ AST, ↑ ALT, ↑ alk phos, ↑ bil, ↓ testosterone, ↓ cortisol.
  < 1%- hemolytic anemia, ↓ platelets, ↓ WBC, ↓ chol, ↑ TG.[6]
  Monitor: Hepatic func baseline & frequently during use.

ketoprofen
  generics only
  Cap-
  propylene glycol,
  Na starch glycolate
  (SR) Cap- starch, sucrose

ANTIARTHRITIC, ANALGESIC, NSAID   See listing for **ibuprofen p 170**
  Drug: May take c̄ food, milk or antacids to ↓ GI irritation.
  Food ↓ rate, but not extent of abs. Swallow SR Cap whole.
  S/Cond: Do not use SR form c̄ ↓ hepatic func.

| **Klonopin**
  clonazepam | ANTIEPILEPTIC, ANTIPANIC | See **Benzodiazepines p 54** |
| **K-Lor, Klor-Con, Klotrix, K-Lyte** | ELECTROLYTE, Potassium Supplement | See **potassium chloride p 260** |

Kombiglyze XR	ANTIDIABETIC, Combination Drug (**saxagliptin**, **metformin**)
Tab- polyethylene glycol	Take once daily c̄ evening meal. Do not crush, chew or cut.
	See lising for **sitagliptin p 293** See **metformin p 210**

Kondremul   LAXATIVE, Lubricant   See **mineral oil p 218**

K-Phos Neutral   ACIDIFIER, PHOSPHOROUS SUPPLEMENT   See **phosphates p 257**

Kristalose   LAXATIVE   See **lactulose p 186**

Krystexxa   TREATMENT OF GOUT REFRACTORY TO CONVENTIONAL TREATMENT,
     Uric acid specific enzyme   See **pegloticase p 248**

K-Tab   ELECTROLYTE, Potassium Supplement   See **potassium chloride p 260**

Kuvan   HYPERPHENYLALANINEMIA TREATMENT in PKU
     See **sapropterin p 287**

Kytril   ANTIEMETIC, ANTINAUSEANT   See **granisetron p 158**

labetalol
  Trandate   ANTIHYPERTENSIVE, Alpha$_1$ & Beta-Blocker   Oral or Parenteral (IV)
  Tab- cornstarch,   **Drug:** Oral- Take c̄ food to ↑ bioavailability.
  lactose   **Diet:** ↓ Na, ↓ cal diet may be recommended. Avoid natural licorice, see p 374.
  Parenteral-   **Oral/GI:** Taste changes, <u>N</u>/V, dyspepsia.
  Generic brands only   **S/Cond:** Limit alcohol. Caution c̄ lactation.

Caution c̄ diabetes- may mask symptoms of & prolong hypoglycemia.
May reduce insulin release in response to hyperglycemia.
Caution c̄ ↓ hepatic func or CHF.
Caution c̄ asthma/bronchospasm. Caution c̄ geriatric.
Pregnancy: Category C, but often prescribed c̄ **methyldopa** for HTN in pregnancy.
Other: ↓ *BP* c̄ possible hypotension, <u>dizziness</u>, <u>fatigue</u>, headache,
visual changes, rash, edema, dyspnea, transient scalp tingling,
flushing c̄ IV. Rare- jaundice, hepatitis, SLE, paresthesias.
Blood/Serum: ↓ WBC, ↑ BUN, ↑ crea, ↑ AST, ↑ ALT, ↑ bil, ↑ LDH,
↑ glucose, + ANA, ↑ prolactin (IV only).
Monitor: BP, hepatic & renal func.

lacosamide
 Vimpat
  Tab
  Parenteral

ANTIEPILEPTIC for Partial-Onset Seizures   Oral or Parenteral (IV)
 Drug: Take s̄ regard to food.
 Oral/GI: Dry mouth, ↓ oral sensation, dyspepsia, <u>N/V</u>, diarrhea, constipation.
 S/Cond: Not c̄ lactation. Caution with severe ↓ renal func.
 Caution c̄ mild ↓ hepatic func. Not c̄ severe ↓ hepatic func.
 Caution c̄ cardiac disease.
 Pregnancy: Category C.
 Other: <u>Dizziness</u>, <u>ataxia</u>, <u>blurred</u> <u>vision</u>, <u>double</u> <u>vision</u>, nystagmus,
 asthenia, fatigue, drowsiness, depression, confusion, irritability, tremor,
 headache, paresthesia. Rare- suicidal thinking & behavior.
 Blood/Serum: ↑ AST, ↑ ALT. Anemia, ↓ neutrophils.
 Monitor: Hepatic func.

lactobacillus
 Lactinex- L. acidophilus
 + L. bulgaricus
  Chew Tab- lactose,
  sucrose, mineral oil
 Granules
 Bacid Cap- L. acidophilis,
  L. bulgaris, B. biffidum, S. thermophilus, maltodextrin

BIOTHERAPEUTIC AGENT, Antidiarrheal, Live microbial supplement
 Drug: Chew chewable tabs well, follow by small amt milk, fruit juice or
 water. Take granules in or c̄ food, cereal, milk, fruit juice or water.
 Take separately from antibiotics by ≥ 2 hr.
 Oral/GI: Burping, vomiting, diarrhea, <u>transient</u> <u>flatulence</u>.
 S/Cond: Not c̄ milk allergy. Not c̄ high fever or severe immunodeficiency.

lactulose
 Soln
 Enulose- soln & rectal supp
 Constulose
 10 g lactulose,
 < 1.2 g lactose,
 < 1.6 g galactose,
 < 1.2 g other sugar/15 mL

 Crystals

LAXATIVE (Hyperosmotic), To Treat ↑ AMMONIA LEVEL (Soln only)
 (To prevent or treat PSE- portal-systemic encephalopathy)
 Synthetic Disaccharide   Oral or Rectal
 Drug: Take c̄ juice, milk, water or mix c̄ sweet food to improve taste.
 Follow c̄ 8 oz water. Dissolve crystals in 4 oz water.
 Diet: High fiber c̄ 1500-2000 mL fluid/day to prevent constipation.
 Not c̄ lactose or galactose restricted diet.
 Do not take concomitantly c̄ antacids, Ca or Mg suppl.
 Caution c̄ **glutamine**- in theory may ↓ antiammonia effect.[93]
 Nutr: Drug ↑ abs of Ca & Mg.[129]
 Oral/GI: N/V, <u>belching</u>, <u>cramps</u>, <u>borborygmi</u>, diarrhea, <u>flatulence</u>.

Kristalose
< 0.3 g lactose +
galactose/10 g

S/Cond: Caution c̄ lactation. Caution c̄ diabetes.
Dilute before use in TF.[6]
Pregnancy: Category B.
Blood/Serum: ↓ NH_3. ↑ glucose in diabetics.
Monitor: Electrolytes in geriatric or debilitated c̄ LT use (> 6 mo).[6]
Glucose in diabetics.

Lamictal   ANTIEPILEPTIC   See **lamotrigine p 188**

Lamisil oral   ANTIFUNGAL   See **terbinafine p 307**

lamivudine (3TC)
  Epivir [a]
  Epivir-HBV [b]
  Heptovir [a] (Canada)
Soln- 200 mg/mL sucrose,
propylene glycol
Tab- Na starch glycolate,
propylene glycol

ANTIRETROVIRAL (HIV/AIDS),[a] To treat Chronic Hepatitis B,[b] NRTI
Drug: Take s̄ regard to food.
Nutr: Anorexia.
Oral/GI: <u>NAUSEA</u>, <u>vomiting</u>, dyspepsia, abdominal cramps, diarrhea.
S/Cond: Caution c̄ alcohol- ↑ risk of pancreatitis.[13] Not c̄ lactation.
Caution c̄ pediatric patients c̄ history or risk of pancreatitis.
Caution c̄ ↓ renal func or ↓ hepatic func or risk factors for hepatic disease.
Caution c̄ geriatric. Obesity ↑ risk of lactic acidosis or hepatotoxicity.
Pregnancy: Category C.
Other: <u>Headache</u>, dizziness, pancreatitis (↑ <u>in children</u>), fatigue,
insomnia, peripheral neuropathy (↑ <u>in children</u>), depression,
muscle/bone pain, cough, nasal congestion, wheezing, sore throat, rash.
Rare- lipodystrophy, lactic acidosis & hepatomegaly c̄ steatosis (can be
fatal). Exacerbation of hepatitis B upon DC of drug.
Blood/Serum: ↓ neutrophils, anemia, ↑ amylase, ↑ lipase, ↑ ALT,
↑ AST, ↑ glucose, ↑ bil, ↓ platelets, ↑ CPK.
Monitor: Renal func. Possibly amylase & hepatic func,
especially in children.[13]

lamotrigine
  Lamictal[a, b]
  Tab- lactose, starch
  Chewable Dispersible
   Tab- calcium carbonate,
   starch, saccharin Na
  ODT- mannitol,
   sucralose
  Lamictal XR[a]
   Tab- lactose

ANTIEPILEPTIC[a], ADJUNCT MOOD STABILIZER in Bipolar Disorder[b]
Dihydrofolate Reductase Inhibitor

Drug: Take s̄ regard to food. Swallow or chew chewable tab c̄ small amount liquid OR disperse in small amount water or fruit juice, wait 1 minute, mix soln & drink.
Nutr: Anorexia, ↓ wt.
Oral/GI: Dry mouth, tooth disorder, <u>N/V</u>, dyspepsia, abdominal pain, diarrhea, constipation.
S/Cond: Avoid alcohol. Not c̄ lactation.
Caution c̄ ↓ hepatic func, ↓ renal func or ↓ cardiac func.[7] DC if rash occurs. Oral clearance was 25% lower in nonwhite pt than in white pt.[10]
Pregnancy: Category C.
Other: <u>DIZZINESS</u>, <u>DOUBLE VISION</u>, <u>ataxia</u>, <u>headache</u>, <u>blurred vision</u>, <u>rash</u> (may be fatal) (↑ <u>incidence in children</u>), drowsiness, photosensitivity, insomnia, tremor, seizure, hot flashes, fever, depression, anxiety, neck or joint pain, dysmenorrhea, pharyngitis, bronchitis, rhinitis, infection, flu-like syndrome, chest pain.
Rare- (can be fatal)- SJS (↑ incidence in children), angioedema, TEN.
Rare- suicidal thinking & behavior.
Blood/Serum: < 1%- dyscrasias. In theory may ↓ Fol.
Urinary: UTI. **Monitor:** Renal & hepatic func.[21]

Lanoxin

CARDIOTONIC, ANTIARRHYTHMIC, CHF TREATMENT   See **digoxin p 110**

lansoprazole
  Prevacid/Prevacid 24/Prevacid I.V./Prevacid Solu-Tab

ANTIULCER, ANTIGERD, ANTISECRETORY

See **Proton Pump Inhibitors p 268**

lanthanum
  Fosrenol
  Chew Tab-
   dextrates (hydrated),
   Ca free

PHOSPHATE BINDER (for use in ESRD)
Drug: Take c̄ or immediately after meals.
Do not swallow tab whole, chew completely.
Diet: Low phosphate diet.
Oral/GI: <u>N/V</u>, <u>abdominal pain</u>, <u>diarrhea</u>, <u>constipation</u>.
S/Cond: Caution c̄ lactation. 99% serum pro bound but little drug is absorbed.
Not for children - drug deposited into developing bone/growth plate.

Caution c̄ acute peptic ulcer, ulcerative colitis, Crohn's or bowel obstruction.
Pregnancy: Category C.
Other: Headache, <u>dialysis graft occlusion</u>, hypotension.
Blood/Serum: ↓ <u>PHOSPHATE</u>, ↓ <u>PTH</u>. **Monitor:** P levels

Lantus
  insulin glargine

ANTIDIABETIC, HYPOGLYCEMIC   See **insulin p 175**
  Long acting form. Do not mix c̄ any other insulin.

lapatinib
  Tykerb
  Tab- lactose

ANTINEOPLASTIC (Advanced Breast Cancer), Kinase Inhibitor
  Used c̄ **capecitabine** for HER-2 & epidermal growth factor
  type 1 positive cancer. Effects are for the combination of both drugs.
  Drug: Take once a day 1 hr before or after a meal
  to allow lower drug dose.
  Diet: Avoid grapefruit/related citrus, see p 390. Avoid SJW, see p 286.
  Oral/GI: <u>NAUSEA/VOMITING</u>, <u>dyspepsia</u>, <u>stomatitis</u>, <u>DIARRHEA</u>.
  S/Cond: Not c̄ lactation. Caution c̄ severe ↓ hepatic func.
  > 99% serum pro bound. Correct hypokalemia or hypomagnesemia
  prior to drug use. **Pregnancy:** Category D.
  Other: <u>PALMAR-PLANTAR</u> <u>ERYTHRODYSESTHESIA</u>, <u>RASH</u>, <u>dry skin</u>,
  <u>musculoskeletal pain/inflammation</u>, <u>back pain</u>, <u>dyspnea</u>, <u>insomnia</u>,
  ↑ QT interval. Rare- hepatotoxicity, ↓ LVEF, interstitial lung disease or
  pneumonitis.
  Blood/Serum: ↓ <u>HEMOGLOBIN</u>, ↓ <u>NEUTROPHILS</u>, ↓ <u>platelets</u>, ↑ <u>ALT</u>, ↑ <u>AST</u>,
  ↑ <u>BILIRUBIN</u>.
  Monitor: Prior to use & periodically- ECG, hepatic func, electrolytes, LVEF,
  CBC c̄ diff. For S/S of pulmonary disease.

Larodopa
  previous brand name

ANTIPARKINSON   See **levodopa p 192**

Lasix
  furosemide

DIURETIC, ANTIHYPERTENSIVE   See **Diuretics, loop p 114**

Latuda

ANTIPSYCHOTIC (Second Generation)   See **lurasidone p 201**

L

Lazanda	ANALGESIC, Narcotic, Opioid	See **fentanyl p 139**

Lescol/Lescol XL
  fluvastatin

ANTIHYPERLIPIDEMIC (to ↓ chol or TG)

See **HMG-CoA Reductase Inhibitors p 164**

letrozole
  Femara

ANTINEOPLASTIC

See **Aromatase Inhibitors p 42**

leucovorin
  folinic acid
  Tab- cornstarch
  Parenteral
  100 mg vial-
  NaCl 80 mg/100
  350 mg vial- 140 mg
  some brands-
  benzyl alcohol

CHEMOTHERAPY RESCUE OR ADJUNCT   Oral or Parenteral (IV or IM)
  Methotrexate (MTX) rescue agent to ↓ side effects.
  5-Fluorouracil (5FU) adjunct to ↑ anti-cancer effect in colorectal cancer.
  Also used to treat megaloblastic anemia due to folic acid def.
  Drug: Do not use oral form c̄ GI toxicity, N/V or diarrhea.
  Diet: MTX rescue- Insure adequate hydration c̄ fluids 3L/day & $NaHCO_3$
  to maintain urine pH ≥ 7.0. **Nutr:** Anorexia.
  Oral/GI: <u>STOMATITIS</u>, <u>N/V</u>, <u>DIARRHEA</u>, constipation.
  S/Cond: Caution c̄ lactation. Not c̄ Vit b_{12} def anemia or Hx of seizures.
  Caution c̄ geriatric. Caution c̄ ↓ renal func.
  Pregnancy: Category C.
  Other: <u>Lethargy/fatigue</u>, syncope, allergic reaction. Rare- seizures.
  Urinary: Maintain pH ≥ 7.0.
  Monitor: CBC c̄ diff & platelets prior to each treatment,
  electrolytes & LFT c̄ **5FU**. Crea & **MTX** level daily, CBC c̄ diff c̄ **MTX**

Leukine
  sargramostim

COLONY STIMULATING FACTOR   See listing for **filgrastim p 142**
  Liquid- 1.1 % benzyl alcohol Pwd- no preservatives Parenteral only (IV)

leuprolide
  Lupron (SC) [a c]
  benzyl alcohol 9 mg/mL
  Lupron Depot (IM) [a b c d]
  D-mannitol
  Eligard (SC) [a]
  Depot

ANTINEOPLASTIC (Prostate Cancer),[a] ENDOMETRIOSIS,[b] CENTRAL
  PRECOCIOUS PUBERTY (CPP)[c] or UTERINE FIBROID TREATMENT[d]
  Hormone Analog of GnRH (Receptor Agonist)
                                          Parenteral only (IM or SC)
  Nutr: <u>Anorexia</u>, ↓ or ↑ wt, ↑ thirst. Fe suppl c̄ use as fibroid treatment.
  Oral/GI: Dry mouth, taste changes, dysphagia, <u>N/V</u>, GI bleeding,
  <u>constipation</u>, diarrhea.
  S/Cond: Not c̄ lactation. **Pregnancy:** Category X.

Other: <u>H</u>ot <u>flashes</u>, ↓ <u>bone density</u>, <u>headache</u>, <u>vaginitis</u>, <u>amenorrhea</u>, <u>peripheral edema</u>, <u>dizziness</u>, <u>bone/joint pain</u>, <u>breast pain</u>, <u>asthenia</u>, <u>insomnia</u>, depression, gynecomastia, testicular pain/atrophy, CHF, arrhythmia, palpitations, ECG changes,[6] phlebitis, muscle pain, dyspnea, anxiety, blurred vision, peripheral neuropathy, mood swings, acne, hair loss, hirsutism. Rare - CHF.[6]

Blood/Serum: ↓ <u>*TESTOSTERONE*</u>, ↓ <u>*ESTROGEN*</u>, <u>anemia</u>, ↓ WBC, ↑ <u>AST</u>, ↑ <u>LDH</u>, ↑ <u>alk phos</u>, ↑ <u>Ca</u>, ↑ <u>TG</u>, ↑ <u>chol</u>, ↑ <u>LDL</u>, ↓ <u>HDL</u>, ↓ glucose, ↑ uric acid.

Urinary: <u>Dysuria</u>, ↑ frequency, obstruction, blood.

Monitor: PSA, testosterone in prostate cancer pt.

levalbuterol
  Xopenex Inhalation Soln
  Xopenex HFA Inhalation Aerosol
	ANTIASTHMA, BRONCODILATOR
	R-isomer of **albuterol**
		See listing for **albuterol p 25**

Levaquin	ANTIBIOTIC, Fluoroquinolone	See **levofloxacin p 194**
Levbid (SR)	ANTISPASMODIC, ANTICHOLINERGIC	See **hyoscyamine p 169**
Levemir **insulin detemir**	ANTIDIABETIC, HYPOGLYCEMIC, Analog	See **insulin p 175**

levetiracetam
  Keppra
  Tab
  Soln-
   maltitol 300 mg/mL,
   K acesulfame
  IV- single use vial

ANTIEPILEPTIC (Adjunctive Treatment)   Oral or Parenteral (IV)

Drug: Take s̄ regard to food. PI states do not crush or chew tab, but crushing tab & mixing c̄ food or enteral formula did not affect levels.[130]

Nutr: Anorexia. **S/Cond:** Not c̄ lactation. Caution c̄ ↓ renal func. Pediatric dose based on body wt.

Pregnancy: Category C.

Other: <u>Drowsiness</u>, <u>asthenia</u>, <u>dizziness</u>, <u>infection</u>, headache, amnesia, anxiety, ataxia, depression, emotional lability, paresthesia, ↑ cough, pharyngitis, rhinitis, sinusitis, double vision, hair loss, pancreatitis. Rare- bone marrow suppression, suicidal thinking & behavior.

Urinary: Alb.

Blood/Serum: ↓ RBC, ↓ Hb, ↓ HCT, ↓ WBC, ↓ neutrophils, ↓ platelets.

Monitor: Baselione CBC & renal func, then as needed.[26]

levocarnitine
  L-carnitine
  Carnitor
  Tab
  Soln- sucrose
  Sugar Free Soln-
    saccharin Na
  Vial- preservative free

NUTRITIONAL SUPPLEMENT to correct carnitine def   Amino Acid Derivative
  Oral (Primary or Secondary Carnitine def or cyclic vomiting treatment)
  Parenteral (IV) (Dialysis-Related Carnitine def)
  IV- PEDIATRIC CARDIOMYOPATHY TREATMENT[26]
    (idiopathic or due to carnitine def)
Drug: Take c̄ or after meals & ingest slowly to ↓ GI effects.
May mix soln c̄ drink or liquid food.
Take in evenly spaced divided doses 3-4X/day.
Warning- D,L-carnitine inhibits L-carnitine & can cause def.[7]
Diet: Treat L-carnitine def c̄ suppl & diet high in CHO & low fat.[41]
Oral/GI: Taste changes, transient N/V, gastritis, cramps, diarrhea.
S/Cond: Manufacturer states not c̄ lactation. Occurs naturally in breast milk.
Caution c̄ seizures. Caution c̄ ↓ hepatic func.[93]
Caution c̄ ESRD- only IV form indicated c̄ dialysis.
Caution c̄ thyroid dysfunction- carnitine acts as a peripheral thyroid hormone.[93]
Pregnancy: Category B.
Other: Drug body odor, HTN, headache, ↑ muscle mass, blurred vision,
hypercalcemia. Rare- seizures.
Blood/Serum: ↑ Ca. IV- Slightly ↓ TG, ↓ chol, ↓ LDL, ↑ HDL.
Monitor: Blood chem, carnitine level, TG,[13] free fatty acids.[13]

levocetirizine
  Xyzal
  Tab- lactose
  Soln- maltitol, saccharin

ANTIHISTAMINE for Allergic Rhinitis or Chronic Urticaria
  Active enantiomer of **cetirizine**   See **cetirizine p 81**

levodopa
  Dopar
  (previous brand name)
  Cap- tartrazine,
   lactose
  Larodopa
  (previous brand name)
  Tab- cornstarch

ANTIPARKINSON, Also for herpes zoster (shingles) pain or restless leg syndrome
Drug: Take at least 1/2 hr before meals to ↑ abs. May take c̄ low pro
food or juice if GI distress occurs. Not directly c̄ high pro food,
amino acids or protein hydolysates. Protein re-distribution diet of 5:1 to
7:1 CHO to pro c̄ most pro in evening, may stabilize
drug effects & ↓ motor fluctuations.[35]
Diet: Limit Pyr to < 5 mg/day (may ↓ drug effect).[1] Take Fe suppl or
MVI c̄ minerals separately (Fe ↓ abs of drug). Caution- Fava beans

contain significant levodopa (content varies by crop conditions).[36]

Nutr: <u>ANOREXIA</u>, ↓ <u>wt</u>, ↑ wt. Aromatic amino acids compete c̄ drug for abs both in the intestine & at the blood/brain barrier.

Oral/GI: <u>Dry mouth</u>, TASTE LOSS, <u>excessive salivation</u>, dark saliva, <u>bitter taste</u>, <u>teeth grinding</u>, <u>dysphagia</u>, NAUSEA/VOMITING (80%), <u>epigastric distress</u>, constipation, diarrhea, flatulence. Rare- GI ulcers & bleeding.

S/Cond: Not c̄ lactation. Caution c̄ ↓ renal func.[58] Not c̄ narrow angle glaucoma. Caution c̄ open angle glaucoma.
Caution c̄ cardiovascular, pulmonary, hepatic or endocrine disease. Caution c̄ geriatric, Alzheimer's, asthma or peptic ulcer.

Pregnancy: Category C.[23]

Other: <u>DYSKINESIA</u> c̄ LT use, FLUSHING, ORTHOSTATIC HYPOTENSION, <u>dizziness</u>, <u>ataxia</u>, <u>neuropathy</u>, <u>headache</u>, <u>weakness</u>, <u>insomnia</u>, <u>fatigue</u>, psychosis, compulsion, depression c̄ suicidal tendencies, rash, ↑ sweating, dark sweat, blurred vision, palpitations, hand tremor.

Blood/Serum: Infrequent- ↓ Hb, ↓ HCT. Transient ↑ BUN, ↑ AST, ↑ ALT, ↑ alk phos, ↑ LDH, ↑ bil, ↓ K, ↓ WBC, ↑ homocysteine, ↑ CPK. Rare- + Coombs' test c̄ LT use.

Urinary: Dark color, blood, WBC. False + glucose ($CuSO_4$) or false negative (glucose oxidase)[6]. <u>Retention</u>, ↑ frequency, UTI.

Monitor: CBC, hepatic, renal & cardiovascular func.

---

levodopa & carbidopa
 Sinemet
 Tab- starch
 Sinemet-CR (SR)
 Tab
 Parcopa (ODT)
 aspartame =
 phenylalanine 3.4 mg in
 10/100 & 25/100 Tabs,
 8.4 mg in 25/250 Tab,
 mannitol

ANTIPARKINSON   See **levodopa above**

Carbidopa c̄ **levodopa** ↑ availability of **levodopa** to the brain by ↓ peripheral decarboxylation of **levodopa** to dopamine. Lower doses of **levodopa** are needed. Lower dose ↓ incidence of <u>N/V</u> (15%), anorexia, constipation & other side effects. **Carbidopa** usually prevents negative Pyr effect with less than 10-25 mg Pyr/day.
Higher doses of Pyr may require extra **carbidopa**.

Drug: May take CR tab c̄ meals, food delays abs, but ↑ peak plasma levels. Do not crush or chew CR tab. May break CR 50/200 tab in half.
Dissolve ODT on tongue c̄ or s̄ liquid, swallow saliva.

Pregnancy: Category C.

L

levofloxacin ANTIBIOTIC, Fluoroquinolone Oral or Parenteral (IV)
  Levaquin L-isomer of **ofloxacin**
  Tab **Drug:** Take tab s̄ regard to food. Take soln 1 hr before or 2 hr after
  IV Vial- eating. Take c̄ 8 oz water. Not c̄ orange juice- ↓ drug levels.[3]
   preservative free **Diet:** Insure liberal fluid intake/hydration. Milk/dairy product does not affect drug.
  Soln- sucrose, sucralose, Take tab or soln at least 2 hr before or 2 hr after antacids, Mg, Ca, Fe or
   ascorbic acid, Zn suppl, MVI c̄ minerals,[3] Ca fortified juice[114] or oral enteral product/TF.[39]
   propylene glycol, **Oral/GI:** Taste loss, <u>N</u>/V, dyspepsia, abdominal pain, <u>diarrhea</u>,
   benzyl alcohol constipation, flatulence. Rare- pseudomembranous colitis.
    S/Cond: Not c̄ lactation. Caution c̄ diabetes[13]- ↑ or ↓ glucose.[7]
    Caution c̄ ↓ renal func or seizures. May crush tab for TF, but
    separate from enteral product by ≥ 2 hr.[39] **Pregnancy:** Category C.
    Other: <u>Headache</u>, insomnia, dizziness, dyspnea, vaginitis, fatigue, rash.
    Rare- confusion, CNS toxicity, tendon rupture, tendonitis, joint pain, seizures,
    allergic reaction, anaphylaxis, SJS, TEN, jaundice, arrhythmias, phototoxicity.
    Blood/Serum: ↓ glucose, ↓ WBC. < 1%- ↑ glucose, ↑ ALT, ↑ AST,
    dyscrasias, ↑ or ↓ K. **Urinary:** False positive opiate tests.
    Monitor: Hepatic & renal func & CBC c̄ diff c̄ LT use. Glucose in diabetic.

levothyroxine THYROID HORMONE (T$_4$) See **thyroid p 313**
  Levothroid, Levoxyl, Synthroid, Unithroid

Levsin previous brand name ANTISPASMODIC, ANTICHOLINERGIC See **hyoscyamine p 169**

Lexapro ANTIDEPRESSANT, SSRI See listing for **citalopram p 86**
  escitalopram Tab S-isomer of **citalopram**
  Soln- sorbitol, propylene glycol

Lexiva ANTIRETROVIRAL (HIV/AIDS), Protease Inhibitor
    See **fosamprenavir p 151**

Lexxel ANTIHYPERTENSIVE, Combination drug
  Tab- lactose, castor oil **felodipine** (SR) & **enalapril** See **felodipine p 137**
    See **Angiotensin Converting Enzyme Inhibitors p 36**

| **Lialda** | ANTIINFLAMMATORY (in ulcerative colitis) | |
| Tab- once daily | | See **mesalamine p 209** |

| **Librium** | ANTIANXIETY | See **Benzodiazepines p 54** |
| chlordiazepoxide | | |

linagliptin ANTIDIABETIC AGENT, Incretin Enhancer
  Tradjenta DPP-4 (dipeptidyl-peptidase-4) Inhibitor
Tab- mannitol, pregelatinized starch, corn starch See listing for **sitagliptin p 293**

linezolid ANTIBIOTIC, Oxazolidinone Oral or Parenteral (IV)
  Zyvox
  Tab- cornstarch,
    Na starch glycolate
  Pwd for Susp-
    sucrose, mannitol,
    xanthan gum,
    aspartame = 20 mg
    phenylalanine/ 5mL,
    8.5 mg (0.4 mEq) Na/5 mL
  IV soln
    Na- 0.38 mg/mL

> **Drug:** Take s̄ regard to food.
> **Diet:** Avoid significant amounts (> 100 mg/meal) of high tyramine food, see p 383.
> Not c̄ SJW, see p 286.
> **Nutr:** Weak MAOI- potential interaction c̄ pressor agents & ↑ BP.
> **Oral/GI:** Oral candidiasis, taste changes, tongue discoloration, dyspepsia,
> N/V, <u>diarrhea</u>, bleeding. Rare- pseudomembranous colitis.
> **S/Cond:** Avoid alcohol.[12] Caution c̄ lactation. Caution c̄ seizures.
> Not c̄ severe ↓ hepatic func.[26] Not c̄ catheter related infection.
> **Pregnancy:** Category C.
> **Other:** <u>Headache</u>, insomnia, dizziness, fever,rash,
> fungal infection/overgrowth, HTN, dyspnea.
> Rare- bone marrow suppression, lactic acidosis, seizures, optic or
> peripheral neuropathy,[26] pancreatitis,[12]
> serotonin syndrome (c̄ antidepressant use).
> **Blood/Serum:** ↓ Hb, ↓ platelets, ↓ WBC, ↓ neutrophils, ↓ K, ↑ <u>AST</u>,
> ↑ <u>ALT</u>, ↑ LDH, ↑ bil, ↑ alk phos, ↑ amylase, ↑ lipase, ↑ BUN.
> **Monitor:** Weekly CBC & platelets, especially c̄ use > 2 wk.

| **Lioresal** | ANTISPASMODIC | See **baclofen p 50** |

| **Lipitor** | ANTIHYPERLIPIDEMIC (to ↓ chol or TG) | |
| atorvastatin | | See **HMG-CoA Reductase Inhibitors p 164** |

liraglutide
Victoza
Pre filled
multi-dose pen

ANTIHYPERGLYCEMIC, Adjunct to Diet & Exercise to Improve Glycemic Control in Adults with Type 2 Diabetes Mellitus
Glucagon like Peptide Receptor Agonist, Incretin Mimetic
Parenteral Only (SC)

Drug: Inject SC in abdomen, thigh, or upper arm once daily s̄ regard to meals.

Diet: Prescribed diabetic diet. ↓ cal if wt loss needed.

Nutr: ↓ appetite, anorexia, ↓ wt.

Oral/GI: ↓ *GASTRIC EMPTYING*, NAUSEA, diarrhea, constipation, vomiting, dyspepsia.

S/Cond: Caution c̄ alcohol, Not c̄ lactation. Not as first line therapy. Not c̄ personal or family Hx of thyroid C-cell tumors, including medullary thyroid carcinoma (MTC), not c̄ Multiple Neoplastic Syndrome Type 2 (MEN 2). Caution c̄ mild to severe ↓ renal or ↓ hepatic func. Caution c̄ pre-existing gastroparesis or pancraetitis. Avoid dehydration. NOT for Type 1 diabetes or diabetic ketoacidosis.

Pregnancy: Category C.

Other: Headache, fatigue, hypoglycemia (may be severe- ↑ risk c̄ sulfonylurea). Rare- acute pancreatitis, acute renal failure requiring dialysis. Production of antiliraglutide antibodies (may affect glycemic response to drug).

Blood/Serum: ↓ *RANDOM FASTING* & *POSTPRANDIAL GLUCOSE*, ↑ *INSULIN* (in response to hyperglycemia), ↓ *POSTPRANDIAL GLUCAGON*, ↑ bil, crea.

Urinary: ↓ *GLUCOSE*.

Monitor: Serum glucose, HbA1_C, renal func, body wt.

---

lisdexamfetamine
Vyvanse Cap

ADHD TREATMENT   See listing for **amphetamines p 33**
pro-drug of **dextroamphetamine**

---

lisinopril
Prinivil/Prinzide
Zestril/Zestoretic

ANTIHYPERTENSIVE   See **Angiotensin Converting Enzyme Inhibitors p 36**
Prinzide & **Zestoretic** also contain **hydrochlorothiazide,** see **p 166**

lithium carbonate (Li)
  Eskalith
  Cap- lactose,
   benzyl alcohol
  Lithobid (SR)
  Tab- Na starch glycolate,
   sorbitol,
   propylene glycol

  lithium citrate
  Syrup- sugar free,
   0.3% alcohol, sorbitol,
   propylene glycol

ANTIMANIC (to treat Bipolar Disorder)
  Drug: Take c̄ meals to ↓ GI distress. Swallow SR tab whole.
  Diet: Drink 2-3 L fluid/day. Na intake affects renal clearance of drug 30-50%.
  Consistent Na intake stabilizes drug levels, see p 8.
  Limit xanthine/caffeine- may ↓ Li level,[9b] see p 379.
  Avoid iodine suppl- ↑ risk of hypothyroidism.
  Nutr: ↑ THIRST, ↑ WT, anorexia, ↓ wt.
  Oral/GI: DRY MOUTH, metallic taste, N/V, bloating, diarrhea.
  S/Cond: Limit alcohol.[9b] Not c̄ lactation.
  Syrup precipitates TF.[8] Caution c̄ ↓ renal func or urinary retention.[17]
  Not c̄ severe cardiac or renal disease or dehydration. Caution c̄ geriatric.
  Pregnancy: Category D.[13]
  Other: FATIGUE, DROWSINESS, WEAKNESS, CONFUSION, HAND TREMOR,
  HEADACHE, EDEMA, DIZZINESS, diabetes insipidus,[31] ↑ muscle irritability,
  ataxia, goiter, hypothyroidism, acne, seizures. Rare- nephrotoxicity,
  hyperthyroidism, hyperparathyroidism, pseudotumor cerebri.
  Blood/Serum: ↑ WHITE BLOOD CELLS, ↑ PLATELETS, ↓ T_4, ↓ T_3, ↑ TSH,
  ↑ Ca, ↑ P, ↑ PTH, ↑ glucose, ↑ Mg, ↑ Na.[31]
  Urinary: POLYURIA, incontinence, pro, glucose.
  Monitor: Baseline ECG. Baseline & during use- thyroid & renal func,
  CBC c̄ diff, platelets, Na, K, Li levels, Ca, P. Urinalysis.[7] Wt.

Livalo
  pitavastatin

ANTIHYPERLIPIDEMIC   See **HMG-CoA Reductase Inhibitors p 164**

Lodine/Lodine XL
  generic equivalents

ANALGESIC, ANTIARTHRITIC, NSAID   See **etodolac p 131**

Lodosyn
  carbidopa
  Tab- starch

ANTIPARKINSON adjunct   See **levodopa** & **carbidopa p 193**
  Prescribed c̄ **levodopa** or c̄ **carbidopa-levodopa** (eg **Sinemet**),
  particularly to ↓ **levodopa** induced N/V.

Loestrin
Loestrin 24 Fe

ORAL CONTRACEPTIVE   See **Oral Contraceptives p 237**

L

| **Lofibra** | ANTIHYPERLIPIDEMIC, Fibrate | See **fenofibrate p 138** |

Lo Loestrin FE — ORAL CONTRACEPTIVE — See **Oral Contraceptives p 237**

lomefloxacin — ANTIBIOTIC, Fluoroquinolone — See listing for **levofloxacin p 194**
  Maxaquin — Tab- lactose — **Other:** Higher incidence of photosensitivity.

Lomotil — ANTIDIARRHEAL — See **diphenoxylate with atropine p 112**

Lo/Ovral 28 — ORAL CONTRACEPTIVE — See **Oral Contraceptives p 237**

loperamide — ANTIDIARRHEAL, Antiperistaltic Agent
  Imodium A-D — Also indicated to reduce volume of discharge from ileostomies.
  Tab — **Diet:** Diarrhea may ↑ fluid & electrolyte needs.
  Imodium A-D — Insure adequate fluid intake/hydration.
  Adult & Children New Liquids **EZ Chews** tab- Take only on empty stomach (1 hr before or 2 hr after meal).
  propylene glycol, — **Oral/GI:** Dry mouth, N/V, abdominal pain, bloating, constipation.
  sucralose, xanthan gum, — **S/Cond:** Caution c̄ lactation. Not c̄ pseudomembranous colitis, or other
  simethicone — enteroinvasive GI infections,[7] ulcerative colitis, fever, blood or mucus in
  Imodium A-D EZ Chews — stool. Caution c̄ ↓ hepatic func- ↑ risk of CNS toxicity.
  Tab- confectioners sugar, — Caution c̄ children or geriatric- may mask dehydration or electrolyte
  sucralose, acesulfame K, — imbalance. 97% serum pro bound.
  dextrose — **Pregnancy:** Category B.
    Other: Drowsiness, dizziness, rash, fatigue.
    Rare- allergic reaction/rash, toxic megacolon.
    Monitor: Fluid & electrolytes.
  Imodium Advanced also contains **simethicone** see p 292
  Chew Tab- simethicone 125 mg, confectionary sugar, dextrates, saccharin, sorbitol
  Tab- simethicone 125 mg, acesulfame K, Na starch glycolate

Lopid — ANTIHYPERLIPIDEMIC, Fibrate — See **gemfibrozil p 155**

lopinavir/ritonavir
Kaletra
Tab
Cap- propylene glycol,
  sorbitol
Soln- 42.4% alcohol,
  acesulfame K,
  corn syrup, menthol,
  peppermint oil,
  propylene glycol,
  saccharin Na, castor oil

ANTIRETROVIRAL (HIV/AIDS), Protease Inhibitors
Drug: Take soln or cap c̄ food to ↑ bioavailability.
Tab may be taken s̄ regard to food, but do not chew, break or crush.
Diet: Avoid SJW, see p 286. Moderate to high fat meal significantly ↑ drug level.
Oral/GI: <u>N/V</u>, dyspepsia, <u>abdominal pain</u>, diarrhea.
S/Cond: Not c̄ lactation. 98-99% serum pro bound. Caution c̄ diabetes
or ↓ hepatic func. **Pregnancy:** Category C.
Other: <u>Headache</u>, <u>asthenia</u>, rash, pancreatitis, edema.
May ↑ risk of lipodystrophy, hepatotoxicity or diabetes.
Blood/Serum: ↑ <u>TG</u>, ↑ <u>chol</u>, ↑ GGT, ↑ <u>ALT</u>, ↑ <u>AST</u>, ↑ bil,
↑ <u>amylase</u>, ↓ platelets, ↓ neutrophils, ↑ glucose, ↑ uric acid, ↓ Na, ↑ P.
Monitor: Baseline & periodic hepatic func, glucose, lipids.

Lopressor   ANTIHYPERTENSIVE   See **metoprolol p 215**

loratadine
Claritin (24 hr)
Tab- lactose, cornstarch
Children's Fruit Flavor
  Syrup- sucrose,
  propylene glycol
Children's Grape Flavor
  Syrup- maltitol,
  propylene glycol, sorbitol,
  sucralose
Children's Chew Tab-

ANTIHISTAMINE   H$_1$-Receptor Antagonist
Drug: Take once a day s̄ regard to food.
Dissolve ODT on tongue c̄ or s̄ liquid, swallow saliva.
Diet: No interaction c̄ grapefruit/related citrus, see p 390.
Nutr: ↑ appetite, ↑ wt, ↑ thirst, anorexia.
Oral/GI: Dry mouth, altered taste, tooth disorder, stomatitis,
abdominal pain, diarrhea.
S/Cond: Not c̄ lactation. 97-99% serum pro bound.
Caution c̄ ↓ hepatic func or ↓ renal func. **Pregnancy:** Category B.
Other: Headache, drowsiness, fatigue, tachycardia, insomnia,
nervousness, hyperkinesia, wheezing, nosebleed. Rash in children.[6]

aspartame = 1.4 mg phenylalanine, mannitol, Na starch glycolate
Claritin Reditabs ODT- mannitol, gelatin
Alavert ODT- aspartame (phenylalanine 8.4 mg/Tab), corn syrup solids, mannitol, modified starch,
Na bicarbonate

lorazepam   ANTIANXIETY   See **Benzodiazepines p 54**
Ativan

L

losartan Cozaar/Hyzaar	ANTIHYPERTENSIVE	See **Angiotensin II Receptor Antagonists p 38** **Hyzaar** also contains **hydrochlorothiazide**, see **p 166**
Lotensin/Lotensin HCT benazapril	ANTIHYPERTENSIVE	See **Angiotensin Converting Enzyme Inhibitors p 36** **Lotensin HCT** also contains **hydrochlorothiazide**, see **p 166**
Lotrel Cap- lactose, cornstarch, potato starch, castor oil **amlodipine** & **benazepril**	ANTIHYPERTENSIVE, ANTIANGINA	See **amlodipine p 32** Combination Ca Channel Blocker & ACE Inhibitor (**benazepril**) See **Angiotensin Converting Enzyme Inhibitors p 36**
lovastatin Altoprev Mevacor	ANTIHYPERLIPIDEMIC	See **HMG-CoA Reductase Inhibitors p 164**
Lovaza	ANTIHYPERLIPIDEMIC to reduce triglyceride levels	See **omega-3 fatty acids p 234**
Lovenox	ANTICOAGULANT, low molecular wt **heparin**	See **enoxaparin p 124**
Low-Ogestrel	ORAL CONTRACEPTIVE	See **Oral Contraceptives p 237**

loxapine **Loxitane** previous brand name Cap- lactose Oral Soln (Canada)- propylene glycol Tab (Canada)- lactose Vial (Canada)- propylene glycol	ANTIPSYCHOTIC, Dibenzoxazepine Oral or Parenteral (IM) **Drug:** Take c̄ food or 8 oz water or milk to ↓ GI distress.[13] Dilute soln in at least 60 mL orange juice.[13] **Nutr:** ↑ or ↓ wt. Polydipsia. **Oral/GI:** <u>Dry mouth</u>, ↑ salivation, N/V, constipation. **S/Cond:** Avoid alcohol. Not c̄ lactation. ↑ risk of dental problems, see p 11 & 15. Caution c̄ seizures or ↓ hepatic func.[13] Caution c̄ cardiac disease or glaucoma. **Pregnancy:** Category C.[13] **Other:** EPS, <u>akathisia</u>, <u>drowsiness</u>, <u>blurred</u> <u>vision</u>, <u>orthostatic</u> <u>hypotension</u>, <u>confusion</u>, HTN, dizziness, tachycardia, insomnia, headache, ataxia, rash, gynecomastia, weakness.[6] ↑ mortality in geriatrics c̄ dementia-related psychosis. <u>Tardive</u> <u>dyskinesia</u> c̄ LT use. Rare- NMS, seizures, galactorrhea, ↑ QT interval. **Blood/Serum:** ↑ alk phos, ↑ AST, ↑ ALT. Rare- dyscrasias, ↑ prolactin. **Urinary:** Retention. **Monitor:** CBC, hepatic func.

Lozol
  indapamide
	ANTIHYPERTENSIVE, DIURETIC See listing for **hydrochlorothiazide p 166**
	    Tab- lactose, cornstarch, starch
	    Blood/Serum: Does **not** cause ↑ chol.

L-thyroxine   THYROID HORMONE (T₄)   See **thyroid p 313**

lubiprostone
  Amitiza
  Cap- medium chain
  triglycerides, sorbitol

CHLORIDE CHANNEL ACTIVATOR for chronic idiopathic constipation
    Drug: Take c̄ food to ↓ nausea.
    Diet: High fiber c̄ 1500-2000 mL fluid/day to prevent constipation.
    Oral/GI: Dry mouth, dyspepsia, ↓ GASTRIC EMPTYING,[9a] NAUSEA, vomiting,
    GERD, abdominal pain, diarrhea, flatulence.
    S/Cond: Not c̄ lactation. 94% serum pro bound. **Pregnancy:** Category C.
    Other: Headache, fatigue, dyspnea, back pain, edema. **Urinary:** UTI.

Lunesta   SLEEP AID, Non-Benzodiazepine   See **eszopiclone p 129**

Lupron   ANTINEOPLASTIC, Hormone   See **leuprolide p 190**

lurasidone
  Latuda
  Tab- mannitol,
  pregelantinized starch

ANTIPSYCHOTIC (Second Generation)
    Drug: Take c̄ food (minimum 350 cal). Food ↑ drug abs. Take c̄ full glass water.
    Diet: Caution c̄ grapefruit/related citrus, see p 390. Avoid SJW, see p 286.
    Nutr: ↓ appetite.**Oral/GI:** N/V, dyspepsia, ↑ salivation, abdominal pain,
    diarrhea, dysphagia, gastritis.
    S/Cond: Avoid alcohol. Caution c̄ lactation. 99% serum pro bound-
    hypoalbuminemia (< 3 g/dL) may ↑ drug effects. Caution c̄ moderate to
    severe ↓ renal or hepatic func. Caution c̄ seizures. Caution c̄ dysphagia.
    Caution c̄ geriatric. ↑ risk of mortality in geriatrics c̄ dementia-related psychosis.
    Pregnancy: Category B. **Other:** SEDATION, EPS, akathisia, agitation,
    anxiety, dizziness, dystonia, insomnia, angina pectoris, tachycardia,
    bradycardia, CVA, HTN, orthostatic hypotension, fatigue, restlessness,
    syncope, pruritis, rash, blurred vision, back pain.
    Blood/Serum: ↑ prolactin, ↑ crea, ↑ CPK, ↑ ALT, ↑ AST, anemia,
    Monitor: Baseline weight then at 4, 8 and 12 wks after initiating or
    changing dose. Baseline BP, FBS, lipids, then at 3 months, then annually.
    Baseline and monthly CBC in pts c̄ hx of drug induced leukopenia/neutropenia.

L

Drug	Classification	Reference
Luride	MINERAL SUPPLEMENT	See **fluoride p 146**
Luvox/Luvox CR (**Luvox** previous brand name)	OCD or SOCIAL ANXIETY DISORDER TREATMENT, SSRI Also used to treat depression	See **fluvoxamine p 149**
Lybrel (stops all menstruation) - 50% have breakthrough bleeding	ORAL CONTRACEPTIVE	See **Oral Contraceptives p 237** First continuous use form
Lyrica **pregabalin** Cap- lactose, cornstarch	ANALGESIC for Diabetic Peripheral Neuropathy or Post Herpetic Neuralgia FIBROMYALGIA TREATMENT, ANTIEPILEPTIC ADJUNCT	See listing for **gabapentin p 152**
Maalox, Liquid	ANTACID, ANTIFLATULENT Combination drug	See **aluminum hydroxide & magnesium hydroxide p 29** See **simethicone p 292**
Maalox Max Liquid	ANTACID, ANTIFLATULENT Combination drug **S/Cond:** Thickens TF.[8]	See **aluminum hydroxide & magnesium hydroxide p 29** See **simethicone p 292**
Maalox Total Stomach Relief	ANTACID, ANTINAUSEANT	See **bismuth subsalicylate p 58**
Macrobid (SR) **Macrodantin**	ANTIBIOTIC, urinary macrocrystals	See **nitrofurantoin p 230**

magnesium
Magonate (Mg Gluconate)
Liquid- 54 mg (4.5 mEq)
 Mg/5 mL, sorbitol,
 3 g CHO/5 mL
Generic Mg gluconate
Tab- 27 mg (2.3 mEq) Mg
Mag-Ox 400 (MgO)
Tab- 241 mg (20.1 mEq) Mg
Slow-Mag (SR MgCl$_2$)
Tab- 64 mg (5.3 mEq) Mg,

MINERAL SUPPLEMENT, ANTACID, LAXATIVE, Osmotic   Oral or Parenteral (IV)
1 g Mg = 83.3 mEq (41.7 mmol) IV- Pre-eclampsia or eclampsia Treatment
Drug: As antacid- take after meals & HS. As Mg suppl- follow PI directions.
As laxative- take c̄ 8 oz water. Swallow SR form whole, do not crush or chew.
Diet: Take fiber, Fol or Fe suppl separately by at least 2 hr.
Do not take c̄ ↑ fiber, ↑ oxalate (see p 357) or ↑ phytate food (see p 358).
See Mg sources, p 386.
UL (mg/day) for <u>supplementary</u> Mg- Children 1-3 yr = **65**. 4-8 = **110**.
>8-70+ = **350**. Lactation = **350**.
Nutr: AI (mg/day) Infant 0-6 mo = **30**. 7-12 mo = **75**.
RDA (mg/day)- Children 1-3 yr = **80**. 4-8 = **130**. 9-13 = **240**.

$CaCO_3$ =
  113 mg Ca/Tab,
  187 mg Cl, starch
IV- Mg Sulfate
1 g = 97.5 mg (8.1 mEq) Mg

Males 14-18 = **410**. 19-30 = **400**. 31-70+ = **420**.
Females 14-18 = **360**. 19-30 = **310**. 31-70+ = **320**. Lactation = **310-360**.
Adequate Mg is essential for abs of Ca & deposition in bone, but
additional Mg does not ↑ Ca abs.[1] High Zn intake ↑ Mg excretion &
↓ Mg balance. [120] Hypomagnesemia from drug therapy may require ↑ doses.
Oral/GI: Chalky taste, N/V, cramps, diarrhea.
S/Cond: Safe for lactation at < 350 mg/day.[93] Caution c̄ ↓ renal func or
cardiac disease. Not c̄ ESRD. High alcohol intake ↑ Mg need by
↑ excretion.[13] Not c̄ hypocalcemia.
Pregnancy: Category B.[23] IV- Category A except last 2 hr before delivery.[26]
RDA = 350-400 mg/day. **UL** (mg/day) of supplementary Mg/day = **350** mg.
Other: ↓ BP in HTN. Hypotension, confusion, flushing, bradycardia.[93]
Blood/Serum: ↑ *Mg*. LT high dose- ↓ P.[1]
Monitor: Mg serum level c̄ use as suppl.

magnesium hydroxide
  Milk of Magnesia (MOM)
  Phillips' MOM
  0.12 mg Na/Tab or tsp
  Tab- sucrose, starch,
    129.7 mg (10.8 mEq)
    Mg/Tab
  Conc- 29% sorbitol,
    8% sucrose, 333.5 mg
    (27.78 mEq) Mg/5mL
  Liquid- original
    167 mg (13.91 mEq) Mg/5 mL

LAXATIVE (Osmotic), ANTACID
Drug: Take each dose c̄ 8 oz water or citrus juice (to improve taste).
Diet: High fiber c̄ 1500-2000 mL fluid/day to prevent constipation.
Take Fe or Fol suppl separately by at least 2 hr.[13]
Nutr: 15-30% of Mg is abs.
Oral/GI: Chalky taste, nausea, cramping, diarrhea.
Laxative dependence c̄ LT use.
S/Cond: Caution c̄ ↓ renal func- ↑ Mg.
Pregnancy: Avoid osmotic laxative use in pregnancy.[2]
Monitor: Electrolytes & Mg c̄ LT use.

maraviroc **Selzentry** Tab- Na starch glycolate, soy lecithin **Celsentri** (Canada)	ANTIRETROVIRAL (HIV/AIDS), CCR5 Antagonist for CCR5-tropic HIV-1 Entry Inhibitor For use c̄ other antiretroviral(s) **Drug:** Take s̄ regard to food. Swallow tab whole, do not chew, split or crush. **Diet:** Avoid SJW, see p 286. Caution c̄ grapefruit/related citrus, see p 390. **Oral/GI:** Stomatitis, esophageal candidiasis, abdominal pain, diarrhea, constipation. Rare- pseudomembranous colitis. **S/Cond:** Not c̄ lactation. Caution c̄ ↓ hepatic func, hepatitis B or C or ↓ renal func. Caution c̄ pt at risk of CV event. **Pregnancy:** Category B. **Other:** <u>URTI</u>, <u>cough</u>, influenza, sinusitis, rhinitis, breathing abnormalities, fever, herpes, dizziness, edema, musculoskeletal/joint symptoms, sleep disorder, rash, paresthesias, sensory abnormalities, lipodystrophy, HTN. Rare- hepatotoxicity, CV disorder, pneumonia, rhabdomyolysis, osteonecrosis, neoplasms, immune reconstitution syndrome. **Blood/Serum:** ↑ AST, ↓ neutrophils, ↑ CPK. **Urinary:** Bladder & urethral symptoms. **Monitor:** Baseline & periodic hepatic func.	
Marinol	ANTIEMETIC	See **dronabinol p 118**
Marplan isocarboxazid	ANTIDEPRESSANT, MAOI Tab- lactose, cornstarch	See listing for **phenelzine p 252**
Mavik trandolapril	ANTIHYPERTENSIVE See **Angiotensin Converting Enzyme Inhibitors p 36**	
Maxalt/Maxalt MLT rizatriptan	ANTIMIGRAINE, Serotonin 5-HT$_1$ Receptor Agonist See **Antimigraine p 39**	
Maxaquin lomefloxacin Tab- lactose	ANTIBIOTIC, Fluoroquinolone **Other:** Higher incidence of photosensitivity.	See listing for **levofloxacin p 194**
Maxipime	ANTIBIOTIC**, cefepime**	See **cephalosporins p 80**
Maxzide/Maxzide 25 Tab	ANTIHYPERTENSIVE, DIURETIC Combination drug	See **triamterene p 322** See **hydrochlorothiazide p 166**

meclizine
  Antivert
  Tab- sucrose, starch
  Bonine
  Chew Tab- lactose,
  saccharin Na

ANTIEMETIC, ANTIVERTIGO, Antihistamine
  Oral/GI: Dry mouth/throat, constipation.
  S/Cond: Avoid alcohol. Caution c̄ lactation. May inhibit lactation.[13]
  Caution c̄ glaucoma.[6]
  Pregnancy: Category B.
  Other: <u>Drowsiness</u>, fatigue, blurred vision.
  Urinary: Retention.

Medrol   CORTICOSTEROID, **methylprednisolone**   See **corticosteroids p 94**

medroxyprogesterone   HORMONE   See **progesterone p 265**

Mefoxin   ANTIBIOTIC, **cefoxitin**   See **cephalosporins p 80**

---

megestrol
  Megace
  Tab- lactose, cornstarch
  (original)
  Susp- sucrose,
  < 0.06% alcohol,
  xanthan gum
  Megace ES (nanocrystals)
  Concentrated Susp-
  < 0.06% alcohol,
  sucrose, docusate Na

APPETITE STIMULANT (Susp), ANTINEOPLASTIC (Tab), Hormone (progestin)
  Advanced Breast or Endometrium Cancer, Also used to treat Hot Flashes
  Drug: Take original Susp c̄ high fat meal- ↑ blood levels 600%
  Take Tab or ES Susp s̄ regard to food. May take c̄ food to ↓ GI distress.
  Nutr: ↑ <u>*APPETITE*</u>, ↑ <u>*WEIGHT*</u> (not from edema).
  Oral/GI: Nausea, dyspepsia.
  S/Cond: Not c̄ lactation. Caution c̄ diabetes, existing diabetes may be
  exacerbated- up to 10 fold ↑ glucose. [83] Caution c̄ ↓ renal func or
  geriatric. Caution c̄ bed-ridden pt- ↑ risk of thromboembolism.
  Pregnancy: Susp- Category X.
  Tab- Category D (not recommended in the first four months).
  Other: <u>EDEMA</u>, depression, headache, drowsiness, weakness, insomnia,
  paresthesia, HTN, thromboembolism/DVT, hot flashes, fever,
  ↓ bone density c̄ LT use. Adrenal suppression/insufficiency.[83]
  Rare- cardiomyopathy, hepatotoxicity,[12] CHF.
  Blood/Serum: ↑ <u>Na</u>, ↑ glucose, ↓ HDL, ↑ LDL, ↑ alk phos, ↑ bil, ↑ AST, ↑ ALT.
  Monitor: Renal func. Glucose in diabetics.

melatonin
  Melatonin
  multiple forms
  available

  Tab, Cap, Liquid,
  SR Tab, Lozenges,
  Tea

HORMONE, Natural Product, FDA orphan drug
To treat Circadian Rhythm Sleep Disorders in the totally blind
(Also used as sleep aid, to combat jet lag- not FDA approved)
Diet: Caffeine ↑ drug levels- generally not clinically significant.[3]
Drug: Take HS. Not for LT use.
Only pharmaceutical grade is available as an orphan drug.
Oral/GI: N/V, stomach discomfort, abdominal cramps.
S/Cond: Avoid alcohol or other sedating drugs/herbs. Not c̄ lactation.
Not for children. Caution c̄ HTN, seizures, depression, ↓ hepatic func
or diabetes (may ↑ glucose).[93] **Pregnancy:** Avoid use.
Other: _DROWSINESS_, "heavy head", dizziness, headache,
mild transient depression, mild anxiety, vivid dreams, tremor,
irritability, confusion, hypotension, hypothermia.
Blood/Serum: ↑ GH, ↓ LH, ↑ or ↓ oxytocin (dose dependent),
↑ or ↓ vasopressin (dose dependent).[93] ↑ glucose in diabetics.

meloxicam
  Mobic
  Tab- lactose
  Susp- sorbitol,
   xylitol, saccharin Na

ANTIARTHRITIC (Osteo or Rheumatoid Arthritis), NSAID
Drug: Take s̄ regard to food, but may take c̄ food
or milk to if GI distress occurs.
Diet: Caution c̄ GI irritants eg K suppl (↑ risk of GI irritation).
Limit caffeine to ↓ GI effects. Avoid or limit natural products which
affect coagulation (eg garlic, ginger, ginkgo, ginseng, horse chestnut).
Oral/GI: Stomatitis, GERD, dyspepsia, nausea, abdominal pain, diarrhea,
colitis, flatulence. GI ulcers & bleeding (may be sudden & serious).
S/Cond: Avoid alcohol. Not c̄ lactation. 99.4% serum pro bound.
Hypoalbuminemia (< 3 g/dL)- may ↑ drug effects.
Do dental care cautiously, see p 11 & 15. Not c̄ aspirin allergy.
Caution c̄ ↓ renal func, ↓ hepatic func, HTN, CHF or edema.
Not c̄ severe ↓ renal func. Not c̄ gastritis/ulcer. Not c̄ dehydration.
Pregnancy: Category C, but not recommended in pregnancy.
Category D in 3rd trimester due to ↑ risk to fetus & mother, including death.
Other: Headache, dizziness, edema, insomnia, confusion, drowsiness,
nervousness, tremor, URTI.

Rare- hepatitis, pancreatitis, syncope, seizures, SJS, TEN.
↑ risk of CV problems, eg HTN, CHF, MI, CVA.
Blood/Serum: ↑ AST, ↑ ALT, ↑ bil, ↑ GGT, ↑ BUN, ↑ crea,
↓ platelet aggregation. Anemia c̄ LT use. **Urinary:** Alb. Hematuria.[10]
Monitor: CBC, blood chem. Hepatic & renal func c̄ LT use.

melphalan
 Alkeran
 Tab

 Parenteral
 Vial-
 0.52 mL ethanol,
 propylene glycol
 6 mL/ 10 mL Vial

ANTINEOPLASTIC (Multiple Myeloma, Ovarian Cancer)
 Alkylating Agent, Nitrogen Mustard   Oral or Parenteral (IV)
 Diet: Insure adequate fluid intake/hydration. Food significantly ↓ bioavailability.
 Oral/GI: Stomatitis (rare), mild N/V, diarrhea.
 S/Cond: Not c̄ lactation. Do dental care cautiously, see p 11 & 15.
 Caution c̄ ↓ renal func or geriatric. **Pregnancy:** Category D.
 Other: BONE MARROW SUPPRESSION, hair loss, hypersensitivity reactions,
 leukemia, rash, ↓ ovarian or testicular func, amenorrhea.
 Rare- nephropathy, hepatitis, jaundice, pulmonary fibrosis, vasculitis.
 Blood/Serum: ↓ WHITE BLOOD CELLS, ↓ PLATELETS, anemia, ↑ uric acid.
 Rare- ↑ ALT, ↑ AST. **Urinary:** ↑ uric acid.
 Monitor: CBC c̄ diff & platelets prior to each dose. Renal func, uric acid.

memantine
 Namenda
 Tab- lactose
 Soln- sorbitol 70%,
 propylene glycol
 Namenda XR
 Cap- sugar spheres,
 polyethylene glycol,
 medium chain triglycerides,
 gelatin

ALZHEIMER'S DISEASE TREATMENT, NMDA Receptor Antagonist
 Moderate to Severe Alzheimer's, Also used to treat Vascular Dementia
 Drug: Take s̄ regard to food. Soln to be given by mouth c̄ syringe,
 do not mix c̄ other liquids. Swallow cap whole. Do not crush, chew
 or divide. Cap may be opened and contents sprinkled on applesauce.
 The entire contents of cap should be consumed. Do not divide dose.
 Diet: Diet or medication resulting in alkaline urine (eg predominantly
 milk/milk products, citrus fruit) ↑ drug blood levels due to ↓ excretion.
 Oral/GI: Vomiting, constipation. (Note- sorbitol in soln may ↑ risk of diarrhea).
 S/Cond: Caution c̄ lactation. Caution c̄ moderate ↓ renal func.
 Not c̄ severe ↓ renal func. **Pregnancy:** Category B.
 Other: Dizziness, confusion, headache, hallucinations, drowsiness,
 fatigue, cough, dyspnea, HTN, back pain.
 Urinary: ↑ pH > 8.0 ↓ drug clearance 80%. **Monitor:** Possibly renal func.

M

Menostar
low dose **estradiol** patch

HORMONE, To Prevent Osteoporosis

See **Hormone Therapy p 165**

meperidine
Demerol
Tab- starch
Syrup- glucose,
saccharin

ANALGESIC, Narcotic, Opioid   Oral or Parenteral (IM or IV)
(often used to prevent or ↓ acute infusion reactions to IV **amphotericin B**)[6]
Drug: Dilute syrup in 1/2 glass water. **Nutr:** Anorexia.
Oral/GI: Dry mouth, <u>N/V</u>, GI pain, <u>constipation</u>.
S/Cond: Avoid alcohol. Not c̄ lactation. May be habit forming c̄ LT use.
Caution c̄ ↓ hepatic func or ↓ renal func. Caution c̄ seizures, obesity,
hypothyroidism, asthma/bronchospasm, ↓ pulmonary func.
Caution c̄ geriatric or debilitated.[84]
Pregnancy: Not for use prior to labor.
Category D for LT high use or close to term.
Other: <u>Respiratory</u> <u>depression</u>, <u>drowsiness</u>, <u>dizziness</u>, <u>sedation</u>,
<u>weakness</u>, <u>hypotension</u>, <u>sweating</u>, headache, visual changes, confusion,
syncope, flushing, restlessness, trembling, tachycardia,
seizures (risk ↑ c̄ ESRD).[58]
Blood/Serum: ↑ amylase, ↑ lipase.
Urinary: Retention.

Mephyton

VITAMIN   See **vitamin K p 342**

meropenem
Merrem I.V.
90 mg (3.92 mEq) Na/g

ANTIBIOTIC, Carbapenem   Parenteral only (IV)
Oral/GI: Oral candidiasis, glossitis, N/V, <u>diarrhea</u>, constipation.
Rare- pseudomembranous colitis, GI bleeding.
S/Cond: Caution c̄ lactation. Caution c̄ ↓ renal func or seizures.
Dosage based on body wt for children < 50 kg.
Pregnancy: Category B.
Other: Headache, rash, apnea.
Rare- seizures, allergic reaction, anaphylaxis, SJS, TEN.
Blood/Serum: Hypoglycemia, anemia/ ↓ Hb/Hct.
< 1%- ↓ WBC, ↑ eosinophils, ↑ or ↓ platelets, ↑ BUN, ↑ crea, ↑ AST,
↑ ALT, ↑ alk phos, ↑ LDH, ↑ bil, ↓ K, ↓ PT/INR, ↓ PTT.
Urinary: RBC. **Monitor:** CBC c̄ diff, renal & hepatic func c̄ LT use.

mesalamine (5 ASA)   ANTI-INFLAMMATORY (in ulcerative colitis or Crohn's)   Oral or Rectal
  Asacol (DR)   **Drug:** Swallow tab/cap whole c̄ 8 oz water.
  Tab- lactose,   Do <u>not</u> break, chew or crush. Use rectal suppository HS.
  Na starch gycolate   **Nutr:** Anorexia, ↓ wt.
  Lialda (DR)   **Oral/GI:** N/V, dyspepsia, abdominal cramps, diarrhea, constipation, flatulence.
  Tab- Na starch gycolate   **S/Cond:** Caution c̄ lactation. Caution c̄ ↓ renal func or ↓ hepatic func.
  Pentasa (SR)   Not c̄ aspirin allergy.
  Cap- starch, sugar,   **Pregnancy:** Category B.
  castor oil   **Other:** <u>Headache</u>, weakness, rash, fever, pharyngitis,
  Canasa (rectal)   acute intolerance syndrome.
  Suppository   Rare- hepatitis, pancreatitis, pericarditis/myocarditis, nephropathy.
  Rowasa (rectal)   **Blood/Serum:** ↑ AST,↑ ALT, ↑ alk phos, ↑ BUN, ↑ crea, ↑ amylase, ↑ lipase.
  Enema   **Monitor:** Baseline & periodic renal func.[7]

Metadate CD/ER   ANTI-ADHD, ANTINARCOLEPSY, Stimulant See **methylphenidate p 214**

Metaglip   ORAL HYPOGLYCEMIC & ANTIHYPERGLYCEMIC AGENT
  Tab   Combination drug   See **sulfonylureas (glipizide) p 299**
    See **metformin p 210**

Metamucil   LAXATIVE, Bulk Forming   See **psyllium p 270**

metaxalone   SKELETAL MUSCLE RELAXANT, Sedative
  Skelaxin   **Drug:** May crush tab & mix c̄ food or liquid.
  Tab- cornstarch   **Nutr:** Anorexia. **Oral/GI:** Dry mouth, GI upset, abdominal pain, N/V.
    S/Cond: Avoid alcohol. Not c̄ lactation.
    Not c̄ anemia, severe ↓ hepatic func or ↓ renal func. Caution c̄ geriatric.[84]
    Pregnancy: Category C.
    Other: <u>Drowsiness</u>, <u>dizziness</u>, headache, confusion, nervousness,
    irritability, paradoxical stimulation, rash. Rare- hepatotoxicity, nephrotoxicity.
    Blood/Serum: ↑ AST, ↑ ALT, ↑ alk phos, ↑ bil, ↑ cephalin flocculation.
    Rare- hemolytic anemia, ↓ WBC.
    Urinary: Retention. Pro. False + glucose ($CuSO_4$).
    Monitor: Baseline & periodic hepatic func.

metformin
  Glucophage
  Tab
  Glucophage XR (SR)
  Tab
  Glumetza (SR)
  Tab
  Riomet
  Soln- saccharin Ca,
   xylitol
  Fortamet (SR)
  Tab

ANTIHYPERGLYCEMIC AGENT, Biguanide
  Potentiates the effect of insulin, ↓ GI glucose abs, ↓ hepatic glucose production.
  Drug: Take c̄ meals to ↓ GI distress.
  Swallow SR form whole c̄ evening meal.
  Diet: Prescribed diabetic diet. ↓ cal if wt loss needed.
  Take guar gum ≥ 6 hr after drug- ↓ drug abs.[3]
  Nutr: Anorexia. Stable wt or ↓ wt. ↓ Fol & Vit B_{12} abs.
  Oral/GI: (↓ % incidence c̄ XR form) metallic taste, dyspepsia,
  <u>NAUSEA/VOMITING</u>, <u>BLOATING</u>, <u>DIARRHEA</u>, <u>FLATULENCE</u>. Constipation c̄ XR form.
  S/Cond: Avoid alcohol- ↑ risk of lactic acidosis. Not c̄ lactation.
  Caution c̄ ↓ hepatic func. Not c̄ severe ↓ hepatic func. Not c̄ ↓ renal func,[58]
  serum crea ≥ 1.5 for male, 1.4 for female or abnormal CrCl.
  Caution c̄ CHF. Not c̄ severe cardiac disease.
  Not c̄ metabolic acidosis or dehydration. Caution c̄ geriatric.
  Does <u>not</u> cause hypoglycemia when used as a single agent.
  Pregnancy: Category B, but use is not recommended.
  Other: Headache, fatigue, muscle pain, dyspnea, rash, ↑ sweating, chills,
  flu syndrome, flushing, chest discomfort, palpitation, dizziness, asthenia.
  Very rare- lactic acidosis (fatal in 50% of cases).
  Blood/Serum: ↓ <u>*GLUCOSE*</u>, ↓ *Hb A1$_C$*, ↓ <u>CHOL</u>, ↓ <u>LDL</u>, ↓ <u>TG</u>, ↑ <u>HDL</u>.
  ↓ <u>Vit B$_{12}$</u> , ↑ <u>homocysteine</u>. Possible- ↓ <u>Fol</u>, anemia c̄ LT use.
  Monitor: Glucose, Hb A1$_c$ q 3mo. Vit B$_{12}$, Fol, renal func.
  Baseline & annual CBC.

methadone
  Dolophine
  Tab- starch
  Methadose
  Conc- 38% sucrose,
   propylene glycol
  Sugar free Conc-
   no sucrose
  Tab- starch

ANALGESIC, Narcotic, Opioid   Oral or Parenteral (IV, IM or SC)
  Drug: Must dissolve **Disket** in 4 oz acidic fruit juice or water.
  May divide **Disket**, but do not chew or swallow.
  Diet: Caution c̄ grapefruit/related citrus, see p 390. Avoid SJW,[9b] see p 286.
  Nutr: Anorexia. **Oral/GI:** Dry mouth, N/V, cramps, <u>constipation</u>.
  S/Cond: Avoid alcohol. Not c̄ lactation. May be habit forming c̄ LT use.
  Caution c̄ ↓ hepatic func or ↓ renal func, ↓ pulmonary func,
  asthma/bronchospasm, obesity, geriatric, seizures or hypothyroidism.
  Not c̄ paralytic ileus.

Diskets Dispersible Tab-
starch
Generic Flavored Conc-
sucrose, sorbitol,
saccharin Na,
propylene glycol

Pregnancy: Category C.
Other: RESPIRATORY DEPRESSION, DROWSINESS, SEDATION, dizziness,
hypotension, headache, confusion, flushing, sweating, edema,
visual changes, nervousness, palpitations, syncope, rash, insomnia.
Rare- ↑ QT interval.
Blood/Serum: ↑ amylase, ↑ lipase.
Urinary: Retention. Urinary acidifiers ↑ drug excretion.

methimazole
Tapazole
Tab- lactose

ANTIHYPERTHYROID   See listing for **propylthiouracil p 267**
Drug: Food may affect bioavailability,
take consistently c̄ or s̄ food each day.[13]

methocarbamol
Robaxin
Tab- Na starch glycolate,
starch, lactose in some
brands

SKELETAL MUSCLE RELAXANT, ADJUNCT to TETANUS TREATMENT
carbamate derivative of guaifenesin   Oral or Parenteral (IV or IM)
Nutr: Anorexia.
Oral/GI: Abnormal taste, dyspesia, N/V.
S/Cond: Avoid alcohol. Oral- Caution c̄ lactation. IV- Not c̄ lactation.[26]
Tab- caution c̄ ↓ renal func. Parenteral- not c̄ ↓ renal func.
Pregnancy: Category C.
Other: Drowsiness, dizziness, lightheadedness, blurred or double vision,
nasal congestion, conjunctivitis, allergic fever, headache, flushing,
amnesia, confusion, hypotension, syncope, insomnia, rash, ataxia,
nystagmus. Rare- jaundice, bradycardia, seizures.
Blood/Serum: Rare- ↓ WBC, ↓ platelets, ↓ K, ↓ Mg.
Urinary: Color change- black, brown or green urine. Interferes c̄
5-HIAA or VMA tests.
Monitor: Renal func c̄ parenteral use for > 3 days.

M

methotrexate (MTX)
  Methotrexate [a]
  Tab- lactose, starch,
  may contain
  cornstarch
  Generic brands IV-
  50 mg (2.18 mEq)
  Na/10 mL,
  161 mg
  (7.0 mEq) Na/1g vial,
  0.9% benzyl alcohol
  in <u>some</u> formulations
  Rheumatrex [b, c]
  Tab- lactose,
  cornstarch

ANTINEOPLASTIC [a], ANTIPSORIATRIC [b], ANTIARTHRITIC [c] (Rheumatoid)
Oral, Intrathecal or Parenteral (IV, IM)
Folic Acid Antagonist (Dihydrofolate Reductase Inhibitor)
Rheumatrex is a low dose oral once a week formulation $\bar{c}$ fewer side effects.
Diet: Encourage ↑ fluid intake to ↑ urine output.
Food delays abs, ↓ peak conc & bioavailability.[7]
Leucovorin (folinic acid) rescue prescribed $\bar{c}$ MTX to ↓ oral & GI effects.[82]
One study- ↑ caffeine ↓ drug effect in arthritis.[3]
Newer study found no interaction $\bar{c}$ caffeine.[121]
Nutr: ↓ abs of Fol.[11] <u>ANOREXIA</u>, ↓ <u>wt</u>, dehydration.
Oral/GI: <u>STOMATITIS</u>, gingivitis, altered taste, <u>N/V</u>, diarrhea,
hemorrhagic enteritis. Interrupt use if diarrhea & ulcerative stomatitis occur.
S/Cond: Avoid alcohol. Not $\bar{c}$ lactation.
Do dental care cautiously, see p 11 & 15.
Caution $\bar{c}$ ↓ hepatic func or ↓ renal func, geriatric, peptic ulcer, colitis.
Not $\bar{c}$ immunodeficiency syndromes.
Pregnancy: Category X.
Other: <u>BONE MARROW SUPPRESSION</u>, <u>infection</u>, <u>nephropathy</u>, <u>hair loss</u>,
hepatotoxicity, headache, fatigue, fever, chills, dizziness, drowsiness, rash,
pulmonary toxicity, pancreatitis, hemorrhage (may be sudden & serious).
Rare- SJS, TEN.
Blood/Serum: ↓ <u>WHITE BLOOD CELLS</u>, ↓ <u>PLATELETS</u>, <u>ANEMIA</u>, ↑ <u>HOMOCYSTEINE</u>,[90]
↑ <u>uric acid</u>, ↑ <u>AST</u>, ↑ <u>ALT</u>, ↑ <u>bil</u>, ↑ <u>BUN</u>.
Urinary: ↑ <u>uric acid</u>.
Monitor: Baseline & periodic CBC $\bar{c}$ diff, platelets, alb, hepatic & renal func,
chest x-ray, uric acid.

methylcellulose
  Citrucel (gluten free)
  Tab- maltodextrin =
  1 g CHO, 5 cal
  Pwd- 18 g CHO, 70 cal
  105 mg K, 3 mg Na,

LAXATIVE, Bulk Forming
Drug: Do not use for > one wk $\bar{s}$ physician's advice.
Tab- Take $\bar{c}$ 8 oz water or other liquid.
May break into pieces to swallow, but do not crush or chew.
Pwd- Do <u>not</u> swallow dry pwd. Mix $\bar{c}$ 8 oz cold water or non-carbonated
liquid. Not $\bar{c}$ milk.

sucrose
Fiber Shake Pwd-
aspartame = phenylalanine
49 mg/scoop, cocoa pwd,
corn syrup, non-fat milk pwd,
soy lecithin, sunflower oil
9 g CHO, 40 cal

Smoothie- Mix c̄ 8 oz cold non-carbonated juice or fruit smoothie.
Shake- Mix c̄ 8 oz milk or water.
Diet: High fiber c̄ 1500-2000 mL fluid/day to prevent constipation.
Oral/GI: ↑ _PERISTALSIS_ & _BOWEL MOTILITY_. Rare- bowel obstruction.
S/Cond: Not c̄ dysphagia. Use sugar free form c̄ diabetes.
Pregnancy: Consult physician.
Bulk forming laxatives are commonly used in pregnancy.[2]

Fiber Smoothie Pwd- sucrose, maltodextrin, 12 g CHO, 55 mg K, 3 g Na, 37 cal/dose
Sugar Free Pwd- maltodextrin, aspartame = 52 mg phenylalanine/dose, 85 mg Ca, 105 mg K, 3 g Na, 24 cal

---

methyldopa
  Aldomet
  (previous brand name)
  Generic Brands
  Parenteral- 16 mg
  Na Bisulfite/vial
  Tab- guar gum,
  contains no sulfites
  Aldoril
  Tab- guar gum,
  propylene glycol
  also contains
  hydrochlorothiazide
  see **p 166**

ANTIHYPERTENSIVE   Oral or Parenteral (IV)

Diet: ↓ Na, ↓ cal may be recommended. Avoid natural licorice, see p 374.
Take Fe suppl separately by 2 hr (↓ abs of drug).[9b]
Nutr: ↑ need for Vit B$_{12}$ & Fol c̄ high dose.[12]
Oral/GI: <u>Dry mouth</u>, sore/black tongue, N/V, diarrhea, flatulence.
S/Cond: Avoid alcohol. Not c̄ lactation.
↑ risk of dental problems, see p 11 & 15. Caution c̄ G6PD def- ↑ risk of
hemolytic anemia. Not c̄ active hepatic disease or history of drug
induced hepatitis. Caution c̄ ↓ hepatic func or ↓ renal func.
Caution c̄ geriatric.[84]
Pregnancy: Category B (oral).
Commonly used for pregnancy induced HTN. Category C (IV).[7]
Other: ↓ _BP_ c̄ possible hypotension, <u>SEDATION</u>, <u>drowsiness</u>, <u>headache</u>,
peripheral edema, <u>fever</u>, blurred vision, asthenia, rash, paresthesias,
Parkinsonism, ↓ mental acuity, depression, nightmares,
lupus-like syndrome, nasal stuffiness, bone marrow suppression.
Rare- CHF, psychosis, hepatitis or pancreatitis (can be fatal).
Blood/Serum: ↑ <u>alk phos</u>, ↑ <u>AST</u>, ↑ <u>ALT</u>, ↑ <u>bil</u>, + Coombs' test,
↑ BUN, ↑ amylase, ↑ K, ↑ Na, ↑ prolactin, hemolytic anemia,
↑ PT/INR, + ANA, ↑ crea.[58] Rare- dyscrasias.
Monitor: BP. Baseline CBC, hepatic func & Coombs' test, then periodically.

M

methylnaltrexone	LAXATIVE, Opioid Antagonist for Severe Opioid-Induced Constipation
Relistor Parenteral (SC)	Does not enter CNS nor reverse analgesic effects of narcotics.
NaCl 3.9 mg/vial	**Drug:** For palliative care in advanced illness.

methylnaltrexone
Relistor Parenteral (SC)
NaCl 3.9 mg/vial

LAXATIVE, Opioid Antagonist for Severe Opioid-Induced Constipation
Does not enter CNS nor reverse analgesic effects of narcotics.
Drug: For palliative care in advanced illness.
Oral/GI: <u>Nausea</u>, vomiting, <u>abdominal pain</u>, <u>flatulence</u>, diarrhea.
S/Cond: Caution c̄ lactation. Caution c̄ severe ↓ renal func.
Not c̄ bowel obstruction. **Pregnancy:** Category B. **Other:** Dizziness.
Monitor: Bowel function.

methylphenidate
Concerta (SR) (1X/day)
Tab- lactose, propylene glycol
Metadate CD (1X/day)
Cap- sugar spheres (sucrose & starch)
(30% IR + 70% SR beads)
Metadate ER (8 hr)
Tab- lactose
Ritalin (2-3X/day)
5 & 10 mg Tab- starch, lactose
20 mg Tab- sucrose
Ritalin SR (8 hr)
Tab- lactose, mineral oil
Ritalin LA (1X/day)
Cap- sugar spheres
(sucrose & starch)
(50% IR + 50% SR beads)
Daytrana
Transdermal patch
for once a day use

ANTI-ADHD, ANTINARCOLEPSY (IR or SR forms), Stimulant
Also used in geriatrics as stimulant, antidepressant
Drug: Take s̄ regard to meals, no later than 6 PM.
Food ↑ extent, but not rate of abs of IR & SR forms.
Swallow SR or ER tab whole- do not divide, chew or crush.
May open LA Cap & sprinkle beads on applesauce- do not chew or crush.
Diet: Insure adequate cal intake. Limit caffeine, see p 379.
Avoid SJW, see p 286.
Nutr: <small>ANOREXIA</small>, ↓ wt, ↓ <small>GROWTH</small> c̄ <u>LT use</u>.
Oral/GI: Dry throat, N/V, <u>abdominal pain</u>, diarrhea.
S/Cond: Avoid alcohol. Caution c̄ lactation.
Caution c̄ HTN or severe CAD. Not c̄ anxiety, tics, Tourette's syndrome,
hyperthyroidism, thyrotoxicosis or glaucoma.
Caution c̄ seizures- drug ↓ seizure threshold.
May be habit forming c̄ LT high dose. **Pregnancy:** Category C.
Other: <small>NERVOUSNESS</small>, <small>INSOMNIA</small>, <u>tachycardia</u>, HTN, hypotension,
rash, palpitations, angina, joint pain,[13] dizziness, dyskinesia, drowsiness,
headache, cough, fever, URTI. Rare- visual disturbances, toxic psychosis.
Blood/Serum: Rare- ↓ platelets, ↓ WBC, anemia.
Monitor: CBC c̄ diff & platelets c̄ LT use. BP. Children's growth.

methylprednisolone

CORTICOSTEROID   See **corticosteroids p 94**

metoclopramide
Reglan
5 mg Tab- lactose,

ANTIEMETIC, ANTIGERD, DIABETIC GASTROPARESIS TREATMENT
Dopamine Antagonist   Oral or Parenteral (IM or IV)
Drug: Take 1/2 hr before meals & HS.

cornstarch
10 mg Tab- mannitol
Syrup- sorbitol
Parenteral-
 preservative free
Metozolv ODT-
 gelatin, mannitol
 acesulfame K

Dissolve ODT on tongue s̄ liquid, swallow saliva.
Oral/GI: Dry mouth, ↑ *GASTRIC EMPTYING*, nausea, diarrhea, constipation.
S/Cond: Avoid alcohol- ↑ alcohol effects. Caution c̄ lactation.
Caution c̄ diabetes- may alter insulin requirements.
Syrup form incompatible c̄ some TF.[32] Caution c̄ HTN, seizures, geriatric
or ↓ renal func. Not c̄ pheochromocytoma- ↑ risk of hypertensive crisis.
Pregnancy: Category B.
Other: Restlessness, drowsiness, fatigue, akathisia, dizziness, insomnia,
headache, mental depression, confusion, visual changes, galactorrhea,
transient edema. Rare- EPS (↑ incidence in children, young adults or ESRD),
HTN, acute CHF, seizures, NMS, tardive dyskinesia c̄ LT use
(↑ incidence in geriatric).
Blood/Serum: ↑ prolactin. Transient ↑ aldosterone.
Urinary: ↑ frequency, incontinence.

metolazone
 Zaroxolyn
 Tab

ANTIHYPERTENSIVE, DIURETIC   See listing for **hydrochlorothiazide p 166**
 Thiazide-like (K-depleting)   Generally prescribed c̄ loop diuretic,
 but the combination may cause severe K depletion & profound diuresis.

metoprolol
 Lopressor
 Tab- lactose,
  Na starch glycolate
 IV 5 mg Vial- NaCl 45 mg
 Toprol XL (SR)
 Tab
 Lopressor HCT
 Tab- lactose, sucrose,
  cornstarch,
  Na starch glycolate
 also contains
 hydrochlorothiazide
 see **p 166**

ANTIHYPERTENSIVE, ANTIANGINA, CHF TREATMENT (XL form only)
 MI TREATMENT Cardioselective Beta-Blocker   Oral or Parenteral (IV)
 Drug: Take tab c̄ food to ↑ bioavailability. May divide XL Tab,
 but do not crush or chew.
 Diet: ↓ Na, ↓ cal may be recommended. Avoid natural licorice, see p 374.
 Oral/GI: Dry mouth, N/V, dyspepsia, flatulence, diarrhea, constipation.
 S/Cond: Caution c̄ lactation. Caution c̄ diabetes- may mask signs of hypoglycemia.
 May reduce insulin release in response to hyperglycemia.[6] Extreme caution c̄
 asthma/bronchospasm. Caution c̄ ↓ hepatic func, hyperthyroidism or geriatric.
 Pregnancy: Category C. **Other:** ↓ *BP* c̄ possible hypotension, confusion,
 fatigue, dizziness, insomnia, depression, rash, peripheral edema,
 bradycardia, palpitations, headache, nightmares, CHF.
 Blood/Serum: Rare-↑ AST, ↑ ALT, ↑ alk phos, ↑ LDH, ↑ K, ↑ TG, ↑ uric acid.
 Monitor: BP, heart rate, ECG c̄ IV.

metronidazole
  Flagyl
    Cap- cornstarch
    Tab
  Flagyl ER (SR)
    Tab- lactose
  Flagyl I.V.
    RTU IV
    322 mg (14.01 mEq)
    Na/100 mL
    Lyophilized IV-
    415 mg mannitol/dose

ANTIBIOTIC, AMEBICIDE, ANTITRICHOMONAL   Oral or Parenteral (IV)
    Often used to treat C. difficile pseudomembranous colitis
    Drug: May take c̄ meals to ↓ GI distress, but food ↓ drug bioavailability.
    Diet: Consider Na content c̄ ↓ Na diet. **Nutr:** <u>Anorexia</u>.
    Oral/GI: Dry mouth, candidiasis, stomatitis, <u>metallic taste</u>, <u>N</u>/V,
    <u>epigastric distress</u>, <u>diarrhea</u>, constipation.
    S/Cond: Avoid <u>all</u> alcohol during use & for three days afterwards
    (disulfiram-like reaction). Not c̄ lactation. ↑ risk of dental problems.
    Caution c̄ severe ↓ hepatic func or severe ↓ renal func,[58] geriatric or seizures.
    Pregnancy: Category B, but contraindicated in first trimester.
    Other: <u>Dizziness</u>, <u>headache</u>, ataxia, fatigue, confusion, rash.
    Rare- hypersensitivity, peripheral neuropathy, pancreatitis, seizures c̄ high dose.
    Blood/Serum: Mild ↓ WBC. Rare- ↓ platelets. False ↓ AST, ↓ ALT,
    ↓ LDH, ↓ TG, glucose c̄ some assays. **Urinary:** Rare- darkened urine, dysuria.
    Monitor: CBC c̄ diff & platelets. Possibly renal & hepatic func in geriatric.

Mevacor
  lovastatin

ANTIHYPERLIPIDEMIC   See **HMG-CoA Reductase Inhibitors p 164**

Miacalcin

Ca REGULATOR, Hormone   See **calcitonin p 68**

Miacalcin Nasal Spray

OSTEOPOROSIS TREATMENT   See **calcitonin p 68**

---

micafungin
  Mycamine

ANTIFUNGAL   See **echinocandins p 120**

Micardis/Micardis HCT
  telmisartan

ANTIHYPERTENSIVE   See **Angiotensin II Receptor Antagonists p 38**
    Micardis HCT also contains **hydrochlorothiazide**, see **p 166**

Microgestin Fe

ORAL CONTRACEPTIVE   See **Oral Contraceptives p 237**

Microzide
  Cap- lactose, cornstarch

ANTIHYPERTENSIVE, DIURETIC   See **hydrochlorothiazide p 166**
  once daily, low dose

---

midazolam
  Versed

ANESTHESIA ADJUNCT, Sedative   See **Benzodiazepines p 54**

miglitol **Glyset** Tab- starch	ANTIDIABETIC AGENT for TYPE 2 DIABETES, Alpha-glucosidase Inhibitor (may be used alone or c̄ sulfonylurea) **Drug:** Take c̄ first bite of each meal. Do not take c̄ digestive enzymes, eg amylase or pancreatin. **Diet:** Adjunct to prescribed diabetic diet. **Nutr:** Delays abs of dietary disaccharides & complex CHO. ↓ abs of Fe. **Oral/GI:** <u>Abdominal pain</u>, DIARRHEA, FLATULENCE. **S/Cond:** Limit alcohol. Not c̄ lactation. Caution c̄ mild to moderate ↓ renal func. Not c̄ severe ↓ renal func. Not c̄ diabetic ketoacidosis or chronic intestinal disease eg IBD. Does <u>not</u> cause hypoglycemia when used as single agent. **Pregnancy:** Category B. **Other:** Transient rash. **Blood/Serum:** ↓ _FASTING GLUCOSE_, ↓ _POSTPRANDIAL GLUCOSE_, ↓ _Hb A1$_c$_, transient ↓ <u>Fe</u>. Does not affect insulin level. **Monitor:** Glucose. Hb A1$_c$ q 3-6 mo. Possibly renal func.[13]
Milk of Magnesia (MOM)	LAXATIVE (Osmotic), ANTACID See **magnesium hydroxide p 203**
milnaciprin **Savella** Tab	FIBROMYALGIA MANAGEMENT, SNRI, Also used as Antidepressant **Drug:** Take BID s̄ regard to food. **Nutr:** ↓ appetite, slight wt loss. **Oral/GI:** Dry mouth, dysgeusia, dyspepsia, GERD, N/V, GI bleeding, abdominal pain, <u>constipation</u>, flatulence. **S/Cond:** Avoid alcohol, Not c̄ lactation. Caution c̄ moderate or severe ↓ renal func or Hx of urinary retention. Not c̄ ESRD. Caution c̄ severe ↓ hepatic func. Not c̄ uncontrolled narrow angle glaucoma. Caution c̄ seizures. **Pregnancy:** Category C. **Other:** <u>Hot flushes</u>, <u>palpitations</u>, <u>tachycardia</u>, <u>dizziness</u>, <u>hypertension</u>, <u>headache</u>, ↑ <u>sweating</u>, migraine, chest pain/discomfort, chills, tremor, paresthesia, URTI, insomnia, anxiety, irritability, rash, itching, fatigue, edema. Rare- suicidal thinking & behavior, seizures, SIADH, SJS, serotonin syndrome. **Blood/Serum:** Mild ↑ ALT/AST. ↑ Na. ↑ chol. ↑ prolactin. **Urinary:** UTI, cystitis. Rare- dysuria, retention. **Monitor:** Baseline & periodic BP & heart rate

mineral oil **Kondremul Plain**	LAXATIVE, Lubricant	

Drug: Take on empty stomach 2 hr apart from food & fat soluble Vit. Do not take HS. Not c̄ stool softener eg- **docusate Na**.
Diet: High fiber c̄ 1500-2000 mL fluid/day to prevent constipation.
Nutr: ↓ wt, anorexia,[14] dehydration.[1] May ↓ abs of fat soluble Vits (A, D, E & K) & Ca, P, K[27]- clinically significant only c̄ LT use.
Oral/GI: Belching, nausea, dyspepsia, cramps, flatulence, diarrhea.
S/Cond: Not c̄ dysphagia, diverticulitis or ulcerative colitis.
Avoid LT continuous use.
Not if bedridden or for children < 6 yr except c̄ Doctor's order- may cause lipid pneumonitis due to oil aspiration.
Pregnancy: Category C.[11] Caution due to ↓ abs of vit.

Minipress **prazosin**	ANTIHYPERTENSIVE	See **Alpha₁ Adrenergic Blockers p 28**

minocycline **Dynacin, Minocin** **Solodyn** (SR)	ANTIBIOTIC Also used as ANTIARTHRITIC (Rheumatoid).	See **Tetracyclines p 310**

MiraLax	LAXATIVE (Osmotic)	See **polyethylene glycol p 259**

Mirapex/Mirapex ER	ANTIPARKINSON, Dopamine Agonist	See **pramipexole p 261**

mirtazapine **Remeron** Tab- cornstarch, lactose **Remeron SolTab** ODT aspartame = phenylalanine 2.6 mg/15 mg drug, mannitol, starch, sucrose	ANTIDEPRESSANT, NaSSa (noradrenergic agonist, specific serotonin antagonist) Presynaptic Alpha-2 Receptor Antagonist	

Drug: Take s̄ regard to food, preferably HS.
Dissolve ODT on tongue c̄ or s̄ liquid, swallow saliva. Do not split tab.
Diet: Avoid SJW, see p 286.
Nutr: ↑ APPETITE, ↑ WEIGHT, ↑ thirst, anorexia.
Oral/GI: Dry mouth, N/V, abdominal pain, constipation.
S/Cond: Avoid alcohol. Caution c̄ lactation.
Caution c̄ ↓ hepatic func or ↓ renal func. Caution c̄ geriatric.
Pregnancy: Category C.
Other: DROWSINESS, dizziness, asthenia, flu-like syndrome,

back, muscle or joint pain, edema, tremor, confusion, dyspnea, HTN, anxiety, rash, cough, vertigo, hyperkinesia or hypokinesia.
Rare- suicidal thinking & behavior, orthostatic hypotension.
Blood/Serum: ↑ chol, ↑ TG, ↑ ALT. < 1%- ↓ WBC, ↓ platelets, anemia.
Urinary: ↑ frequency.
Monitor: Possibly CBC c̄ diff & platelets.

mitoxantrone
Novantrone
3.2 mg (0.14 mEq) Na/mL

ANTINEOPLASTIC, (ANLL Leukemia, Prostate Cancer), MULTIPLE SCLEROSIS TREATMENT, Anthracenedione Antibiotic   Parenteral only (IV)
Diet: Insure adequate fluid intake/hydration to ↑ uric acid excretion.
Nutr: Anorexia.
Oral/GI: STOMATITIS, MUCOSITIS, NAUSEA/VOMITING, abdominal pain, GI bleeding, DIARRHEA.
S/Cond: Not c̄ lactation. Do dental care cautiously, see p 11 & 15.
Caution c̄ ↓ hepatic func or cardiac disease.
Pregnancy: Category D.
Other: BONE MARROW SUPPRESSION, ASTHENIA, FEVER, INFECTIONS, HAIR LOSS, AMENORRHEA, headache, cough, dyspnea, petechiae, jaundice, nail changes, skin discoloration or fungus, edema, seizures, HTN, acute myelogenous leukemia (AML), acute CHF (may be delayed for years), arrhythmias, tachycardia, ↓ LVEF.
Blood/Serum: ↓ PLATELETS, ↓ WHITE BLOOD CELLS, ↑ glucose, anemia, ↑ ALT, ↑ AST, ↑ LDH, ↑ bil, ↑ GGT, ↓ K, ↑ crea, ↑ uric acid.
Urinary: ↑ uric acid, pro, blue-green color.[13] UTI.
Monitor: Baseline & before each dose CBC, platelets.
Renal & hepatic func, uric acid. Possibly cardiac func, chest x-ray.

Moban   ANTIPSYCHOTIC, Dihydroindolone   See **molindone p 220**

Mobic   ANTIARTHRITIC, NSAID   See **meloxicam p 206**

moexipril
Univasc/Uniretic

ANTIHYPERTENSIVE   See Angiotensin Converting Enzyme Inhibitors p 36
Uniretic also contains **hydrochlorothiazide**, see **p 166.**

molindone
Moban
All Tabs- lactose,
50 mg Tab-
 also contains
 Na starch glycolate

ANTIPSYCHOTIC, Dihydroindolone
Drug: Take c̄ food or 8 oz milk or water to ↓ GI distress.
Nutr: Anorexia, ↓ wt.
Oral/GI: <u>Dry mouth</u>, <u>nausea</u>, GI upset, <u>constipation</u>.
S/Cond: Avoid alcohol. Caution c̄ lactation. Caution c̄ seizures.[23]
↑ risk of dental problems, see p 11 & 15. Not c̄ severe CNS depression.
Pregnancy: Category C.
Other: <u>DROWSINESS</u>, <u>restlessness</u>, <u>headache</u>, <u>blurred vision</u>, <u>EPS</u>,
<u>tardive dyskinesia</u> c̄ LT use, depression, euphoria, dizziness,
orthostatic hypotension, insomnia, amenorrhea.
↑ mortality in geriatrics c̄ dementia-related psychosis.
Rare- NMS, galactorrhea, hyperactivity.
Blood/Serum: ↑ prolactin. Rare- ↑ or ↓ WBC. **Urinary:** Retention.

mometasone
Nasonex Nasal Spray
Asmanex Twisthaler
Pwd-
 anhydrous lactose (contains milk pro)

ANTI-ALLERGIC RHINITIS   See listing for **beclomethasone p 51**
Spray also indicated TO TREAT NASAL POLYPS
Corticosteroid, Nasal Spray or Inhaler

Monopril

ANTIHYPERTENSIVE   See **Angiotensin Converting Enzyme Inhibitors p 36**

montelukast
Singulair
Tab- lactose
Chew Tab- mannitol,
4 mg tab-
 aspartame = 0.674 mg
 phenylalanine
5 mg tab-
 aspartame = 0.842 mg
 phenylalanine
Oral Granules-
 mannitol

ASTHMA Prophylaxis & Chronic Treatment (not for acute attacks)
    ALLERGIC RHINITIS, Exercise-induced bronchoconstriction (EIB)
                                        Leukotriene Receptor Antagonist
Drug: For asthma take in the evening s̄ regard to food.
For EIB take 2 hr before exercise. Chew chew tab well.
Take granules directly in mouth or mix c̄ cold or room temp applesauce,
ice cream, carrots, rice, breast milk or formula.
Diet: No interaction c̄ grapefruit/related citrus, see p 390.
Oral/GI: Dyspepsia, diarrhea.
S/Cond: Caution c̄ lactation. > 99% serum pro bound.
Caution c̄ severe ↓ hepatic func. **Pregnancy:** Category B.
Blood/Serum: < 1%- ↑ AST, ↑ ALT.

morphine
　MS Contin (SR)
　Tab- lactose
　Avinza (SR)
　Cap (IR & SR beads)
　sugar starch spheres,
　fumaric acid
　Kadian (SR) Cap
　(100% SR beads)-
　sucrose, cornstarch
　Roxanol Oral Conc
　DepoDur (SR)
　liposome injection

ANALGESIC, Narcotic, Opioid　　　　　Oral, Parenteral or Rectal Suppository

Drug: May take c̄ food to ↓ GI distress. Swallow SR tab whole. Insure adequate fluid intake/hydration.
Swallow SR cap whole or open & sprinkle beads on applesauce-swallow s̄ chewing. Rinse mouth immediately, swallow water.
Nutr: Anorexia ↓ wt, ↑ thirst, dehydration.
Oral/GI: <u>Dry mouth</u>, taste changes, dysphagia, dyspepsia, ↓ <u>gastric motility</u>, <u>N/V</u>, <u>CONSTIPATION</u>, impaction, <u>diarrhea</u>.
S/Cond: Avoid alcohol, especially c̄ **Avinza** or **Kadian**. Alcohol ↑ drug release from SR beads - potentially fatal. Not c̄ lactation. ↑ risk of dental problems, see p 11 & 15. May be habit forming c̄ LT use. Not c̄ paralytic ileus. Caution c̄ dysphagia, ↓ hepatic func, ↓ renal func, morbid obesity, seizures, depression, geriatric, asthma, or severe ↓ pulmonary func.
TF- Do not use SR beads in NG tube, see PI for use in PEG tube.
Pregnancy: Category C.
Other: <u>RESPIRATORY DEPRESSION</u>, <u>APNEA</u>, <u>EUPHORIA</u>, <u>DROWSINESS</u>,
↓ <u>COUGH REFLEX</u>, <u>DEPRESSION</u>, <u>hypotension</u>, <u>sedation</u>, <u>sweating</u>, <u>dizziness</u>,
<u>dyspnea</u>, <u>paresthesia</u>, <u>asthenia</u>, <u>back pain</u>, <u>flu syndrome</u>,
blurred or double vision, headache, confusion, anxiety, rash, edema, histamine release (flushing, red eyes, sweating, itching, ↓ BP), hypothermia,[26] bradycardia, syncope, tremor, seizure, insomnia, hiccups.
Blood/Serum: ↑ amylase, ↑ lipase.[13] Anemia, ↓ platelets.
Urinary: <u>RETENTION</u> (↑ in males), <u>OLIGURIA</u>, <u>UTI</u>.

Motrin　　　　　ANTIARTHRITIC, ANALGESIC, NSAID　　　See **ibuprofen p 170**

Movana　　　　HERBAL PRODUCT (Not FDA approved)　　　See **St. John's wort p 286**

moxifloxacin
   Avelox
   Tab- lactose
   IV- preservative free
	ANTIBIOTIC, Fluoroquinolone
	   Oral or Parenteral (IV)
	 Diet: Take oral drug at least 4 hr before <u>or 8 hr after</u> Mg, Fe or Zn suppl, MVI c̄ minerals or Al/Mg antacids, oral enteral product or TF.[19]
	 S/Cond: No dosage adjustment needed for ↓ renal func. Not for UTI.
	 Other: Rare- ↑ QT interval.
		See listing for **ciprofloxacin p 85**

MS Contin	ANALGESIC, Narcotic, Opioid	See **morphine p 221**
Mucinex	ANTITUSSIVE	See **guaifenesin p 159**

Mucinex D (SR)
   Tab- Na starch glycolate
	ANTITUSSIVE, DECONGESTANT
	   Combination drug
		See **guaifenesin p 159**
		 See **pseudoephedrine p 269**

Multaq	ANTIARRHYTHMIC	See **dronedarone p 118**
Myambutol	TUBERCULOSIS TREATMENT	See **ethambutol p 130**
Mycamine micafungin	ANTIFUNGAL	See **echinocandins p 120**
Mycelex	ANTIFUNGAL	See **clotrimazole p 90**

mycophenolate mofetil
   CellCept
   Cap- starch
   Tab-
     ethyl & methyl
     alcohol
   Susp- aspartame =
     0.56 mg
     phenylalanine/mL,
     sorbitol,
     soy lecithin,
     xanthan gum
   IV Pwd
	IMMUNOSUPPRESSANT (To prevent renal, hepatic or cardiac transplant rejection)
	   Used c̄ **cyclosporine** & corticosteriods Oral or Parenteral (IV)
	 Drug: Take on an empty stomach, 1 hr before or 2 hr after food.
	 Swallow whole. Do not open or crush.
	 Diet: Take Mg suppl/antacid separately from drug.
	 Nutr: Anorexia c̄ hepatic transplant.
	 Oral/GI: Oral candidiasis, stomatitis, <u>dyspepsia</u>, <u>N/V</u>, <u>GI hemorrhage</u>, <u>abdominal pain</u>, colitis, <u>diarrhea</u>, constipation.
	 S/Cond: Not c̄ lactation. 97% serum pro bound.
	 Caution c̄ severe ↓ renal func. Caution c̄ GI disease, eg ulcer(s).
	 Caution c̄ soy allergy c̄ susp. **Pregnancy:** Category D.
	 Other: <u>Infection</u>, <u>chest pain</u>, <u>cough</u>, <u>dyspnea</u>, <u>HTN</u>, <u>edema</u>, <u>headache</u>, <u>asthenia</u>, thrombosis, insomnia, arrhythmia,

mycophenolic acid	back/joint/muscle pain, tremor, dizziness, paresthesia, rash, acne.
Myfortic (SR)	Rare- lymphoma, skin cancer, pancreatitis. Rare- pure red cell aplasia (PRCA)
Tab- lactose, starch	**Blood/Serum:** <u>Anemia</u>, ↓ platelets, ↓ WBC, ↓ neutrophils, ↑ or ↓ K, ↑ chol, ↓ P, ↑ glucose. > 1% in cardiac pt- ↑ LDH, ↑ AST, ↑ ALT, ↓ Mg, ↑ BUN, ↑ crea. **Urinary:** Hematuria, UTI.

Monitor: Weekly CBC for 1st mo, 2X/mo for 2nd & 3rd mo, then 1X/mo through 1st yr.

Mycostatin	ANTIFUNGAL	See **nystatin** p 232
Myfortic	IMMUNOSUPPRESSANT	See **mycophenolate above**

Mylanta	ANTACID, ANTIFLATULENT	See **aluminum hydroxide &**
Mylanta Maximum Strength	contain **simethicone**, see p 292	**magnesium hydroxide** p 29
	S/Cond: Mylanta Maximum Strength thickens some TF.[8]	

Mylanta Gas	ANTIFLATULENT	See **simethicone** p 292
Mylicon	ANTIFLATULENT	See **simethicone** p 292

| **Mysoline** | ANTIEPILEPTIC | See listing for **phenobarbital** p 252 |
| **primidone** Tab- lactose, Na starch glycolate | Metabolized to **phenobarbital** & **phenylethylmalonamide** (PEMA) | |

nadolol
  Corgard
  Tab- cornstarch
  Nadolol
  Tab- lactose, starch

ANTIHYPERTENSIVE, ANTIANGINA, Non-selective Beta-Blocker
Drug: Take $\bar{s}$ regard to food.
Diet: ↓ Na, ↓ cal may be recommended. Avoid natural licorice, see p 374.
S/Cond: Limit alcohol. Not $\bar{c}$ lactation. Caution $\bar{c}$ diabetes- may mask symptoms of & prolong hypoglycemia. May reduce insulin release in response to hyperglycemia. Caution $\bar{c}$ ↓ hepatic func[6] or ↓ renal func or CHF. Not $\bar{c}$ asthma/bronchospam.
Pregnancy: Category C.
Other: ↓ <u>*BP*</u> $\bar{c}$ possible hypotension, dizziness, fatigue, depression, drowsiness, heart failure, bradycardia, palpitations, peripheral vascular insufficiency.
Monitor: BP, heart rate.

nafcillin ANTIBIOTIC, Penicillin (penicillinase resistant)   Oral or Parenteral (IM or IV)
Parenteral- 67-90 mg (2.92-3.92 mEq) Na/g depending upon brand   See listing for **penicillin p 249**

naltrexone ALCOHOL DEPENDENCE TREATMENT[a], NARCOTIC OPIOID ANTAGONIST[b]
  ReVia[a] [b] Oral or Parenteral (IM)
Tab- lactose **Drug:** May take tab $\bar{c}$ food to ↓ GI distress.
  Vivitrol[a] **Nutr:** Anorexia, ↓ wt, ↑ thirst.
Parenteral IM **Oral/GI:** N/V, abdominal pain, cramps, constipation, diarrhea.
Once a month **S/Cond:** Avoid alcohol. Oral- caution $\bar{c}$ lactation. IM- not $\bar{c}$ lactation.
  Caution $\bar{c}$ ↓ hepatic func or moderate to severe ↓ renal func.
  Pregnancy: Category C.
  Other: Insomnia, anxiety, muscle/joint pain, fatigue, headache, chills,
  rash, depression $\bar{c}$ suicidal thinking & behavior, irritability, nervousness,
  drowsiness, dizziness. Hepatotoxicity $\bar{c}$ high dose.
  Blood/Serum: Rare- ↑ AST, ↑ ALT. **Monitor:** Hepatic func.

Namenda/Namenda XR ALZHEIMER'S DISEASE TREATMENT, NMDA Receptor See **memantine p 207**

naproxen ANTIARTHRITIC, ANALGESIC, NSAID
  Naprosyn **Drug:** Take $\bar{c}$ food or milk to ↓ GI irritation.
Susp- 30 mg (1.5 mEq) Swallow SR & EC tab whole, do not break, crush or chew.
Na/5 mL, sorbitol, sucrose, **Diet:** Consider Na content $\bar{c}$ ↓ Na diet.
Tab Caution $\bar{c}$ GI irritants eg K suppl (↑ risk of GI irritation). Limit caffeine
  EC-Naprosyn (DR) to ↓ GI effects. Avoid or limit natural products which affect coagulation
Tab (eg garlic, ginger, ginkgo, ginseng or horse chestnut). **Nutr:** ↑ thirst.
  Oral/GI: Stomatitis, dry mouth, dysphagia, N/V, dyspepsia,
  GI pain, constipation, colitis, diarrhea, flatulence.
naproxen sodium GI ulcers & bleeding (may be sudden & serious).
  Anaprox **S/Cond:** Avoid alcohol. Not $\bar{c}$ lactation. > 99% serum alb bound.
275 mg Tab- Caution $\bar{c}$ ↓ hepatic func or mild ↓ renal func. Not $\bar{c}$ moderate or
  25 mg (1.09 mEq) Na severe ↓ renal func. Not $\bar{c}$ aspirin allergy. Caution $\bar{c}$ geriatric,
550 mg Tab- IBD, colitis, Crohn's, HTN, CHF or edema. Not $\bar{c}$ gastritis/ulcer.
  50 mg (2.18 mEq) Na **Pregnancy:** Category C, but not recommended in pregnancy.
  Aleve

Tab- 20 mg (0.87 mEq) Na
Naprelan (SR) Tab
375 mg Tab-
 37 mg (1.61 mEq) Na
500 mg Tab-
 50 mg (2.18 mEq) Na

Category D in 3rd trimester due to ↑ risk to fetus & mother including death.
Other: Dizziness, drowsiness, headache, peripheral edema, dyspnea,
blurred vision, rash, flu syndrome, ↑ BP, palpitations, paresthesia,
tinnitus, vertigo, sweating. Rare- jaundice & hepatitis, SJS, TEN.
↑ risk of CV problems, eg HTN, CHF, MI, CVA.
Blood/Serum: ↑ ALT, ↑ AST, ↑ alk phos, ↑ LDH, ↑ BUN, ↑ crea,
↑ K, ↑ glucose, ↓ platelet aggregation. Rare- dyscrasias.
Urinary: UTI, cystitis. **Monitor:** CBC, hepatic & renal func c̄ LT use.

naratriptan
 Amerge

ANTIMIGRAINE, Serotonin 5-HT$_1$ Receptor Agonist
 See **Antimigraine p 39**

Nardil

ANTIDEPRESSANT, MAOI
 See **phenelzine p 252**

Nasacort AQ

ANTIASTHMA, Corticosteroid
 See **triamcinolone p 322**

Nascobal
 vitamin B$_{12}$

VITAMIN, ANTIANEMIC
 Intranasal Gel & Nasal Spray
 See **vitamin B$_{12}$ p 333**

Nasonex
 mometasone

ANTIALLERGIC RHINITIS
 Corticosteroid, Nasal
 See listing for
 beclomethasone p 51

Natazia

ORAL CONTRACEPTIVE
 See **Oral Contraceptives p 237**

nateglinide
 Starlix
 Tab- lactose

ORAL HYPOGLYCEMIC for TYPE 2 Diabetes, Meglitinide
 (Monotherapy or c̄ **metformin**, **pioglitazone** or **rosiglitazone**)
 Drug: Take 1-30 minutes before meals. Omit if meal is skipped.
 Diet: Prescribed diabetic diet, exercise. ↓ cal if wt loss needed.
 Nutr: *STIMULATES INSULIN RELEASE*.
 S/Cond: Limit alcohol. Not c̄ lactation. 98% serum alb bound.
 Caution c̄ ↓ hepatic func or severe ↓ renal func.
 Not c̄ Type 1 diabetes or diabetic ketoacidosis. **Pregnancy:** Category C.
 Other: Hypoglycemia, flu symptoms, URTI, dizziness, joint disorder.
 Blood/Serum: ↑ *INSULIN*, ↓ *FASTING GLUCOSE*, ↓ *POSTPRANDIAL GLUCOSE*,
 ↓ *Hb A1$_C$*, ↑ uric acid. **Monitor:** FBS & Hb A1$_C$ periodically.

Navelbine	ANTINEOPLASTIC	See **vinorelbine** p 335

nebivolol
  Bystolic
  Tab- lactose, starch

ANTIHYPERTENSIVE, Beta 1 Blocker, Cardioselective
  Drug: Take s̄ regard to food.
  Diet: ↓ Na, ↓ cal may be recommended. Avoid natural licorice, see p 374.
  Oral/GI: Nausea, diarrhea. **S/Cond:** Not c̄ lactation. 98% serum pro bound.
  Caution c̄ severe ↓ renal func or moderate ↓ hepatic func or CHF.
  Not c̄ severe ↓ hepatic func. Not c̄ asthma/bronchospasm, severe
  bradycardia, severe heart conditions (see PI).
  Caution c̄ diabetes- may mask signs of hypoglycemia.
  May reduce insulin release in response to hyperglycemia.
  Pregnancy: Category C.
  Other: ↓ _BP_ c̄ possible hypotension, headache, fatigue, dizziness,
  insomnia, chest pain, bradycardia, rash, dyspnea, peripheral edema.
  Blood/Serum: ↑ BUN, ↑ uric acid, ↑ TG, ↓ HDL, ↓ chol, ↓ platelets.
  Monitor: BP, heart rate.

nelfinavir (NFV)
  Viracept
  Pwd- sucrose,
    maltodextrin
    aspartame =
    phenylalanine 11.2 mg/g
  Tab

ANTIRETROVIRAL (HIV/AIDS), Protease Inhibitor
  Drug: Take c̄ food to ↑ blood level & AUC 2-3X.
  Mix pwd c̄ small amount water, milk, soy milk, infant formula,
  dietary supplement, pudding or ice cream.[6]
  Do not mix pwd c̄ acidic food or liquid, causes bitter taste.[7]
  Can crush tab & mix c̄ pudding or in water.
  Rinse & drink water mix several times.[5]
  Diet: Avoid SJW, see p 286. **Nutr:** Anorexia.
  Oral/GI: Nausea, abdominal pain, flatulence, DIARRHEA.
  S/Cond: Not c̄ lactation. > 98% serum pro bound.
  Caution c̄ diabetes- ↑ glucose. Caution c̄ ↓ mild hepatic func.
  Not c̄ moderate to severe ↓ hepatic func. Caution c̄ hemophilia- ↑ bleeding time.
  Pregnancy: Previously category B.
  Other: Rash (↑ in women). Fat redistribution.
  Bloods/Serum: ↑ glucose, ↑ alk phos, ↑ ALT, ↑ AST, ↑ CPK, ↑ amylase,
  ↑ LD, ↑ GGT, ↑ chol.

| **Neoral** | IMMUNOSUPPRESSANT | See **cyclosporine p 96** |

Neulasta
  pegfilgrastim
   prefilled syringe- sorbitol 30 mg

COLONY STIMULATING FACTOR   See listing for **filgrastim p 142**
      Longer acting than **filgrastim**   Parenteral only (SC)

| **Neumega** | PLATELET GROWTH FACTOR | See **oprelvekin p 236** |

| **Neupogen** | COLONY STIMULATING FACTOR | See **filgrastim p 142** |

| **Neurontin** | ANTIEPILEPTIC | See **gabapentin p 152** |

nevirapine (NVP)
  Viramune
  Tab- lactose,
   Na starch glycolate
  Susp- sorbitol,
   sucrose
  Viramune XR
  Tab- (SR)- lactose

ANTIRETROVIRAL (HIV/AIDS), NNRTI
    Drug: Take s̄ regard to food. Swallow XR tab whole.
    Do not crush, chew or divide XR tab
    Diet: Not c̄ SJW, see p 286.
    Oral/GI: Stomatitis, <u>N/V</u>, abdominal pain, diarrhea.
    S/Cond: Not c̄ lactation. Caution c̄ mild ↓ hepatic func.
    Not c̄ moderate to severe ↓ hepatic func.
    Caution c̄ severe ↓ renal func requiring dialysis.
    Additional dose needed after dialysis.
    Pregnancy: Category C.
    Other: <u>Rash</u>, life threatening skin reactions (SJS, TEN)/hypersensitivity
    reactions, fever, headache, fatigue, muscle or joint pain, drowsiness,
    paresthesia, hepatotoxicity (↑ risk in women &/or c̄ ↑ CD4 counts)-
    may be fatal.
    Blood/Serum: ↑ GGT, ↑ <u>ALT</u>, ↑ <u>AST</u>, ↑ <u>alk phos</u>.
    Pediatrics- ↑ bil, ↑ <u>amylase</u>, ↑ <u>MCV</u>, ↓ <u>platelets</u>, ↓ <u>neutrophils</u>, ↓ <u>Hb</u>.
    Monitor: Hepatic func prior to & during therapy.

| **Nexavar** | ANTINEOPLASTIC, Multikinase Inhibitor | See **sorafenib p 295** |

Nexium/Nexium I.V.
  esomeprazole

ANTIULCER, ANTISECRETORY, ANTIGERD, Proton Pump Inhibitor
    s-isomer of **omeprazole**   See **Proton Pump Inhibitors p 268**

niacin (Vit B$_3$) B COMPLEX VITAMIN, ANTIHYPERLIPIDEMIC, ANTIPELLAGRA
  nicotinic acid Two major forms are nicotinic acid & nicotinamide (niacinamide)
  Niaspan (SR)- Tab **Drug:** Only nicotinic acid form (1- 6 g/day) will ↓ lipids. Take c̄ food or
  Niacor milk to ↓ GI distress. Swallow SR tab whole HS after ↓ fat snack.
  Tab- vegetable oil Not c̄ hot liquids, spicy foods or alcohol (↑ flushing/itching).[7]

May take c̄ **aspirin** or NSAID, 30 min before taking **niacin**, to help ↓ flushing.[1]
Diet: Antipellagra dose- 200-400 mg daily[52] + 5 mg each Thi, Rib, Pyr.
As antihyperlipidemic- ↓ fat, ↓ chol diet.
Nutr: AI infants 0-6 mo = **2** mg/day preformed niacin
7-12 mo = **4** mg/day niacin equivalents.

  nicotinamide **RDA** (mg/day niacin equivalents)
  (niacinamide) Children 1-3 yr = **6**. 4-8 = **8**. 9-13 = **12**.
  Generic brands Female 14-70+ = **14**. Male 14-70+ = **16**. Lactation = **17**.
UL (mg/day) Children 1-3 yr = **10**. 4-8 = **15**. 9-13 = **20**. 14-18 = **30**.
Adult = **35**. Lactation = **30-35**. 60 mg dietary tryptophan = 1 mg niacin.
Fe, Zn, Pyr or Rib def ↓ conversion of tryptophan to niacin.[47]
Oral/GI: Dry mouth, <u>N/V</u>, peptic ulcer, dyspepsia, <u>cramps</u>,
<u>diarrhea</u>, <u>flatulence</u>.
S/Cond: Not c̄ lactation as antihyperlipidemic.
Caution c̄ diabetes- ↑ glucose. Not c̄ significant ↓ hepatic func.
Caution c̄ ↓ renal func, peptic ulcer, arrhythmias, IBD,
migraines or gout.[47] ↑ need in alcoholism.
Def S/S (pellagra)- dementia, dermatitis, diarrhea, pigmented rash, vomiting,
constipation, red tongue, depression, apathy, headache, fatigue.[47c]
Pregnancy: RDA = **18** mg/day niacin equivalents. **UL** = **30-35** mg/day.
Category C for antihyperlipidemic dose.
Other: <u>FLUSHING</u> (↓ c̄ SR form or c̄ aspirin 30 min before dose), <u>HEADACHE</u>
(nicotinic acid only). <u>ITCHING</u>, rash, hypotension, dizziness,
arrhythmias, muscle pain, gout, jaundice & hepatotoxicity
(↑ c̄ SR form at dose as low as 500 mg daily).
Blood/Serum: High dose- ↑ <u>glucose</u>, ↑ Hb A1$_C$,[93] ↑ <u>homocysteine</u>,[1]
↑ alk phos, ↑ AST, ↑ ALT, ↑ bil, ↑ LDH, ↑ uric acid, ↑ CPK.
Rare- ↓ alb, ↓ P, ↑ PT/INR, ↓ platelets.

Nicotinic acid only- ↓ *CHOL*, ↓ *TG*, ↓ *VLDL*, ↓ *LDL*, ↑ *HDL*, ↓ *LP(a)*.
Urinary: False + glucose (CuSO$_4$).[13]
Monitor: c̄ high dose- hepatic func, glucose, lipids, uric acid.
Possibly PT/INR, platelets, P.

nicotinic acid	ANTIHYPERLIPIDEMIC, B Complex Vitamin See **niacin above**

nifedipine
Adalat
(previous brand name)
All Caps-peppermint oil
10 mg Cap- saccharin
Adalat CC (SR)
Tab- lactose,
cornstarch
Procardia
All Caps- peppermint oil
10 mg Cap- saccharin Na
Procardia XL (SR)
Tab
Nifedipine ER (SR)
Tab

ANTIANGINA, ANTIHYPERTENSIVE (SR form), Ca Channel Blocker
Drug: Swallow SR tab whole- do not chew, divide or crush.
Do not use sublingually for HTN emergencies.
Take **Adalat CC** on an empty stomach.
Diet: Not c̄ grapefruit/related citrus, see p 390.
↓ Na, ↓ cal may be recommended. Avoid natural licorice, see p 374.
Avoid ginger, ginkgo, ginseng,[9b] SJW, see p 286 or melatonin,[4] see p 206.
Oral/GI: Sore throat, nausea, dyspepsia, constipation, diarrhea, flatulence.
S/Cond: Avoid alcohol.[9b] Not c̄ lactation. 92-98% serum pro bound.[6]
Caution c̄ ↓ hepatic func or geriatric. **Pregnancy:** Category C.
Other: ↓ *BP* c̄ possible hypotension, flushing, peripheral edema, dizziness,
headache, muscle cramps, chills, sweating, cough, weakness, tremor,
palpitations, fatigue, blurred vision, nervousness, dyspnea, muscle/joint pain.
Blood/Serum: ↑ alk phos, ↑ AST, ↑ AlT, ↑ LDH, ↑ CPK, + ANA.
Rare- dyscrasias. **Monitor:** BP

Niferex
iron polysaccharide
Elixir- 100 mg Fe/5 mL, 10% alcohol, sorbitol
150 Cap- 150 mg Fe, sucrose, starch, castor oil
150 Forte Cap- 150 mg Fe, 1 mg folic acid, 25 µg Vit B$_{12}$, 60 mg Vit C, starch

SUPPLEMENT, ANTIANEMIC, elemental iron
See listing for **ferrous salts p 140**

Niravam
alprazolam

ANTIANXIETY, ANTIPANIC See **Benzodiazepines p 54**

nisoldipine
Sular Tab (SR)- lactose

ANTIHYPERTENSIVE, Ca Channel Bocker See listing for **nifedipine above**
Drug: Do not take c̄ high fat meal- affects drug kinetics.
Take on empty stomach 1 hr before or 2 hr after a meal.

N

| **Nitro-Dur** | ANTIANGINA | See **nitroglycerin below** |

nitrofurantoin — ANTIBIOTIC, Urinary Tract Infection (Acute Cystitis) Treatment/Prophylaxis only

Macrobid (SR)
25% macrocrystals
75% immediate release
Cap- lactose,
 cornstarch, sugar
Macrodantin
(macrocrystals)
Cap- lactose,
 starch
Furadantin
Oral Susp- saccharin,
 sorbitol

Drug: Take c̄ food or milk to ↓ GI distress & ↑ bioavailability 40%. Swallow SR cap whole.
Diet: Adequate cal, pro, Vit B complex.[13] Mg suppl ↓ abs- take separately by at least 2 hr. **Nutr:** Anorexia.
Oral/GI: N/V, dyspepsia, abdominal pain, diarrhea, constipation, flatulence. Rare- pseudomembranous colitis.
S/Cond: Avoid alcohol.[12] Not c̄ lactation. Caution c̄ G6PD def- risk of hemolytic anemia. Not c̄ ↓ renal func, GFR < 60.[58]
Caution c̄ geriatric.[84] Caution c̄ Vit B def, anemia, diabetes, electrolyte imbalance, pulmonary disease or debilitating disease.
Pregnancy: Category B until 38th wk. Do not use after 37th wk.
Other: Headache, pneumonitis. Rare- allergic reaction, SJS, lupus-like syndrome, hepatitis, peripheral neuropathy, pseudotumor cerebri, pancreatitis, optic neuritis, pulmonary reactions (can be fatal).
Blood/Serum: ↑ AST, ↑ ALT, ↑ P.
Rare- ↓ Hb, dyscrasias including hemolytic anemia.
Urinary: False + glucose ($CuSO_4$), dark color.
Monitor: Pulmonary, renal & hepatic func c̄ LT use.

nitroglycerin — ANTIANGINA — Oral, Parenteral (IV), patch, spray, ointment

Cap (SR) may contain
 lactose, sucrose
Nitro-Dur- patch
Nitrostat- sublingual
Tab- lactose, starch
Nitrolingual Pump Spray-
 medium-chain triglycerides,
 dehydrated alcohol,
 peppermint oil

For relief of acute attack- sublingual tab, lingual spray only.
Drug: Consult pharmacist for proper administration.
Take SR forms on empty stomach c̄ full glass of water, 1 hr before or 2 hr after meals. Swallow SR forms whole.
Oral/GI: Dry mouth, N/V, abdominal pain.
S/Cond: Avoid alcohol. Caution c̄ lactation. Caution c̄ CHF. Not c̄ severe HTN or severe anemia. **Pregnancy:** Category C.
Other: Headache, dizziness, hypotension, weakness, syncope, palpitation, blurred vision, flushing, tachycardia, rash, restlessness.
Blood/Serum: Rare- methemoglobinemia. **Monitor:** BP & heart rate.

nizatidine **Axid/Axid AR**	ANTIULCER, ANTIGERD, ANTISECRETORY	See **Histamine H$_2$ Receptor Antagonists** p 162
Nizoral	ANTIFUNGAL	See **ketoconazole** p 184
NoDoz/No-Doz	STIMULANT	See **caffeine** p 67
Nordette 28	ORAL CONTRACEPTIVE	See **Oral Contraceptives** p 237
Norinyl	ORAL CONTRACEPTIVE	See **Oral Contraceptives** p 237
Norpramin **desipramine**	ANTIDEPRESSANT	See **Tricyclic Antidepressants** p 323
nortriptyline **Pamelor**	ANTIDEPRESSANT	See **Tricyclic Antidepressants** p 323
Norvasc	ANTIHYPERTENSIVE, Ca Channel Blocker	See **amlodipine** p 32
Norvir	ANTIRETROVIRAL (HIV/AIDS), Protease Inhibitor	See **ritonavir** p 281
Novantrone	ANTINEOPLASTIC	See **mitoxantrone** p 219
Novolin/Novolog	ANTIDIABETIC, HYPOGLYCEMIC	See **insulin** p 175
Noxafil	ANTIFUNGAL, Aspergillus, Candida	See **posaconazole** p 259
NPH Insulin	ANTIDIABETIC, HYPOGLYCEMIC	See **insulin** p 175
Nplate	IDIOPATHIC THROMBOCYTOPENIC PURPURA TREATMENT	See **romisplostim** p 284
Nucynta/Nucynta ER	ANALGESIC, Opioid & Norepinephrine Reuptake Inhibitor	See **tapentadol** p 303
Nulojix	IMMUNOSUPPRESSANT, Prophylaxis of Organ Rejection in Kidney Transplant	See: **belatacept** p 52
NuvaRing	CONTRACEPTIVE, Vaginal Insert	See listing for **Oral Contraceptives** p 237

Nydrazid
previous brand name

TUBERCULOSIS TREATMENT

See **isoniazid p 180**

nystatin

ORAL CANDIDIASIS TREATMENT, Antifungal

Mycostatin previous brand name **Drug:** Take oral susp as directed. Retain oral drug in mouth as long as possible.
Generic brands
Susp- $\leq$ 1% alcohol,
3.0 g sucrose/5 mL,
propylene glycol

Oral/GI: GI distress, N/V, stomach pain, diarrhea. No GI absorption.
S/Cond: Do dental care cautiously, see p 11 & 15. Caution $\bar{c}$ lactation.
Pregnancy: Category C.

Nytol

SLEEP AID

See **diphenhydramine p 112**

octreotide
Sandostatin (SC or IV)
mannitol 45 mg/mL
lactic acid 3.4 mg/mL
Sandostatin LAR Depot
(IM only- monthly
intragluteal injection)
mannitol 15 mg/syringe

ANTIDIARRHEAL (in carcinoid tumor, VIPoma, HIV)   Parenteral only
ANTIACROMEGALY (To ↓ GH, ICF-I)
   Also used for acute bleeding esophageal varices treatment
   somatostatin-like action   Parenteral only (SC, IM or IV)
Drug: Inject between meals & HS to ↓ GI effects.
Diet: ↓ fat may ↓ GI side effects.[6]
Nutr: May cause fat & fat soluble Vit malabsorption & delay gallbladder emptying. Alters insulin, growth hormone, thyroid hormone & glucagon levels.
Oral/GI: N/V, ABDOMINAL PAIN, bloating, diarrhea, steatorrhea, constipation, flatulence.
S/Cond: Caution $\bar{c}$ lactation. Caution $\bar{c}$ diabetes- ↑ or ↓ glucose. Caution $\bar{c}$ severe ↓ renal func or gallbladder disease.
IV incompatible $\bar{c}$ TPN solutions.[26] **Pregnancy:** Category B.
Other: GALLBLADDER ABNORMALITIES, BILIARY SLUDGE, BRADYCARDIA, arrhythmias, hypothyroidism, goiter, headache, dizziness, edema, fatigue, fever, flushing, weakness. Rare- ↑ QT interval, pancreatitis, hepatitis.
Blood/Serum: ↓ T_4, ↓ TSH, hyperglycemia, hypoglycemia, ↓ Vit B_{12}.[7] Abnormal Schilling's test.
Monitor: Blood glucose. LT use- baseline & periodic- gallbladder by ultrasound, 72 hr fecal fat & carotene, thyroid func, electrolytes, Vit B_{12}.

Ofirmiv

ANALGESIC, ANTIPRYRETIC

See **acetaminophen p 22**

Oforta	ANTINEOPLASTIC , Antimetabolite (Leukemia)	See **fludarabine p 145**
Ogen	HORMONE	See **Hormone Therapy p 165**

olanzapine
  Zyprexa
  Tab- lactose
  Zyprexa Zydis
  ODT- gelatin, mannitol,
  aspartame = 0.35-0.45mg
  phenylalanine/tab
  Zyprexa Relprevv (IM)
  Vial- mannitol

ANTIPSYCHOTIC (Second Generation)   Oral or Parenteral (IM)
    ANTIMANIC (Bipolar Disorder Treatment)
    ACUTE AGITATION TREATMENT (IM), Dibenzothiazepene Derivative
Drug: Take s̄ regard to food. Swallow **Zydis** tab c̄ or s̄ liquid.
Dissolve **Zydis** ODT on tongue c̄ or s̄ liquid, swallow saliva.
Nutr: ↑ <u>APPETITE</u>, ↑ <u>WEIGHT</u>, <u>obesity</u>, ↓ wt, ↑ thirst.
Oral/GI: <u>Dry</u> <u>mouth</u>, ↑ salivation, <u>dyspepsia</u>, N/V, flatulence, <u>constipation</u>.
Rare- dysphagia, impaction.
S/Cond: Avoid alcohol. Not c̄ lactation. 93% serum pro bound.
Hypoalbuminemia (< 3 g/dL) may ↑ drug effects.
Caution c̄ diabetes- ↑ glucose. Caution c̄ geriatric, Parkinson's[21] or
history of seizures. Not c̄ Alzheimer's. ↑ risk of dental problems, see p 11 &15.
Pregnancy: Category C.
Other: <u>DIABETES</u>, <u>DROWSINESS</u>, <u>dizziness</u>, <u>agitation</u>, <u>weakness</u>, akathisia,
rhinitis, URTI, personality disorder, accidental injury, abnormal gait, HTN,
postural hypotension, edema, tachycardia, nervousness, chest pain, paresthesia,
back or joint pain, headache, fever, cough, neck rigidity, visual disturbances,
tremor, twitching, rash, stuttering, insomnia, tardive dyskinesia, EPS.
Rare- NMS, seizures. ↑ mortality in geriatrics c̄ dementia-related psychosis.
Blood/Serum: ↑ <u>GLUCOSE</u>, ↑ <u>TRIGLYCERIDES</u>,[1] ↑ <u>PROLACTIN</u>,[21] ↑ ALT, ↑ AST,
↑ GGT, ↓ WBC, ↑ eosinophils. < 1%- ↑ alk phos, ↑ bil, ↑ CPK, ↑ or ↓ K,
↓ or ↑ Na, ↑ uric acid, ↓ glucose, ↑ chol.
Urinary: Hematuria, UTI, incontinence, retention.
Monitor: Baseline wt & BP, then monthly.
Baseline FBS, Hb A1$_C$ & lipids, then at 12 wk, then at least annually.[1]

Oleptro	ANTIDEPRESSANT, Heterocyclic	See **trazodone p 321**

olmesartan
  Benicar/Benicar HCT

ANTIHYPERTENSIVE   See **Angiotensin II Receptor Antagonists p 38**
   Benicar HCT also contains **hydrochlorothiazide**, see **p 166**.

olsalazine
  Dipentum- Cap

ANTI-INFLAMMATORY (in ulcerative colitis)   See listing for **mesalamine p 209**
   Drug: Take c̄ food. **S/Cond:** 99% serum pro bound.

N/O

Omacor (original brand name)ANTIHYPERLIPIDEMIC to reduce triglyceride levels
  (brand name now **Lovaza** in USA)   See **omega-3 fatty acids p 234**

omalizumab   ANTIASTHMA   Parenteral (SC)
  Xolair   **Drug:** Dose based on pretreatment IgE & body wt, see PI.
  Vial   **S/Cond:** Caution c̄ lactation. Dose must be adjusted for significant wt change.
  14.5 mg sucrose   Dosing table is for wt ≤ 150 Kg (330 lb). Not c̄ parasitic infection.
                       Pregnancy: Category B.
                       Other: Pain- muscle/arm/leg, fatigue, dizziness, itching, dermatitis,
                       earache, injection site reaction, hair loss. Rare- anaphylaxis (may be delayed).
                       Blood/Serum: ↓ platelets.
                       Monitor: For S/S of anaphylaxis, including a delayed reaction.

omega-3 fatty acids   ANTIHYPERLIPIDEMIC to reduce Triglyceride levels in adult c̄ TG ≥ 500 mg/dL.
  Lovaza (USA)   (for prescription drug **Lovaza** or **Omacor**)
  Omacor (other countries)   Also used as an Anticoagulant, Antiarrhythmic,[122] Antidepressant[93]
  fish oil,   or Anti-inflammatory
  (omega-3- Acid Ethyl Esters)   EPA (eicosapentaenoic acid) & DHA (docosahexaenoic acid)
  Cap- > 900 mg omega-3   **Drug:** Take c̄ meals 1-3X/day. Swallow cap whole, do not open or crush.
  fatty acid, ethyl esters   **Diet:** Drug is adjunct to low fat, low sugar (low cal if needed) diet.
  465 mg EPA, 375 mg DHA,   **Oral/GI:** Taste changes/after taste, belching, dyspepsia.[9]
  4 mg α-tocopheral   Enteric coated form may ↓ upper GI effects. Diarrhea c̄ high dose.
  (= 6 IU Vit E), soybean oil   **S/Cond:** Limit or avoid alcohol. Caution c̄ lactation.
  Optimum Omega   Caution c̄ ↓ hepatic func. Caution c̄ fish or soy allergy.
  (dietary suppl)   May ↑ risk of ventricular fibrillation/tachycardia in pts c̄
  Cap- 150 mg EPA,   implantable defibrillators.[30] Weight loss (if needed) & exercise
  100 mg DHA, 50 mg   advised to ↓ TG levels. No effect on blood glucose c̄ prescribed dose.
  other omega-3 fatty acids,   **Pregnancy:** Category C. **Other:** Rash, flu-like syndrome, infection, mild ↓ BP.[1]
  5 IU Vit E,   **Blood/Serum:** ↓ _TG_, ↓ _chol_, ↓ _VLDL_, ↑ _HDL_, but slightly ↑ _LDL_.
  1 mg deodorized garlic oil   ↑ ALT. Large dose ↑ PT/INR, ↓ platelet aggregation, ↑ bleeding time.
  MarineOmega-3 (dietary suppl) **Monitor:** Baseline & periodic lipid panel, ALT. Possibly PT/INR.
  Cap- 300 mg EPA, 200 DHA, 5 IU Vit E, 1 g fat (0.25 sat fat), 11 cal.
  Fisol (dietary suppl) enteric coated cap- 150 mg EPA, 100 DHA, 1 IU Vit E, 5 cal, 0.5 g fat

| omeprazole
Prilosec/Zegerid | ANTIULCER, ANTIGERD | See **Proton Pump Inhibitors p 268** |

| **Omnaris**
ciclesonide | ANTIALLERGIC RHINITIS
Nasal Spray | See **beclomethasone p 51** |

| **Omnicef** | ANTIBIOTIC, Cephalosporin (oral) | See **cefdinir p 76** |

| **Oncovin** previous brand name | ANTINEOPLASTIC, Vinca Alkoloid | See **vincristine p 334** |

ondansetron
  Zofran
  Tab- lactose,
  starch
  Soln- sorbitol
  Zofran ODT
  Tab-
  aspartame = < 0.03 mg
  phenylalanine,
  mannitol, gelatin
Vial premixed- preservative free

ANTIEMETIC, ANTINAUSEANT (Post Operative or Chemotherapy)
  serotonin $5HT_3$ receptor antagonist   Oral or Parenteral (IV or IM)
Drug: Take initial dose 1/2 hr before chemotherapy.
Dissolve ODT on tongue $\bar{c}$ or $\bar{s}$ liquid, swallow saliva.
Oral/GI: Dry mouth, abdominal pain, constipation, diarrhea.
S/Cond: Caution $\bar{c}$ lactation. Caution $\bar{c}$ ↓ hepatic func.
Pregnancy: Category B.
Other: Headache, fatigue, dizziness, hypoxia, fever/chills, flushing,
hiccups, rash, drowsiness.
Blood/Serum: Transient ↑ AST, ↑ ALT, ↑ bil. Rare- ↓ K. **Urinary:** Retention.

| **Onfi** | ANTIEPILEPTIC (Lennox Gastaut Syndrome) | See **Benzodiazepines p 54** |

| **Onglyza**
saxagliptin
Tab- lactose | ANTIDIABETIC AGENT, Incretin Enhancer
DPP-4 (dipetidyl-peptidase-4) Inhibitor | See listing for **sitagliptin p 293** |

| **Onsolis** Buccal Soluble Film | ANALGESIC Narcotic, Opioid | See **fentanyl p 139** |

| **Opana/Opana ER**
Oxymorphone | ANALGESIC, Narcotic, Opioid
Opana Tab- lactose, starch
Opana ER Tab- only 40 mg strength contains lactose | See listing for **morphine p 221** |

O

oprelvekin
  Neumega
  preservative free

PLATELET GROWTH FACTOR (to prevent thrombocytopenia c̄ chemotherapy)
  Also used to treat Crohn's disease   Parenteral only (SC)
Nutr: Dehydration.
Oral/GI: <u>Oral</u> <u>candidiasis</u>, <u>N/V</u>, <u>pharyngitis</u>, <u>mucositis</u>, <u>diarrhea</u>.
S/Cond: Not c̄ lactation. Caution c̄ severe ↓ renal func, CHF, edema, HTN.
Pregnancy: Category C.
Other: <u>EDEMA</u>, <u>fever</u>, <u>tachycardia</u>, <u>palpitations</u>, <u>syncope</u>, <u>vasodilitation</u>,
<u>weakness</u>, <u>atrial</u> <u>fibrillation</u>, <u>dizziness</u>, <u>insomnia</u>, <u>shortness</u> <u>of</u> <u>breath</u>,
<u>cough</u>, <u>rhinitis</u>, <u>rash</u>, headache, visual changes, paresthesia,
pleural effusion. Rare- allergic reaction, possible anaphylaxis.
Blood/Serum: ↑ *<u>PLATELETS</u>*, ↑ <u>PLASMA</u> <u>VOLUME</u>, ↑ <u>FIBRINOGEN</u>.
Due to ↑ volume- ↓ <u>Hb</u>, ↓ <u>HCT</u>, ↓ <u>alb</u>, ↓ <u>pro</u>, ↓ <u>Ca</u>.
Monitor: CBC c̄ platelets prior to chemotherapy & regularly during use.
Fluid balance, electrolytes.

Optimum Omega

ANTIHYPERLIPIDEMIC to reduce triglyceride levels
See omega-3 fatty acids p 234

Oracea

ANTIBIOTIC, **doxycycline**   See **Tetracyclines p 310**

Oral Contraceptives   HORMONE, Estrogen/Progestin, Birth Control (also Antiacne* & to regulate menstrual cycle)
Drug: To ↓ nausea take c̄ food at same time each day. **Diet:** ↑ food high in Mg,[86] Fol, Pyr, Rib.
Limit caffeine[13]- caffeine levels ↑ 30-40%, see p 379. Caution c̄ grapefruit/related citrus,[136] see p 390.
Avoid SJW or saw palmetto.[93] **Nutr:** ↑ or ↓ wt, appetite changes. Affects Fol, Pyr, Rib, Vit A, Fe, Cu, Mg,
Zn, Ca,[93] possibly Vit B$_{12}$.[131] **Oral/GI:** N/V, bloating, cramps, diarrhea.
S/Cond: Limit alcohol. Not c̄ lactation. Caution c̄ diabetes- may ↑ insulin resistance.
Caution c̄ ↓ hepatic func, edema, HTN, migraines or CAD. Ethinyl estradiol is 95-97% serum alb bound.
Pregnancy: Category X. **Other:** Edema, ↑ BP, depression, dizziness, weakness, headache, migraine, rash,
cholestatic jaundice, visual disturbances, vaginal candidiasis, breakthrough bleeding/spotting (↑ c̄ **Lybrel**),
amenorrhea, breast changes, melasma, thromboembolism/thrombosis (↑ risk in smokers & > 35 years old).
Beyaz, **Safyral**, **Yaz** contains drospirenone- less edema, ↓ BP. Rare- gallbladder disease (dose related), hepatic tumor.
Blood/Serum: ↑ glucose, ↑ insulin, ↓ Fol, ↓ Pyr, ↓ Rib, ↑ Vit A, ↑ or ↓ alb, ↑ transferrin, ↑ TIBC, ↑ Fe,
↑ ceruloplasmin, ↑ prothrombin, ↑ Cu, ↓ Mg, ↓ Zn, ↑ Ca, ↑ alk phos, ↑ bil, ↑ GGT, ↑ AST, ↑ ALT, ↑ LDL,
↓ HDL, ↑ TG. Rare- abnormal thyroid func tests. Temporary or false ↓ Vit B$_{12}$.[131]
Monitor: BP, hepatic func, TSH. Possibly glucose, lipid panel.

All brands are Tabs. Days 22-28 of 28 day products are placebos which contain no hormones.

Aviane- lactose, cornstarch
Beyaz- lactose polyethylene glycol
Cyclessa- Days 1-21- Vit E, starch, lactose
 Days 22-28- lactose, cornstarch
Desogen- lactose, cornstarch, Vit E
Estrostep Fe*- Days 22-28- sucrose, Fe fumarate 75 mg
Femcon Fe Chew Tab- lactose, Na starch glycolate, sucralose
 Fe Fumarate Tab- Na starch gycolate, sugar
Kariva- lactose, cornstarch, Vit E
Loestrin 24- lactose, sugar, starch
 Days 22-28- Fe fumarate 75 mg, Na starch glycolate, sugar
Loestrin Fe- Days 22-28- Fe fumarate 75 mg
Lo Loestrin Fe- Days 1-26 mannitol, Na starch glycolate, Vit E, lactose.
 Days 27-28 Fe fumarate, 75 mg mannitol, Na starch glycolate, sucralose
Lo/Ovral 28- lactose
Low-Ogestrol- lactose
Lybrel 365 day regimen- lactose
Microgestin Fe- lactose, ethyl alcohol
 Days 22-28- starch, Fe fumarate 75 mg

Natazia- maize starch, pregelatinized maize starch
Nordette 28- lactose, starch
Norinyl- lactose, starch
Ortho-Cept- Vit E, lactose, cornstarch
Ortho-Cyclen 28- lactose, cornstarch
Ortho-Novum- lactose, starch
Ortho Tri-Cyclen*- lactose, cornstarch
Ortho Tri-Cyclen Lo- lactose, 22-28- + starch
Ovcon 35 Chewable- starch, lactose, cornstarch, sucralose
Safyral- lactose, polyethylene glycol
Seasonale/Seasonique 91 day regimen- lactose
Sprintec- lactose, cornstarch
TriNessa 28 day c̄ 7 inert green tabs
Tri-Norinyl 28 Day- lactose, starch
Tri-Sprintec- lactose
Trivora-21 & 28- lactose, cornstarch
Yasmin-28- lactose, cornstarch, starch, 22-28 starch free
Yaz*- lactose, cornstarch (also indicated for PMDD)
* Antiacne indication also

Orapred	CORTICOSTEROID, **prednisolone**	See **corticosteroids p 94**
Orencia	ANTIARTHRITIS, Rheumatoid Arthritis	See **abatacept p 19**

orlistat
   Xenical
   (120 mg **orlistat**)
   Cap- Na starch glycolate
   Alli (OTC)
   (60 mg **orlistat**)
   Cap- Na starch glycolate

WEIGHT CONTROL AGENT, Lipase Inhibitor
Drug: Take 1 cap c̄ or within 1 hr of each main meal containing fat.
Diet: Adjunct to reduced cal c̄ ≤ 30% of cal from fat.
Distribute fat among 3 main meals.
MVI essential, take 2 hr before or after drug (eg HS).[7]
Psyllium may help ↓ GI side effects.[1] Avoid **Olestra** fat sub.
Nutr: ↓ _WEIGHT_. ↓ _FAT ABS_ 30%. ↓ _ABS OF FAT SOLUBLE VITS_ (A, D, E, K).
↓ Vit E abs 60%, ↓ beta-carotene abs 33%.
Oral/GI: Tooth/gum disorder, abdominal pain, fecal urgency,
↑ defecation, OILY SPOTTING, fatty stool, fecal incontinence, FLATULENCE.
S/Cond: Not c̄ lactation. > 99% serum pro bound, but drug is minimally
abs from intestine. Not c̄ chronic malabsorption, pancreatitis or cholestatsis.
Not for transplant pt. **Pregnancy:** Category B.
Other: Headache, back pain, anxiety, fatigue, URTI, UTI,
influenza, slightly ↓ BP. Rare- hepatic injury, jaundice.
Blood/Serum: ↓ Vit D. Slightly ↓ chol, ↓ LDL, ↑ HDL, ↑ TG,
↓ fasting insulin. LT use > 1 yr- ↓ Vit A, K, E, beta-carotene.
Urinary: ↑ oxalate, UTI. **Monitor:** PT/INR. Possibly hepatic func, Vit D.

Ortho-Cept	ORAL CONTRACEPTIVE	See **Oral Contraceptives p 237**
Ortho-Cyclen 28	ORAL CONTRACEPTIVE	See **Oral Contraceptives p 237**
Ortho Evra	CONTRACEPTIVE, Patch	See listing for

Ortho Evra — **S/Cond:** Patch effect ↓ if wt > 198 lbs (90 kg)   **Oral Contraceptives p 237**
Other: ↑ risk of blood clots (venous thromboemboli) than c̄ birth control pills.

Ortho-Novum	ORAL CONTRACEPTIVE	See **Oral Contraceptives p 237**
Ortho Tri-Cyclen	ORAL CONTRACEPTIVE, ANTI-ACNE	See **Oral Contraceptives p 237**
Os-Cal	MINERAL SUPPLEMENT	See **calcium carbonate p 70**

oseltamivir **Tamiflu** Cap- starch Susp- sorbitol, saccharin Na, xanthan gum	INFLUENZA TREATMENT OR PROPHYLAXIS (for pt older than 1 yr) Neuraminidase Inhibitor **Drug:** Take $\bar{s}$ regard to food, but taking $\bar{c}$ food may ↓ GI upset. **Oral/GI:** <u>N/V</u>. **S/Cond:** Caution $\bar{c}$ lactation. Caution $\bar{c}$ ↓ renal func. **Pregnancy:** Category C. **Other:** Rare- neurological problems in children eg hallucinations, convulsions.

Ovcon 35	ORAL CONTRACEPTIVE	See **Oral Contraceptives p 237**

oxaliplatin
Eloxatin
Vial

ANTINEOPLASTIC, Metastatic Colorectal Cancer   Parenteral only (IV)
  Used $\bar{c}$ **5FU/leucovorin**
  Drug: Pre & post treatment $\bar{c}$ Mg & Ca may ↓ neurotoxiciy.[26]
  Do not reconstitute or dilute $\bar{c}$ NaCl soln.[26]
  Diet: Avoid cold drinks & use of ice to ↓ neurotoxicity.[26]
  Insure adequate fluid intake/hydration to ↑ urinary output.
  Nutr: <u>ANOREXIA</u>, dehydration.
  Oral/GI: <u>Altered</u> <u>taste</u>, <u>stomatitis</u>, <u>mucositis</u>, dysphagia, reflux,
  <u>NAUSEA/VOMITING</u>, <u>abdominal</u> <u>pain</u>, flatulence, colitis, <u>DIARRHEA</u>, <u>CONSTIPATION</u>.
  S/cond: Not $\bar{c}$ lactation. Do dental care cautiously, see p 11 & 15.
  Caution $\bar{c}$ ↓ renal func.
  Pregnancy: Category D.
  Other: <u>ACUTE</u> <u>PERIPHERAL</u> <u>NEUROPATHY</u> (↑ $\bar{c}$ exposure to cold), <u>PERSISTENT</u>
  <u>PERIPHERAL</u> <u>NEUROPATHY</u>, ↓ <u>SENSE</u> <u>OF</u> <u>BODY</u> <u>ORIENTATION</u>, <u>BONE</u> <u>MARROW</u>
  <u>SUPPRESSION</u>, <u>FEVER</u>, <u>FATIGUE</u>, dyspnea, <u>URTI</u>, coughing, rhinitis, dizziness,
  edema, <u>headache</u>, chest/back/joint pain, <u>rigors</u>, <u>rash</u>, <u>insomnia</u>,
  hiccups, nose-bleed, flushing, thromboembolism, hand-foot syndrome,
  tearing, visual changes, hepatotoxicity.
  Rare- anaphylactic like allergic reaction, pulmonary fibrosis (may be fatal).
  Blood/Serum: <u>ANEMIA</u>, ↓ <u>PLATELETS</u>, ↓ <u>neutrophils</u>, ↓ <u>WBC</u>, ↑ <u>bil</u>,
  ↑ <u>ALT</u>, ↑ <u>AST</u>, ↑ <u>crea</u>, ↓ K. **Urinary:** ↓ output.
  Monitor: CBC $\bar{c}$ diff, platelets, blood chemistry,
  pulmonary func before each dose.

oxandrolone
  Oxandrin
    Tab- cornstarch,
    lactose

ANTIWASTING, Anabolic Steroid
    To promote wt gain after surgery, trauma, infection.
    To ↓ bone pain in osteoporosis. To offset Pro catabolism c̄ corticosteroids.
    Diet: Requires adequate cal & pro intake for anabolic effect.
    Possibly ↓ Na.
    Nutr: ↑ _APPETITE_, ↑ _WT_, ↑ _LEAN BODY MASS_, ↑ _PROTEIN SYNTHESIS_.
    Oral/GI: N/V, diarrhea.
    S/Cond: Not indicated as appetite stimulant.
    Not c̄ lactation. 94-97% serum pro bound.[12]
    Not c̄ severe ↓ hepatic func, hypercalcemia, breast cancer,
    nephrosis, prostatic cancer or hypertrophy.
    Caution c̄ CAD or diabetics on insulin/oral hypoglycemics- ↓ glucose.
    Caution c̄ ↓ renal func or ↓ heptic func.[12]
    Pregnancy: Category X.
    Other: Acne, virilism in females/prepubertal males, menstrual or
    testicular changes, excitation, insomnia, edema, chills, muscle cramps,
    depression, jaundice, skin discoloration. Hypercalcemia in females.
    ↑ bone maturation & ↓ growth in children c̄ LT use.
    Rare, but may be fatal, peliosis hepatis, hepatocellular tumor.
    Blood/Serum: ↑ CPK, ↑ chol, ↑ LDL, ↓ HDL, ↑ crea, ↑ PT/INR,
    ↓ clotting factors, ↑ glucose, ↑ Ca, ↑ P, ↑ K, ↑ Na, ↑ Cl, ↑ bil, ↑ ALT,
    ↑ AST, ↑ alk phos, ↓ LH, ↓ FSH.
    Urinary: ↑ crea. Bladder irritability.
    Monitor: Glucose in diabetics. Lipid panel. Hepatic func.
    Hb/HCT c̄ high dose. Wt. Ca. Bone growth in children c̄ LT use.

oxaprozin
  Daypro

ANTIARTHRITIC, NSAID
    Tab- starch

See listing for **ibuprofen p 170**

oxazepam
  Serax (previous brand name)

ANTIANXIETY

See **Benzodiazepines p 54**

oxcarbazepine
 Trileptal
 Tab
 Susp- 10 mg ascorbic acid/mL,
  ethanol, saccharin Na,
  sorbitol, propylene glycol

ANTIEPILEPTIC   See listing for **carbamazepine** p 72
 Drug: Take s̄ regard to food.
 Diet: Fluid restriction if hyponatremia occurs.
 S/Cond: Caution c̄ ↓ renal func.
 Pregnancy: Category C. **Other:** <u>HYPONATREMIA</u> (30%).
 Monitor: Unlike **carbamazepine**, CBC c̄ diff not necessary.[21]

oxybutynin
 Ditropan/Ditropan XL
 Oxytrol, Gelnique Topical Gel

ANTIMUSCARINIC   See **Bladder Control Agents p 61**

oxycodone
 OxyContin (SR)
 Tab- lactose
 Oxecta
 Tab- IR
 Roxicodone
 Tab- 15 & 30 mg tabs-
  Na starch glycolate,
  cornstarch, lactose

ANALGESIC, Narcotic, Opioid
 Drug: May take c̄ food or milk to ↓ GI distress. Swallow SR form whole.
 Do not chew, crush or break. Peak plasma conc of 160 mg SR tab ↓ 25%
 when taken c̄ a high fat meal. **Oxecta**- immediate release tab not
 amenable to crushing and dissolving to deter abuse. Swallow whole.
 Do not administer via any type of feeding tube- may clog tube.
 Diet: Caution c̄ grapefruit/related citrus, see p 390. **Nutr:** <u>Anorexia</u>.
 Oral/GI: <u>Dry</u> <u>mouth</u>, dyspepsia, gastritis, <u>N/V</u>, diarrhea <u>constipation</u>.
 S/Cond: Avoid alcohol. Not c̄ lactation. May be habit forming c̄ LT use.
 Caution c̄ ↓ hepatic func or ↓ renal func, hypothyroidism or
 ↓ pulmonary func. Not c̄ paralytic ileus, acute or severe asthma
 or respiratory depression.
 Pregnancy: Category B, but not in labor.[7]
 Other: <u>DROWSINESS</u>, <u>sedation</u>, <u>fatigue</u>, <u>dizziness</u>, <u>weakness</u>, <u>itching</u>,
 <u>sweating</u>, fever/chills, hypotension (may be severe),
 respiratory depression, headache, nervousness, confusion, euphoria,
 insomnia, rash, twitching, hiccups. Rare- SIADH.
 Blood/Serum: ↑ amylase, ↑ lipase. < 1%- ↓ Na. **Urinary:** Retention.

oxymorphone
 Opana/Opana ER

ANALGESIC, Narcotic, Opioid   See **morphine p 221**
 Opana Tab- lactose, starch
 Opana ER Tab- only 40 mg strength contains starch

| **Oxytrol** | ANTIMUSCARINIC | See **Bladder Control Agents p 61** |
| oxybutynin | | |

| **Pacerone** | ANTIARRHYTHMIC | See **amiodarone p 31** |

paclitaxel
  Taxol
  castor oil EL (Cremaphor),
   50 % dehydrated alcohol
  Abraxane
  protein bound **paclitaxel**
  900 mg human albumin/vial

ANTINEOPLASTIC (Taxol- Breast, Ovarian, Lung Cancer or Kaposi's Sarcoma),
   Abraxane for breast cancer only
Pretreatment corticosteroid, antihistamine & H$_2$ Antagonist given c̄ **Taxol**
Antimitotic Agent   Parenteral only (IV)
Oral/GI: MUCOSITIS, NAUSEA/VOMITING, DIARRHEA.
S/Cond: Avoid alcohol- high alcohol content may lead to
intoxication, particularly c̄ low BW. Not c̄ lactation.
Do dental care cautiously, see p 11 & 15. 89-98 % serum pro bound.
Caution c̄ moderate to severe ↓ hepatic func. Caution c̄ CHF, recent MI,
cardiac conduction abnormalities. Therapy should not be started
c̄ severe ↓ neutrophils < 1500 cells/mm³ or < 1000 in Kaposi's Sarcoma.
Pregnancy: Category D. Can have adverse reproductive effects in males
resulting in teratogenic effects - avoid conception.
Other: BONE MARROW SUPPRESSION, PERIPHERAL NEUROPATHY, EDEMA,
INFECTION, ALLERGIC REACTION (can be fatal, may be due to castor oil
in **Taxol**), MUSCLE/JOINT PAIN, HAIR LOSS, ASTHENIA, hypotension, fever,
fatigue, rash, itching, bradycardia, arrhythmias, HTN, visual changes.[6]
Rare- SJS, TEN.
Blood/Serum: ↓ WHITE BLOOD CELLS, ANEMIA, ↓ PLATELETS, ↑ ALK PHOS,
↑ AST, ↑ bil, ↑ crea in HIV pt.[6] Transient ↑ TG.
Monitor: Baseline & frequent CBC c̄ diff, platelets, ECG.[26]

palifermin
  Kepivance
  50 mg mannitol,
  25 mg sucrose/vial

ORAL MUCOSITIS TREATMENT, Human Keratinocyte Growth Factor
                           Parenteral only (IV)
Oral/GI: Taste changes, mouth/tongue thickness or discoloration.
Oral or perioral dysesthesia (numbness, tingling, pain, burning).
S/Cond: Caution c̄ lactation. **Pregnancy:** Category C.
Other: Rash, edema, fever, muscle pain, transient ↑ BP.
Blood/Serum: ↑ amylase, ↑ lipase. **Urinary:** Pro.

paliperidone
Invega
Tab SR- propylene glycol
+ lactose in 3 mg Tab only
Invega Sustenna (SR)
Parenteral only (IM)

ANTISYCHOTIC, Second Generation
metabolite of **risperidone**

See listing for **risperidone p 280**
Causes moderate ↑ QT interval

Drug: IM starting dose, then 1/2 dose one wk later, then maintenance
dose q mo.

palonosetron
Aloxi
207.5 mg mannitol/vial
Cap

ANTIEMETIC, ANTINAUSEANT (Acute or Delayed N/V c̄ Chemotherapy)
serotonin 5HT₃ receptor antagonist   Oral or Parenteral (IV)

$5HT_3$ receptor antagonist

Drug: Use IV 1/2 hr before chemotherapy.
Take cap 1 hr before chemotherapy s̄ regard to food.
Diet: Maintain adequate hydration.
Oral/GI: <u>Constipation</u>, diarrhea.
S/Cond: Not c̄ lactation. Caution c̄ ↑ cardiac conduction intervals,
hypomagnesemia or hypokalemia.
Pregnancy: Category B.
Other: <u>Headache</u>, dizziness, hypotension, anxiety, weakness,
tachycardia, bradycardia. <1%- ↑ QT interval.
Blood/Serum: ↑ K. <1%- ↑ ALT, ↑ AST, ↑ bil.

Pamelor
nortriptyline

ANTIDEPRESSANT

See **Tricyclic Antidepressants p 323**

pamidronate
Aredia

HYPERCALCEMIA TREATMENT, PAGET'S DISEASE TREATMENT,
ADJUNCT TO TREATMENT OF BONE METASTASES

See **Bisphosphonates, Parenteral p 60**

O/P

pancrelipase (pancreatin)
  Creon (SR)
   Cap
  Pancrease
   Cap- cornstarch, sugar,
   Na starch glycolate
  Pancrease MT 4, 10, 16
   EC microtablets
  Pancrecarb (DR)
   microspheres in
   EC Cap-
   Na carboxymethyl starch
  Pancrelipase (DR, EC)
   Cap- castor oil
  Ultrase
   Cap microspheres-
   simethicone
  Ultrase MT 12 or 20
   Cap- minitablets,
   simethicone, castor oil
  Viokase
   Tab- lactose
   Pwd- lactose
  Zenpep (DR)
   pwd in Cap- castor oil

PANCREATIC ENZYME (mixture of porcine lipase, amylase & protease)
To treat steatorrhea due to pancreatic insufficiency (eg cystic fibrosis (CF), alcoholic pancreatitis, GI surgery)
Drug: Must take c̄ food. Take c̄ meal or snack & fluid. Preferably swallow Cap whole but may open cap & mix contents c̄ small amount acidic food (eg applesauce or gelatin) on spoon, take immediately- DO NOT chew or crush. Follow by glass of water or juice.
Mix **Zenpep** c̄ food c̄ < 4.5 pH. Do not mix cap contents c̄ food c̄ pH >5.5 for other brands. DO NOT INHALE PWD.
Dose based on symptoms/steatorrhea/g fat ingestion & actual wt.
Diet: Insure adequate hydration/fluid intake.
Pt c̄ pancreatic enzyme insufficiency- high calorie diet c̄ unrestricted fat intake, as appropriate for age & symptomology.
Not c̄ $CaCO_3$ or MgOH.[13] Take Fe or Fol separately.
Nutr: Enzymes ↓ Fe & Fol abs.[7, 13]
Oral/GI: N/V, stomach cramps, bloating, constipation, diarrhea, flatulence. Rare- intestinal obstruction, fibrosing colonopathy in CF or stenosis. Oral/esophageal membrane irritation if chewed.
S/Cond: Caution c̄ lactation. Not c̄ pork allergy. Not c̄ acute pancreatitis. Caution c̄ gout, ↑ uric acid, or ↓ renal func.
Pregnancy: Pancrease- Category B.
Zenzep, Creon, Ultrase, Pancrecarb, Pancrease MT, Viokase- Category C.
Other: Rare- allergic reaction.
Blood/Serum: ↓ Fe, ↓ Fol, ↑ uric acid c̄ very high dose.
Urinary: ↑ uric acid c̄ very high dose.

panitumumab **Vectibix** preservative free	ANTINEOPLASTIC, (Colorectal Cancer) Parenteral (IV) Epidermal Growth Factor Inhibitor, NOT for *KRAS* mutations in codon 12 or 13 **Diet:** ↑ Mg, ↑ Ca &/or suppl. **Oral/GI:** <u>S</u>tomatitis, <u>mucositis</u>, <u>NAUSEA</u>/<u>vomiting</u>, <u>ABDOMINAL</u> <u>PAIN</u>, <u>DIARRHEA</u>, <u>CONSTIPATION</u>. **S/Cond:** Not c̄ lactation. Not c̄ pulmonary fibrosis. **Pregnancy:** Category C. **Other:** <u>SKIN</u> <u>TOXICITY</u>- <u>INFLAMMATION</u>, <u>ACNEFORM RASH</u>, <u>ITCHING</u>, <u>EXFOLIATION</u>, <u>FISSURES</u>, <u>dry</u> <u>skin</u>, <u>FATIGUE</u>, <u>cough</u>, <u>edema</u>, <u>nail</u> <u>disorder</u>/<u>INFECTION</u>, <u>eye</u> <u>disorders</u>, <u>eyelash</u> <u>growth</u>, infusion reaction, pulmonary toxicity, angioedema. **Blood/Serum:** ↓ <u>MAGNESIUM</u>, ↓ Ca. **Monitor:** Periodic & for 8 wk after use- Electrolytes, Ca, Mg.
Panixine DisperDose	ANTIBIOTIC, Cephalosporin See **cephalexin p 79**
pantoprazole **Protonix/Protonix I.V.**	ANTIGERD, ANTISECRETORY See **Proton Pump Inhibitors p 268**
Parcopa	ANTIPARKINSON See **levodopa & carbidopa p 193**
paricalcitol **Zemplar** IV- 20% alcohol, 30% propylene glycol Cap- medium chain triglycerides (from coconut & palm kernel oils), alcohol	PREVENTION & TREATMENT OF SECONDARY HYPERPARATHYROIDISM in ESRD synthetic **Vitamin D** Oral & Parenteral (IV) See listing for **calcitriol p 68**
Parlodel	ANTIPARKINSON See **bromocriptine p 64**
Parnate **tranylcypromine**	ANTIDEPRESSANT, MAOI See listing for **phenelzine p 252** Tab- lactose

paroxetine HCl
  Paxil[a b c d e f]

Tab- Na starch glycolate
Susp- sorbitol,
  saccharin Na,
  simethicone,
  propylene glycol
Paxil CR[a d e g] (SR)
Tab- lactose

paroxetine mesylate
  Pexeva[a b c d]

Tab- Na starch glycolate

ANTIDEPRESSANT[a], ANTIANXIETY[b], TREATMENT of OCD[c],
  PANIC DISORDER[d], SOCIAL ANXIETY[e] or PTSD[f], PMDD[g]   SSRI
  Diet: Take s̄ regard to food. Avoid tryptophan suppl- may ↑ drug side
  effects.[3] Avoid SJW, see p 286.
  Nutr: ↑ APPETITE, ↑ WEIGHT.[37] ↓ appetite, ↓ wt.
  Oral/GI: Dry mouth, TASTE CHANGES (↓ SWEET & BITTER THRESHOLDS),[21]
  nausea, dyspepsia, constipation, diarrhea, flatulence. Rare- upper GI bleeding.
  S/Cond: Avoid alcohol. Caution c̄ lactation. 93-95% serum pro bound.
  Hypoalbuminemia (< 3 g/dL)- may ↑ drug effects.
  Caution c̄ geriatric- drug conc ↑ 70-80%- ↑ risk of hyponatremia.[21]
  Caution c̄ history of seizures. Not c̄ active seizure disorder.
  Caution c̄ severe ↓ hepatic func or ↓ renal func. Not for pt < 18 years old.
  Pregnancy: Category D.
  Other: Weakness, insomnia, drowsiness, dizziness, sweating, tremor,
  blurred vision, nervousness, confusion, paresthesia, palpitations,
  tachycardia, headache, syncope, chills, cough, muscle pain, edema,
  HTN, rash, sexual dysfunction. Withdrawal symptoms upon DC of drug.
  Rare- SIADH, akathisia, serotonin syndrome, suicidal thinking & behavior.
  Blood/Serum: ↓ Hb, ↓ HCT, ↓ Na, ↑ chol, ↓ WBC.[13]
  Urinary: ↑ frequency, hesitancy.

Paxil/Paxil CR

ANTIDEPRESSANT, ANTIANXIETY, TREATMENT of OCD, PANIC DISORDER,
  SOCIAL ANXIETY or PTSD   **See paroxetine HCl above**

pazopanib
  Votrient
Tab- starch

ANTINEOPLASTIC (Renal CA), Multi-Tyrosine Kinase Inhibitor
  Drug: Take s̄ food 1 hr before or 2 hr after a meal. Do not crush tab.
  Diet: Not c̄ grapefruit/related citrus, see p 390. Avoid SJW, see p 286.
  Nutr: Anorexia, ↓ weight.
  Oral/GI: Dysgeusia, dyspepsia, N/V, diarrhea, abdominal pain.
  Rare- GI perforation or fistula.
  S/Cond: Not c̄ lacataion. > 99% serum pro bound. Caution c̄ mild to
  moderate ↓ hepatic func. Not c̄ severe ↓ hepatic func.
  Caution c̄ Hx of ↑ QT interval or cardiac disease. Caution c̄ geriatric.

Pregnancy: Category D.
Other: <u>HYPERTENSION</u>, <u>hemorrhagic events</u> (rarely may be fatal), <u>headache</u>, <u>rash</u>, <u>hand-foot</u> <u>syndrome</u>, <u>fatigue</u>, <u>asthenia</u>, <u>hair</u> <u>loss</u>, hair color changes, myocardial event, possible slow wound healing, facial edema, skin color loss, ↑ QT interval, hypothyroidism.
Rare- ↑ torsades de pointes, pancreatitis.
Blood/Serum: ↑ <u>BILIRUBIN</u>, ↑ <u>ALT</u>, ↑ <u>AST</u>, ↓ <u>PHOSPHORUS</u>, ↑ <u>glucose</u>, ↓ <u>glucose</u>, ↓ <u>Na</u>, ↓ <u>Mg</u>, ↓ <u>WHITE BLOOD CELLS</u>, ↓ <u>NEUTROPHILS</u>, ↓ <u>LYMPHOCYTES</u>, ↓ <u>PLATELETS</u>.
Urinary: <u>Pro</u>.
Monitor: Baseline hepatic func, then q 4 wk for at least 4 mo, then periodically. BP, ECG, electrolytes. Thyroid func. Urinalysis for pro.

PCE	ANTIBIOTIC	See **erythromycin p 128**
Pediaflor	MINERAL SUPPLEMENT	See **fluoride p 146**
Pegasys	CHRONIC HEPATITIS C TREATMENT	See **interferon alfa-2A p 177**

pegfilgrastim   COLONY STIMULATING FACTOR   See listing for **filgrastim p 142**
  Neulasta   Longer acting than **filgrastim**   Parenteral only (SC)
prefilled syringe- sorbitol 30 mg, preservative free

peginterferon alfa-2a   CHRONIC HEPATITIS C TREATMENT   See listing for **interferon alfa-2b p 177**
  Pegasys   Once-weekly Parenteral (SC) fixed dose.
              Often used c̄ **Copegus** (oral **ribavirin**)

peginterferon alfa-2b   CHRONIC HEPATITIS C TREATMENT   See listing for **interferon alfa-2b p 177**
  Peg-Intron   Once-weekly Parenteral (SC) dose based on body wt.
              Often used c̄ **Rebetrol** (oral **ribavirin**)

pegloticase
Krytexxa
IV solution
single vial,
preservative free

TREATMENT OF GOUT REFRACTORY TO CONVENTIONAL TREATMENT,
Uric acid specific enzyme   Parenteral only (IV)
    Drug: Administer as IV infusion. Do not administer as IV bolus.
Premedicate c̄ antihistamines and corticosteroids.
    Oral/GI: <u>N</u>, vomiting. constipation.
    S/Cond: Not c̄ lactation. Not c̄ G6PD def- risk of hemolysis or
methemoglobinemia. Caution c̄ CHF.
    Pregnancy: Category C.
    Other: <u>INFUSION REACTIONS</u>, (<u>anaphylaxis</u>, <u>urticaria</u>, <u>dyspnea</u>,
<u>chest discomfort</u>, <u>erythema</u>, <u>pruritis</u>), <u>contusion</u>, <u>ecchymosis</u>,
<u>nasopharyngitis</u>, gout flares, chest pain.
    Blood/Serum: ↓ *uric acid*.
    Monitor: Uric acid level before each infusion. Higher risk of infusion
reaction after ≥ 2 consecutive pretreatment uric acid levels > 6mg/dL.
S/S of hypersensitivity/anaphylaxis after each infusion.

pemetrexed
Alimta
500 mg mannitol/vial

ANTINEOPLASTIC, Antifolate (Lung Cancer, Mesothelioma)   Parenteral (IV)
    Drug: Given IV daily in 21 day cycles c̄ **cisplatin** for mesothelioma.
    Diet: Insure adequate fluid intake/hydration.
Pt must take low dose Fol (eg 400 mcg) or MVI + Fol. At least 5 daily
doses must be taken during the 7 day period prior to use, daily during
use & for 21 days after last dose of cycle. In addition IM Vit B_{12},
1000 mcg, must be given once during the wk before the first dose.
Repeat Vit B_{12} at the start of every third cycle.
    Nutr: <u>ANOREXIA</u>, <u>dehydration</u>.
    Oral/GI: <u>STOMATITIS/PHARYGITIS</u>, <u>dysphagia</u>, <u>swallowing pain</u>,
<u>NAUSEA/VOMITING</u>, <u>CONSTIPATION</u>, <u>DIARRHEA</u>.
    S/Cond: Not c̄ lactation. Do dental care cautiously, see p 11 & 15.
Therapy should not be started c̄ severe ↓ neutrophils < 1500 cells/mm³,
platelets < 100,000 cells/mm³ or CrCl < 45 mL/minute.
Caution c̄ ↓ hepatic func or ↓ renal func. **Pregnancy:** Category D.
    Other: <u>BONE MARROW SUPRESSION</u>, <u>FATIGUE</u>, <u>DYSPNEA</u>, <u>CHEST PAIN</u>,
<u>RASH</u> (↓ c̄ use of corticosteroid pretreatment), <u>fever</u>, <u>sensory neuropathy</u>,

depression, <u>infection</u>, <u>thrombosis/embolism</u>, <u>allergic reaction</u>, <u>renal failure</u>.
Blood/Serum: ↓ <u>WHITE BLOOD CELLS</u>, <u>ANEMIA</u>, ↓ <u>PLATELETS</u>, ↑ <u>CREA</u>.
Monitor: Baseline CBC c̄ diff, platelets. CrCl, hepatic func.
CrCl prior to each cycle. Hepatic func periodically.
CBC, platelets, before each cycle & on days 8 & 15 of each cycle.

penicillin   ANTIBIOTIC   Oral or Parenteral
   Drug: Pen VK- Take 1 hr before or 2 hr after food to ↑ abs.[6] May take c̄ food if GI distress occurs.
   Diet: Caution c̄ K suppl c̄ pen VK. Some parenteral forms have high Na content.
   Guar gum ↓ oral **penicillin** abs- take separately by several hr.[4] **Nutr:** Anorexia.
   Oral/GI: Black hairy tongue, dry mouth, taste changes, <u>oral</u> <u>candidiasis</u>, <u>N/V</u>, <u>epigastric distress</u>,
   <u>diarrhea</u>, flatulence. Rare- pseudomembranous colitis.
   S/Cond: Caution c̄ lactation. Caution c̄ ↓ renal func. Consider K or Na content c̄ ↓ renal func.
   Pregnancy: Category B. **Other:** <u>Allergic reaction</u> (can be fatal), <u>rash</u>, anaphylactic shock.
   Rare- angioedema.[6] Neuropathy or nephropathy c̄ high dose parenteral.
   Blood/Serum: Dyscrasias. ↑ <u>K</u> (especially c̄ pen G, pen K IV). ↓ K c̄ penicillin G sodium.[93]
   ↑ <u>Na</u> (pen G Na IV). Positive Coombs' test.
   Urinary: False + glucose (CuSO$_4$) or false ↑ steroids (method dependent) c̄ pen G. ↑ K c̄ penicillin G sodium.[93]
   Monitor: c̄ LT or high dose IV- CBC c̄ diff, renal func, electrolytes. K or Na especially c̄ pen G.

Oral forms-
penicillin V potassium (pen VK) generic only
   101 mg (2.59 mEq) K/g- Tab
   Pwd for soln- saccharin, sugar

Parenteral forms-
penicillin G benzathine (IM only)
   Bicillin L-A- lecithin,
   10 mg (0.44 mEq) Na/5 mL Susp
penicillin G benzathine & **penicillin G procaine**
   Bicillin C-R (IM only)
penicillin G sodium (IV or IM) generic only
   46 mg (2 mEq) Na/1 million units

penicillin G potassium (IM, IV, Intrathecal)
Pfizerpen
   7 mg (0.31 mEq) Na/1 million units
   66 mg (1.69 mEq) K/1 million units

penicillin G procaine (IM only) generic only

Pentasa	ANTI-INFLAMMATORY (in ulcerative colitis)	See **mesalamine p 209**

pentoxifylline
  Trental
  SR Tab

PERIPHERAL VASCULAR DISEASE TREATMENT, Synthetic Xanthine Derivative
  (Reduction of Symptoms of Intermittent Claudication)
  Drug: Take c̄ meals to ↓ GI irritation. Swallow whole.
  Do NOT crush, break or chew.
  Diet: ↓ cal, ↓ chol may be recommended. Limit xanthine/caffeine, see p 379.
  Avoid or limit natural products which affect coagulation (eg garlic, ginger,
  ginkgo or horse chestnut).
  Oral/GI: N/V, dyspepsia, abdominal discomfort, belching, flatulence, bloating.
  S/Cond: Not c̄ lactation. Caution c̄ ↓ hepatic func or ↓ renal func.[13]
  Caution c̄ geriatric. **Pregnancy:** Category C.
  Other: Dizziness, agitation, flushing, arrhythmia/palpitation, blurred vision.
  Blood/Serum: ↓ VISCOSITY, IMPROVED CAPILLARY FLOW. ↓ FIBRINOGEN.

Pepcid/Pepcid AC
  famotidine

ANTIULCER, ANTIGERD, ANTISECRETORY

See **Histamine H$_2$ Receptor
  Antagonists p 162**

Pepcid Complete (OTC)
Tab- 800 mg CaCO$_3$ (Ca 320 mg), 165 mg (Mg 70 mg) MgOH,
cornstarch, corn syrup solids, lactose, mineral oil, sucralose

ANTACID

  Drug: Chew completely. Do not swallow whole.

See **Histamine H$_2$ Receptor
  Antagonists p 162**
See **calcium carbonate p 70**

Pepto-Bismol	ANTIDIARRHEAL	See **bismuth subsalicylate p 58**

Percocet
  Tab- cornstarch

ANALGESIC, Narcotic, Opioid
  Combination drug

See **oxycodone p 241**
See **acetaminophen p 22**

Percodan
  Tab- cornstarch

ANALGESIC, Narcotic, Opioid
  Combination drug

See **oxycodone p 241**
See **aspirin p 44**

Perdiem Overnight Relief	LAXATIVE, Stimulant	See **senna p 290**

Perforomist
  formoterol

ANTIASTHMA (not for acute symptoms), COPD TREATMENT, EIB
  Inhalation Aerosol Soln- preservative free See listing for **salmeterol p 286**

| **Periactin** | ANTIHISTAMINE, Also used as an Appetite Stimulant | |
| previous brand name | | See **cyproheptadine p 97** |

Peri-Colace LAXATIVE (Stimulant), STOOL SOFTENER
Tab 50 mg **docusate sodium** Combination drug See **docusate sodium p 115**
8.5 mg sennosides, 20 mg Ca, 4 mg Na See **senna p 290**

perindopril ANTIHYPERTENSIVE See **Angiotensin Converting Enzyme Inhibitors p 36**
Aceon

Periostat ANTIBIOTIC, Adjunct to periodontitis treatment See **Tetracyclines p 310**
doxycycline

perphenazine ANTIPSYCHOTIC, ANTIEMETIC See **Phenothiazines p 254**
Trilafon previous brand name

Persantine ANTIPLATELET See **dipyridamole p 113**

Pexeva ANTIDEPRESSANT, SSRI See **paroxetine mesylate p 246**

Phazyme ANTIFLATULENT See **simethicone p 292**

phenazopyridine URINARY ANALGESIC, Azo Dye
Pyridium **Drug:** Take c̄ food to ↓ GI upset.
Tab- sucrose, lactose, **Oral/GI:** Dyspepsia, stomach cramps/pain. RED-ORANGE FECES.
Na starch glycolate **S/Cond:** Not c̄ ↓ renal func. Not c̄ severe hepatitis.
DC if skin becomes yellow.
Caution c̄ G6PD def- risk of hemolytic anemia.[13]
Pregnancy: Category B.[13]
Other: Dizziness, headache, rash, itching, staining of contact lenses.
Rare- renal or hepatotoxicity, anaphylactoid-like reaction,
skin discoloration.
Blood/Serum: Rare- hemolytic anemia, methemoglobinemia.
Urinary: RED-ORANGE COLOR. (May interfere c̄ urinalysis based on
spectrometry or color reaction).

P

phenelzine
Nardil
Tab- Ca CO3, mannitol,
cornstarch, sucrose
gluten free

ANTIDEPRESSANT, MAOI
Drug: Do not take in the evening (to avoid insomnia).
Diet: <u>Avoid foods high in tyramine & other pressor amines</u> during drug use & for 2 wk after DC,[7] to prevent hypertensive crisis, see p 383. Limit licorice see p 374, caffeine, see p 379. Avoid tryptophan suppl. Avoid SJW, see p 286. Avoid ginseng.[93]
Nutr: ↑ <u>appetite</u>, ↑ <u>wt</u>.
Oral/GI: <u>Dry mouth</u>, N/V, <u>constipation</u>.
S/Cond: Avoid alcohol. Not c̄ lactation. Caution c̄ diabetes- ↓ glucose. Caution c̄ ↓ hepatic func or ↓ renal func.[13] Caution c̄ seizures.[6] Not c̄ HTN, cardiovascular disease. Caution c̄ slow acetylators.[7]
Pregnancy: Category C.[13]
Other: <u>INSOMNIA</u>, <u>HTN</u> or <u>hypotension</u>, <u>dizziness</u>, <u>drowsiness</u>, <u>blurred vision</u>,[7] tremor, hyperexcitability, headache, edema, SIADH, muscle pain, weakness. Rare- rash, hepatotoxicity, peripheral neuropathy, suicidal thinking & behavior.
Blood/Serum: ↑ AST, ↑ ALT, ↑ Na, ↓ glucose in diabetes. Rare- dyscrasias.
Urinary: Retention.
Monitor: BP, CBC, hepatic func.

Phenergan

ANTIHISTAMINE, ANTIVERTIGO See **promethazine p 266**

phenobarbital
Phenobarbital
Elixir-
13% alcohol,
0.63 g sucrose/5 mL
Tab- lactose,
cornstarch,
Na starch glycolate

SEDATIVE, HYPNOTIC, ANTIEPILEPTIC, Barbiturate
Oral or Parenteral (IM or IV)
Diet: ↑ Vit D & ↑ Ca intake.
Limit xanthine/caffeine, counteracts sedative effect of drug,[13] see p 379.
May need Vit D, Ca, Vit B_{12} & Fol suppl c̄ LT use.
Limit or avoid quinine- may ↑ drug level.[3a]
One study (5 pts)- ↓ drug level c̄ 200 mg concurrent Pyr.[115]
Nutr: ↑ rate of metabolism of Vit D & Vit K, possibly Fol.
Avoid SJW,[93] see p 286.
Oral/GI: N/V, constipation.
S/Cond: Avoid alcohol. Not c̄ lactation. May be habit forming c̄ LT use.

Caution $\overline{c}$ ↓ hepatic func or ↓ renal func. Caution $\overline{c}$ geriatric.
Not $\overline{c}$ manifest or latent porphyria.

Pregnancy: Category D. ↓ Vit K in fetus- suppl 10 mg/day for the last
month of pregnancy, Vit K indicated for neonate immediately after birth.[93]

Other: <u>Dizziness</u>, <u>drowsiness</u>, <u>ataxia</u>, <u>mental depression</u>, <u>hyperactivity</u>
(especially in children & geriatric), headache, confusion, rash.
Osteomalacia, rickets, ↓ bone mineral density $\overline{c}$ LT use.
<u>Mild respiratory depression</u>, hypotension $\overline{c}$ IV.

Blood/Serum: ↓ <u>BIL</u>, ↓ <u>Fol</u>, ↑ <u>CHOL</u>, ↑ <u>LDL</u>, ↑ <u>LIPOPROTEIN(a)</u>, ↑ HDL,
↑ homocysteine,[60] ↑ NH_3, ↓ Ca, ↓ <u>Vit D</u>,[11] ↓ Mg.[27] ↓ carnitine.[93]
Rare- ↓ Vit B_{12}, dyscrasias or megaloblastic anemia.

Monitor: $\overline{c}$ LT use- Fol, Vit B_{12}, CBC $\overline{c}$ diff, hepatic & renal func,
drug levels, Vit D.

Phenothiazines   ANTIPSYCHOTIC, ANTIEMETIC, ANTIANXIETY   Oral or Parenteral (IM, IV)

Aliphatic Phenothiazines eg **chlorpromazine** cause <u>more</u> sedation, anticholinergic effects & hypotension but <u>less</u> EPS than Piperazine Phenothiazines eg **fluphenazine**, **perphenazine**, **prochlorperazine**.

Drug: May take $\overline{c}$ food or 8 oz milk or water to ↓ GI distress.
Dilute oral conc in at least 2 oz drink, syrup or soft food.

Diet: Take Mg suppl separately by 2 hr.[13] Limit caffeine, see p 379.

Nutr: ↑ <u>APPETITE</u>, ↑ <u>WEIGHT</u>.[17] ↑ need for Rib.[41] May ↓ abs of Vit B_{12}.

Oral/GI: <u>DRY MOUTH</u>, drooling, N/V, <u>CONSTIPATION</u>.

S/Cond: Avoid alcohol. Not $\overline{c}$ lactation. Conc precipitates tube feedings.[8]
↑ risk of dental problems, see p 11 & 15. 90% serum pro bound. Caution $\overline{c}$ ↓ hepatic func or ↓ renal func.
Caution $\overline{c}$ Parkinson's or seizures- drug ↓ seizure threshold.

Pregnancy: Category C.[7] Generally contraindicated in 1st trimester, particularly in wk 6-10.
Discontinue 5-10 days before delivery.[6]

Other: <u>*SEDATION*</u>, <u>EXTRAPYRAMIDAL SYMPTOMS</u>, <u>BLURRED VISION</u>, <u>DRY EYES</u>, ↓ <u>SWEATING</u>, <u>restlessness</u>, drowsiness, <u>dizziness</u>, hives, <u>tachycardia</u>, <u>galactorrhea</u>, <u>menstrual changes</u>, gynecomastia, headache, photosensitivity, edema, jaundice, rash, fever (↑ $\overline{c}$ IM, IV), ↓ cough reflex, syncope, hypotension (↑ $\overline{c}$ IM, IV). ↑ mortality in geriatrics $\overline{c}$ dementia-related psychosis.
Rare- NMS, temperature regulation dysfunction, ↑ QT interval.
Ocular changes, skin pigmentation, tardive dyskinesia $\overline{c}$ LT use.

Blood/Serum: Dyscrasias, ↓ WBC, ↑ bil, ↑ AST, ↑ ALT, ↑ LDH, ↑ alk phos, ↑ or ↓ glucose, ↓ HDL, ↑ TG, ↑ <u>chol</u>, ↑ <u>prolactin</u>. **Urinary:** <u>Retention</u>, glucose, dark color. ↑ <u>Rib</u>.
False + PKU, amylase, pregnancy test. **Monitor:** Hepatic func. CBC $\overline{c}$ diff. BP.

PHENOTHIAZINES

chlorpromazine	fluphenazine HCl	perphenazine	prochlorperazine
Tab- lactose, cornstarch	**Prolixin**	**Trilafon**	**Compazine**
Syrup- sucrose	(previous brand name)	(previous brand name)	(previous brand name)
Conc- saccharin	Tab- lactose, cornstarch	Tab- lactose, sugar,	Tab- lactose, starch
Rectal Suppository-	Elixir- 3 g sucrose/5 mL	potato starch	Syrup- sucrose
coconut & palm kernel oils	Elixir & Conc- 14% alcohol	Parenteral (IM, IV)	Parenteral (IM, IV)
Thorazine previous brand name	Parenteral (IM)- 1.2% benzyl	Na bisulfite	0.75% benzyl
Parenteral (IM, IV) sulfites,	alcohol, sesame seed oil		alcohol, saccharin
benzyl alcohol 2%			Rectal Suppository-
in multidose vials			coconut & palm kernel oils

phentermine
Adipex-P
Cap- lactose, cornstarch
Tab- cornstarch, lactose,
sucrose
Suprenza
ODT- mannitol,
sucralose, citric acid

APPETITE SUPPRESSANT, ANTIOBESITY
Drug: For pt c̄ BMI ≥ 30 or ≥ 27 c̄ other risk factors (e.g., HTN,
diabetes, hyperlipidemia). Do not take HS. Take HCl form before
breakfast or 1-2 hr after breakfast.
Place ODT (Suprenza) on tongue where it will dissolve.
Then swallow c̄ or s̄ water.
Diet: Adjunct to ↓ cal. Avoid caffeine, see p 67.
Nutr: ANOREXIA, ↓ *APPETITE*, ↓ *WT*.
Oral/GI: <u>Dry</u> <u>mouth</u>, <u>unpleasant</u> <u>taste</u>, N/V, diarrhea, constipation.
S/Cond: Avoid alcohol. Not c̄ lactation.
Caution c̄ diabetes- may alter insulin or sulfonylurea effects.
Not c̄ HTN, cardiovascular disease, seizures.[23]
May be habit forming c̄ LT use. Not for < 16 years old.
Pregnancy: Category C.
Other: <u>INSOMNIA</u>, <u>restlessness</u>, ↑ <u>BP</u>, <u>tremor</u>, <u>tachycardia</u>, <u>dizziness</u>,
euphoria, headache, rash.

phenylephrine
Sudafed PE

NASAL DECONGESTANT

See listing for
pseudoephedrine p 269

P

phenytoin
Dilantin
Cap (SR)- lactose,
confectioner's sugar
125 Susp- $\leq$ 0.6% alcohol,
sucrose

Infatab (chew tab)-
saccharin, sucrose

Phenytek
Cap (SR)

ANTIEPILEPTIC, Hydantoin   Oral or Parenteral (IV or IM)
Drug: Take consistently c̄ or s̄ food. May take c̄ food or milk to ↓ GI irritation. Food effect on different formulations/brands varies.[116]
Chew chew tab well. Swallow SR cap whole- do not crush or chew.
Diet: 1 mg Fol daily, often started c̄ **phenytoin**.[89] May need Ca, Vit D &/or Thi suppl. Ca or Mg suppl or antacids may ↓ abs- take separately by 2 hr. Separate susp by $\geq$ 2 hr from oral enteral suppl.[25] Avoid SJW,[93] see p 286.
Nutr: Fol intake of $\geq$ 1 mg/day ↑ drug metabolism & ↓ blood level in 15-50% of pts.[89] Conversely, drug ↓ Fol levels. Drug level must be closely monitored if Fol is added. Drug ↑ metabolism of Vit D & K, especially in children,[11] may cause rickets or osteomalacia.
Oral/GI: <u>GUM HYPERPLASIA</u>, altered taste, dysphagia, <u>N/V</u>, <u>constipation</u>.
S/Cond: Avoid alcohol- acute ingestion ↑ drug levels, but chronic abuse ↓ drug level. Not c̄ lactation. Caution c̄ diabetes- ↑ glucose. Do dental care cautiously. Enteral feedings ↓ bioavailability of **phenytoin** susp- stop TF for $\geq$ 2 hr & flush c̄ $\geq$ 30 mL water or saline before & after drug (closely monitor drug level).
> 90% serum pro bound. Hypoalbuminemia (< 3 g/dL)- may ↑ drug effects. Caution c̄ ↓ hepatic func or ↓ renal func or geriatric.
Caution c̄ Asian pt positive for human leukocyte antigen (HLA) allele, HLA-B*1502- ↑ risk of serious skin reactions.
Pregnancy: Category D.[17] ↓ Vit K in fetus- suppl 10 mg/day for the last month of pregnancy. Vit K to neonate immediately after birth.[93]
Other: <u>ATAXIA</u>, <u>rash</u>, <u>drowsiness</u>, <u>dizziness</u>, <u>confusion</u>, insomnia, motor twitching, tremor, headache, visual changes, edema, hirsutism, enlargement of facial features. Rare- hepatitis, jaundice, rickets, osteomalacia, lymph node hyperplasia, lupus-like syndrome, SJS/TEN, periarteritis nodosa, Peyronie's disease. Peripheral polyneuropathy c̄ LT use.
Blood/Serum: ↓ <u>Fol</u>, ↑ homocysteine, ↓ <u>Vit D</u>, ↓ <u>Ca</u>, ↓ <u>P</u>, ↓ <u>T₄</u>, ↓ biotin,[11] ↓ Thi,[11] ↑ glucose, ↑ alk phos, ↑ GGT, ↑ <u>HDL</u>.[34] Rare- dyscrasias or megaloblastic anemia. ↓ carnitine.[93] **Urinary:** ↑ biotin,[11] ↓ Rib.[41]
Monitor: Drug level, CBC c̄ diff, platelets,[17] hepatic func, Ca, thyroid func, alb. Possibly Fol, Vit D &/or Vit K, especially in children. Possibly prior to use genetic testing for Asian pt.

Phillips' MOM Milk of Magnesia	LAXATIVE, ANTACID	See **magnesium hydroxide p 203**
PhosLo	PHOSPHATE BINDER	See **calcium acetate p 69**

phosphates   URINARY ACIDIFIER (to reduce renal calculi or treat UTI), PHOSPHORUS SUPPLEMENT
Drug: Take at meals & HS to ↓ GI irritation & laxative action. Dissolve **K-Phos** tab in 8 oz water.
Diet: Avoid Ca, Vit D suppl or salt subs. Caution c̄ K suppl. Take Fe, Mg or Zn suppl or Al antacid
separately by 2 hr. Do not take c̄ high oxalate (see p 381) or high phytate (see p 382) foods- ↓ abs.
Insure adequate fluid intake/hydration.
Nutr: ↑ thirst, ↑ wt. Phosphorus **AI** (mg/day) Infants 0-6 mo = **100** (3.2 mM). 7-12 mo = **275** (8.9 mM).
RDA (mg/day) Children 1-3 yr = **460** (14.8 mM). 4-8 = **500** (16.1 mM). 9-18 = **1250** (40.3 mM).
Adult 19-70+ = **700** (22.6 mM). **Lactation**- RDA & UL for age of mother.
UL (g/day) Children 1-8 yr = **3** (96.8 mM). 9-18 = **4** (130 mM). Adult 19-70 = **4** (130 mM).
70+ = **3** (96.8 mM). **Oral/GI:** N/V, stomach pain, <u>diarrhea</u>.
S/Cond: Caution c̄ lactation. Consider Na &/or K content c̄ ↓ K or ↓ Na diet.
Caution c̄ ↓ renal func, cardiac disease or severe ↓ hepatic func.
Pregnancy: Category C. **RDA** = RDA for age of mother. **UL** = **3.5** g (112.9 mM)/day.
Other: Edema, dizziness, headache, confusion, fatigue, muscle cramps, osteomalacia c̄ LT use.
Blood/Serum: ↓ <u>Ca</u>, ↑ <u>P</u>, ↑ K, ↑ Na. **Urinary:** ↓ <u>pH</u>, ↓ <u>CALCIUM</u>, ↓ output, ↑ <u>P</u>.
Monitor: Electrolytes, Ca, P, renal func.

potassium phosphate
UroPhos K	Tab (SR) 155 mg (5 mM, 10 mEq) P		312.5 mg (8 mEq) K/tab

sodium phosphate & potassium phosphate
K-Phos Neutral	250 mg (8 mM, 16.13 mEq) P,	45 mg (1.15 mEq) K,	298 mg (12.96 mEq) Na/tab
Phos-NaK pwd	250 mg (8 mM, 16.13 mEq) P,	280 mg (7.12 mEq) K	160 mg (6.96 mEq) Na/pkt
sugar free, mannitol, sucralose			

phytonadione (K$_1$)	VITAMIN, To Treat HYPOPROTHOMBINEMIA	See **vitamin K p 342**

P

pilocarpine HCl	ANTI-XEROSTOMIA or SJÖGREN'S SYNDROME TREATMENT

pilocarpine HCl
  Salagen
  Tab

ANTI-XEROSTOMIA or SJÖGREN'S SYNDROME TREATMENT
  Cholinergic to treat dry mouth due to radiation treatment or Sjögren's
  Drug: High fat meal ↓ rate of abs & maximum conc.
  Diet: Insure adequate fluid intake/hydration.
  Oral/GI: ↑ *SALIVATION*, taste changes, dysphagia, N/V, dyspepsia, diarrhea.
  S/Cond: Not c̄ lactation. Caution c̄ moderate ↓ hepatic func, CVD, COPD, bronchitis, asthma. Not c̄ severe ↓ hepatic func or uncontrolled asthma.
  Pregnancy: Category C.
  Other: ↑ *SWEATING*, flushing, double/blurred vision, chills, dizziness, weakness, muscle pain, headache, edema, rash, HTN, tachycardia, tremor, rhinitis, nosebleed, ↑ cough, voice changes.
  Urinary: ↑ frequency, incontinence.

pioglitazone
  Actos

ANTIDIABETIC AGENT for Type 2 Diabetes   See **thiazolidinediones p 312**

piperacillin sodium
  Pipracil (previous brand name) 42.5 mg (1.85 mEq) Na/g

ANTIBIOTIC, penicillin   See listing for **penicillin p 249**
Parenteral only (IM or IV)

piroxicam
  generic brand
  Feldene

ANTIARTHRITIC, NSAID   See listing for **ibuprofen p 170**
  Cap- lactose, cornstarch
  Cap- lactose, starch

pitavastatin
  Livalo

ANTIHYPERLIPIDEMIC   See **HMG-CoA reductase inhibitors p 164**
  Tab- lactose

Plaquenil

ANTIARTHRITIC, ANTIMALARIAL   See **hydroxychloroquine p 168**

Platinol-AQ

ANTINEOPLASTIC, Alkylating Agent   See **cisplatin p 86**

Plavix

PLATELET AGGREGATION INHIBITOR   See **clopidogrel p 89**

Plendil
  previous brand name

ANTIHYPERTENSIVE, Ca Channel Blocker   See **felodipine p 137**

Pletal

REDUCTION OF SYMPTOMS OF INTERMITTENT CLAUDICATION
    See **cilostazol p 84**

polyethylene glycol
  Glycolax
  Pwd
  MiraLax
  Pwd
  17 g/dose

LAXATIVE, Osmotic
  Drug: Dissolve each dose of pwd in 8 oz water, juice, soda, coffee or tea.
  Diet: High fiber c̄ 1500-2000 mL fluid/day to prevent constipation.
  Nutr: Not absorbed from GI tract.[13]
  Oral/GI: Nausea, bloating, cramps, flatulence.
  Diarrhea, ↑ stool frequency c̄ high dose.
  S/Cond: Rule out bowel obstruction before use.
  Pregnancy: Category C.

posaconazole
  Noxafil
  Susp- simethicone,
   xanthan gum, glucose

ANTIFUNGAL, Prophylaxis of invasive Aspergillus & Candida
  Treatment of oropharyngeal candidiasis
  Drug: Take c̄ full meal or liquid supplement to ↑ drug level 3-4 X.
  Nutr: Anorexia, ↓ wt, dehydration.
  Oral/GI: Taste changes, dry mouth, N/V, dyspepsia, abdominal pain,
  diarrhea, constipation, flatulence.
  S/Cond: Not c̄ lactation. Caution c̄ ↓ hepatic func or severe ↓ renal func.
  98% serum pro bound.
  Pregnancy: Category C.
  Other: Headache, dizziness, fatigue, weakness, tremor, blurred vision,
  rash, fever, insomnia, drowsiness. Rare- ↑ QT interval.
  Blood/Serum: ↑ AST, ↑ ALT, ↑ alk phos, ↑ bil, ↑ GGT, ↓ platelets, ↓ K,
  ↑ crea, ↓ neutrophils, anemia.
  Monitor: Baseline & periodic hepatic func.

potassium chloride (KCl)   ELECTROLYTE, Mineral Supplement   Oral or Parenteral (IV)
Drug: Take $\bar{c}$ meals & 8 oz liquid. Mix liquid, pwd, granule or effervescent tab in 4-6 oz water or other liquid. Drink slowly, preferably over 5-10 minutes.[13] Swallow SR form whole, do not crush or chew except **K-Dur** may disperse in 4 oz water, drink $\bar{s}$ chewing beads.
Diet: Not $\bar{c}$ salt subs.[13] See K sources table, p 388.
Nutr: No RDA. Minimum adult K requirement = 1600 - 2000 mg (40-50 mEq). Children = 78 mg (2 mEq)/100 cal.[47]
Oral/GI: GI irritation, N/V, abdominal pain, diarrhea, flatulence. Rare- ulceration or stenosis $\bar{c}$ solid forms.
S/Cond: Some liquid/syrup forms precipitate TF.[8] Caution $\bar{c}$ ↓ renal func. Not $\bar{c}$ ESRD or GI ulcer.
Caution $\bar{c}$ dysphagia, cardiac disease, bedridden patient, geriatric.
Pregnancy: Category C. **Blood/Serum:** ↑ _K_, ↑ _Cl_. **Urinary:** ↑ K, ↓ Mg. **Monitor:** Serum K, Cl, Mg, renal func.

K-Dur (SR) generics only 10 mEq Tab- 390 mg K/Tab.   20 mEq Tab- 780 mg K/Tab.
K-Lor Pwd 20 mEq pkt- 780 mg K/dose, saccharin, maltodextrin.
Klor-Con 8 (SR) 312 mg K/Tab.   **Klor-Con 10** (SR) 390 mg K/Tab, propylene glycol, castor oil.
Klotrix (SR) 10 mEq Tab- 390 mg K/Tab.
K-Lyte generics only 25 mEq effervescent Tab- 975 mg K, saccharin, dextrose, docusate Na.
K-Lyte DS generics only 50 mEq effervescent Tab- 1950 mg K, saccharin, lactose, docusate Na.
K-Tab (SR) 10 mEq Tab- 390 mg K/dose, castor oil, Vit E.
Parenteral- KCl in dextrose. KCl in NaCl 20 mEq K, 77 mg Na; 40 mEq K, 154 mg Na

potassium citrate

Urocit-K

Tab
 5 mEq Tab = 195 mg K
 10 mEq Tab = 390 mg K

URINARY ALKALINIZER (to treat or ↓ risk of Ca stones, manage renal tubular necrosis or uric acid lithiasis)

Drug: Take $\bar{c}$ meals or snack. Do not crush, split/break, chew or suck tab.
Diet: ↓ Na $\bar{c}$ fluids of ≥ 2,000 mL/day. **Nutr:** Not $\bar{c}$ K suppl or salt sub.
Oral/GI: N/V, abdominal pain, diarrhea. Rare- ulceration/bleeding.
S/Cond: Caution $\bar{c}$ lactation. Not $\bar{c}$ significant ↓ renal func, CHF, UTI, peptic ulcer, dysphagia, ↓ gastric motility or GI obstruction.
Correct hyperkalemia before use. Not $\bar{c}$ uncontrolled diabetes.
Pregnancy: Category C.
Other: Hyperkalemia.
Blood/Serum: ↑ _POTASSIUM_.
Urinary: ↑ _pH_, ↑ _CITRATE_. Transient ↓ Ca.
Monitor: Baseline & q 4 mo- urinary pH &/or citrate, serum electrolytes, crea, CBC.

potassium gluconate
0.17 mg K/g = 83.45 mg (2.14 mEq) K/500 mg Tab

ELECTROLYTE, Mineral Supplement

See **potassium chloride above**

potassium phosphate
UroPhos K

URINARY ACIDIFIER
PHOSPHORUS SUPPLEMENT

See **phosphates p 257**

Potiga

ANTIEPILEPTIC, Adjunctive Treatment of Partial Onset Seizures in Adults
See **ezogabine p 135**

Pradaxa

PREVENTION of STROKE/SYSTEMIC EMBOLISM in NONVALVULAR
ATRIAL FIBRILLATION   See **dabigatran p 98**

pramipexole
Mirapex
Tab- mannitol,
  cornstarch
Mirapex ER
Tab- corn starch

ANTIPARKINSON, RESTLESS LEG SYNDROME TREATMENT
Dopamine Receptor Agonist, Nonergot
Drug: Take c̄ food if nausea occurs. Food ↓ rate, but not extent of abs.
Swallow ER tab whole. Do not crush, chew or divide.
Diet: Caution c̄ quinine- ↓ drug clearance 20%.
Nutr: Anorexia, ↓ wt, thirst.
Oral/GI: Dry mouth, dysphagia, nausea, constipation.
S/Cond: Not c̄ lactation. Caution c̄ ↓ renal func.
Pregnancy: Category C.
Other: Hallucinations, insomnia, weakness, edema, fever, dizziness,
drowsiness, headache, confusion, amnesia, visual abnormalities,
postural hypotension, EPS, dyskinesias, paranoia, delusions.
Rare- sleep attacks, compulsive behavior, melanoma.
Blood/Serum: ↑ CPK.
Urinary: ↑ frequency, retention, incontinence.
Monitor: Possibly skin exams.

pramlintide
  Symlin
  D-mannitol
 	
  SymlinPen
	ANTIHYPERGLYCEMIC, Hormone, Types 1 or 2 Diabetes Parenteral only (SC)
	  Synthetic analog of human amylin for use $\bar{c}$ **insulin**. Amylin is
	  co-secreted $\bar{c}$ **insulin** by pancreatic beta cells in response to food intake.
	  Drug: Inject prior to meals containing $\geq$250 cal or 30 g of CHO.
	  Dose is titrated up depending upon nausea.
	  DO NOT mix $\bar{c}$ **insulin**, inject $\geq$ 2″ away from insulin injection site.
	  Insulin dose generally must be $\downarrow$ when combined $\bar{c}$ **pramlintide**.
	  Diet: Adjunct to CHO controlled diabetic diet.
	  Nutr: $\downarrow$ _APPETITE_, $\uparrow$ _SATIETY_, $\downarrow$ _FOOD INTAKE_. <u>Anorexia</u>. $\downarrow$ _WEIGHT_.
	  Oral/GI: <u>NAUSEA</u>, vomiting, abdominal pain. $\downarrow$ _RATE OF GASTRIC EMPTYING_.
	  S/Cond: Avoid alcohol. Caution $\bar{c}$ lactation. Not $\bar{c}$ gastroparesis.
	  Not $\bar{c}$ HbA1$_C$ > 9 or for pt $\bar{c}$ hypoglycemic unawareness. Not for children.
	  Pregnancy: Category C. **Other:** <u>Headache</u>, <u>allergic reaction</u>, coughing,
	  pharyngitis, fatigue, muscle pain.
	  Blood/Serum: $\downarrow$ _POSTPRANDIAL GLUCAGON PRODUCTION_.
	  $\uparrow$ <u>RISK OF HYPOGLYCEMIA</u> due to **insulin** (**pramlintide** alone does not cause
	  hypoglycemia). $\downarrow$ _GLUCOSE_, $\downarrow$ _HbA1$_C$_.
	  Monitor: Glucose before & after every meal & HS. HbA1$_C$, body wt.

Prandiment
  Tab- sorbitol
	ANTIHYPERGLYCEMIC AGENT & ORAL HYPOGLYCEMIC Type 2 DM
	  Combination drug See **metformin p 210**
	                                            See **repaglinide p 276**

Prandin	ORAL HYPOGLYCEMIC, Meglitinide See **repaglinide p 276**

prasugrel
  Effient
  Tab- mannitol, lactose
	ACUTE CORONARY SYNDROME TREATMENT
	  Platelet Aggregation Inhibitor, Thienopyridine Prodrug
	  Drug: Must be taken $\bar{c}$ **aspirin**. Take $\bar{s}$ regard to food. Do not break tab.
	  Oral/GI: Nausea, diarrhea.
	  S/Cond: Caution $\bar{c}$ lactation. Caution $\bar{c}$ BW < 60 kg- lower dose needed.
	  Not $\bar{c}$ pt > 75 yr old. Caution $\bar{c}$ severe $\downarrow$ hepatic func. Not $\bar{c}$ Hx of CVA
	  or TIA. Not $\bar{c}$ conditions which $\uparrow$ bleeding e.g. peptic ulcer.
	  Do dental care cautiously, $\uparrow$ risk of bleeding. 98% serum pro bound.

Pregnancy: Category B.
Other: <u>Headache</u>, <u>back pain</u>, bradycardia, atrial fibrillation, dizziness, cough, dyspnea, bleeding (can be fatal), bruising, fever, rash, edema.
Blood/Serum: ↑ <u>BLEEDING TIME</u>, ↓ <u>PLATELETS</u>, ↑ chol, anemia, ↓ WBC.

pravastatin **Pravachol**	ANTIHYPERLIPIDEMIC (to ↓ chol)	See **HMG-CoA Reductase Inhibitors p 164**
prazosin **Minipress**	ANTIHYPERTENSIVE	See **Alpha₁ Adrenergic Blockers p 28**
Precose	ANTIDIABETIC AGENT	See **acarbose p 20**
prednisolone	CORTICOSTEROID	See **corticosteroids p 94**
prednisone	CORTICOSTEROID	See **corticosteroids p 94**

pregabalin ANALGESIC for Diabetic Peripheral Neuropathy,
  Lyrica ANTIEPILEPTIC ADUNCT, POSTHERPETIC NEURALGIA TREATMENT
  Cap- lactose, cornstarch FIBROMYALGIA TREATMENT
  Soln- lactose See listing for **gabapentin p 152**

Prelone	CORTICOSTEROID, **prednisolone**	See **corticosteroids p 94**
Premarin	HORMONE, Estrogen	See **Hormone Therapy p 165**
Premphase **Prempro**	HORMONES Combination drug	See **Hormone Therapy p 165** See **progesterone p 265**

Prevacid/Prevacid 24 hr ANTIULCER, ANTIGERD, ANTISECRETORY
Prevacid I.V.
  lansoprazole See **Proton Pump Inhibitors p 268**

Prevpac ANTIULCER combination- **lansoprazole (Prevacid)**, **p 268**
  clarithromycin (Biaxin), **p 87** & **amoxicillin (Trimox)**, **p 32**
  To eradicate H. Pylori & prevent recurrence of duodenal ulcer

Prezista ANTIRETOVIRAL (HIV/AIDS), Protease Inhibitor See **darunavir p 102**

Prilosec ANTIULCER, ANTISECRETORY, ANTIGERD See **Proton Pump Inhibitors p 268**
  omeprazole

Primaxin ANTIBIOTIC See **imipenem/cilastatin p 172**

primidone ANTIEPILEPTIC See listing for **phenobarbital p 252**
  Mysoline Metabolized to **phenobarbital** & **phenylethylmalonamide (PEMA)**
Tab- lactose, Na starch glycolate

Prinivil/Prinzide ANTIHYPERTENSIVE See **Angiotensin Converting Enzyme Inhibitors p 36**
  Prinzide also contains **hydrochlorothiazide**, see p 166

Pristiq ANTIDEPRESSANT, SNRI See listing for **venlafaxine p 331**
  desvenlafaxine Tab 100 mg- dextrose

probiotic BIOTHERAPEUTIC AGENT See listing for **lactobacillus p 186**

Procardia/Procardia XL ANTIANGINA, ANTIHYPERTENSIVE, Ca Channel Blocker See **nifedipine p 229**

prochlorperazine ANTIEMETIC, ANTINAUSEANT, ANTIPSYCHOTIC, ANTIANXIETY
  Compazine previous brand name See **Phenothiazines p 254**

Procrit RECOMBINANT HUMAN ERYTHROPOIETIN, ANTIANEMIC
See **epoetin alfa p 126**

progesterone	HORMONE (to treat menstrual disorders), CONTRACEPTIVE (IM or SC),

progesterone
medroxyprogesterone
  Provera
  Tab- lactose, sucrose,
   cornstarch, mineral oil
  Depo-Provera (IM)
  (long acting contraceptive)
  Depo-subQ Provera 104 (SC)
  (contraceptive, endometriosis)
 micronized progesterone
 Prometrium
  Cap- peanut oil, lecithin

HORMONE (to treat menstrual disorders), CONTRACEPTIVE (IM or SC),
ANTINEOPLASTIC (IM), ENDOMETRIOSIS TREATMENT (SC)
Oral or Parenteral (IM or SC)
Drug: May take **medroxyprogesterone** c̄ food to ↓ GI distress.
Food ↑ bioavailability 18-33%. Take **Prometrium** HS.
Avoid LT use of **Depo-Provera** (> 2 yr).
Nutr: ↑ APPETITE, ↑ WEIGHT, ↓ wt.
Oral/GI: Dry mouth, N/V, dyspepsia, bloating, constipation, diarrhea.
S/Cond: Caution c̄ lactation. Caution c̄ diabetes c̄
medroxyprogesterone- ↑ glucose. Not c̄ severe ↓ hepatic func.
Caution c̄ ↓ hepatic, ↓ renal func or CHF. **Prometrium**- Not c̄ peanut allergy.
Pregnancy: medroxyprogesterone- Category X. **Prometrium**- Category B.
Other: EDEMA, headache, cramps, musculoskeletal pain, depression,
vision changes, drowsiness, weakness, insomnia, hot flashes, palpitation,
fever, ↓ bone density, irregular bleeding, amenorrhea, menstrual changes,
breast pain (especially c̄ **Depo-Provera**). Dizziness c̄ **Prometrium**.
Rare- thromboembolism, jaundice.
Blood/Serum: ↑ Na, ↓ insulin, ↑ HDL, ↓ LDL, ↓ chol, ↑ TG, ↑ alk phos,
↑ bil, ↑ AST, ↑ ALT, ↑ PBI, ↓ T$_3$ uptake, ↑ prothrombin factors, ↓ LH, ↓ FSH.

Prograf

IMMUNOSUPPRESSANT (Prevent Organ Rejection)   See **tacrolimus p 301**

Prolia

TREATMENT OF POSTMENOPAUSAL WOMEN WITH OSTEOPOROSIS AT
HIGH RISK FOR FRACTURE. TO INCREASE BONE MASS IN MEN AT HIGH
RISK FOR FRACTURE RECEIVING ANDROGEN DEPRIVATION THERAPY
FOR NONMETASTATIC PROSTATE CANCER. TO INCREASE BONE MASS
IN WOMEN RECEIVING ADJUVANT AROMATASE INHIBITOR THERAPY
FOR BREAST CANCER.   See **denosumab p 104**

Prolixin (previous brand name) ANTIPSYCHOTIC   See **Phenothiazines p 254**
  fluphenazine

Promacta

IDIOPATHIC THROMBOCYTOPENIC PURPURA TREATMENT
See **eltrombopag p 122**

promethazine   ANTIHISTAMINE, ANTIVERTIGO, ANTIEMETIC, SEDATIVE
  Generic brands   Phenothiazine derivative   Oral, Rectal Suppository or Parenteral (IM or IV)
  Syrup-   **Drug:** Take c̄ meals or HS c̄ 8 oz water or milk to ↓ GI irritation.
   plain- 7.1% alcohol,   **Nutr:** ↑ need for Rib.[41] **Oral/GI:** Dry mouth, N/V, constipation.
   37.4% sugar, gluten free   **S/Cond:** Avoid alcohol. Not c̄ lactation.
      ↑ risk of dental problems, see p 11 & 15. 76-93% serum pro bound.[6]
  Phenergan   Caution c̄ ↓ hepatic func or cardiovascular disease.
  Parenteral ampule-   Caution c̄ seizures- ↓ threshold. Not for children < 2 years old.
  0.25 mg Na metabisulfite/mL   **Pregnancy:** Category C.
  Tabs- lactose   **Other:** DROWSINESS, SEDATION, blurred vision, dizziness, confusion,
   12.5 & 25 mg- saccharin Na   ↑ or ↓ BP, photosensitivity, rash. Rare- EPS, jaundice, NMS.
      Blood/Serum: ↑ glucose. Rare- dyscrasias.
      Urinary: ↑ Rib.

Prometrium   HORMONE   See **progesterone p 265**

Propecia   MALE PATTERN BALDNESS TREATMENT   See **finasteride p 142**

propofol   ANESTHESIA, SEDATIVE   Parenteral Only (IV)
  Diprivan   ICU Sedation for intubated and/or mechanically ventilated adults
  10% soy oil   **Diet:** Use > 72 hr- Low fat diet, low fat enteral feeding or low fat TPN
  (100 mg/mL),   (subtract drug fat cal from TPN fat requirements- fat free TPN often used).
  1.1 cal/mL,   **Nutr:** IV infusion rate of 30 mL/hr (300 mg/hr) provides 790 cal fat/day.[40]
  1.2% egg lecithin   **S/Cond:** Avoid alcohol. Not c̄ lactation. Not for pediatric ICU use.
      Not c̄ egg or soy allergy. Caution c̄ hyperlipidemia, acute pancreatitis,
      lipid nephrosis.[40] Caution c̄ diabetes, cardiac disease, HIV/AIDS,
      ↓ renal func, ↓ hepatic func, seizures, geriatric or anemia.
      Pregnancy: Category B.
      Other: HYPOTENSION, bradycardia, agitation, ↓ pulmonary func.
      Rare- anaphylaxis, pulmonary edema.
      Blood/Serum: ↑ TRIGLYCERIDES, ↑ CHOL.
      Urinary: ↑ Zn. Green color.
      Monitor: TG, lipid panel, serum turbidity, vital signs.

propranolol
  Inderal
    Tab- lactose
  Inderal LA (SR)
    Cap
  InnoPran XL (SR)
    Cap- sugar spheres
    (sucrose & starch)
  Propranolol
    Soln- saccharin, orbitol

ANTIARRHYTHMIC, ANTIANGINA, ANTIHYPERTENSIVE, ANTIMIGRAINE
    HYPERTROPHIC SUBAORTIC STENOSIS
    Also used to Treat Aggression, Tremor & as Antianxiety Adjunct
        Non-selective Beta-Blocker   Oral or Parenteral (IV)
    Drug: InnoPran XL- Take HS, at same time each night.
    Take $\bar{c}$ food to enhance bioavailability.[7] Swallow SR cap whole.
    May mix soln $\bar{c}$ liquid or semi-solid food & consume immediately.
    Diet: ↓ Na, ↓ cal may be recommended. Avoid natural licorice, see p 374.
    Oral/GI: Dry mouth, N/V, epigastric distress, diarrhea, constipation, flatulence.
    S/Cond: Avoid alcohol- may ↓ drug effect.[9b] Caution $\bar{c}$ lactation.
    Caution $\bar{c}$ diabetes- may mask symptoms of & prolong hypoglycemia.
    May reduce insulin release in response to hyperglycemia.
    93% serum pro bound. Hypoalbuminemia (< 3 g/dL) may ↑ drug effects.
    Caution $\bar{c}$ CHF, ↓ hepatic func, ↓ renal func or hyperthyroidism.
    Not $\bar{c}$ asthma/bronchospasm or severe COPD. **Pregnancy:** Category C.
    Other: ↓ _BP_ $\bar{c}$ possible hypotension, BRADYCARDIA, dizziness, drowsiness,
    fatigue, insomnia, weakness, depression, ataxia, confusion.
    Blood/Serum: ↑ AST, ↑ ALT, ↑ alk phos, ↑ LDH, ↑ or ↓ T_4, ↑ or ↓ T_3,
    ↑ K, ↑ TG, ↑ VLDL, ↓ HDL.[34] Rare- dyscrasias.
    ↑ BUN $\bar{c}$ severe heart disease.[7] Possible ↓ CoQ10.[11]
    Monitor: BP, hepatic & renal func.

propylthiouracil (PTU)
  Generic brands
    Tab

ANTIHYPERTHYROID (To treat over active thyroid)
    Drug: Take $\bar{s}$ regard to food. **Nutr:** Anti-vitamin K effect- ↑ PT/INR.
    S/Cond: Not $\bar{c}$ lactation. Not $\bar{c}$ moderate to severe ↓ hepatic func.
    Not $\bar{c}$ pediatrics unless intolerant/allergy to **methimazole**.
    Pregnancy: Category D.
    Other: Rare- hepatotoxicity (eg- jaundice, hepatitis), bleeding,
    lupus-like syndrome.
    Blood/Serum: _Normalized TSH, T_4, T_3._
    Rare- agranulocytosis, aplastic anemia, ↓ platelets, ↑ PT/INR.
    Monitor: Baseline & periodic thyroid func, CBC. Possibly PT/INR.
    Baseline hepatic func & periodically for ≥ 6 mo.

R

Proquin XR	ANTIBIOTIC	See **ciprofloxacin p 85**
Proscar	BPH TREATMENT, Androgen Hormone Inhibitor	See **finasteride p 142**

Proton Pump Inhibitors (PPI) ANTIULCER, ANTIGERD, ANTISECRETORY   Oral or Parenteral (IV)
   (**esomeprazole** indicated only as ANTIULCER or ANTIGERD).
   (**pantoprazole** indicated only as ANTIGERD or ANTISECRETORY).
         Although serum half-life is 2-4 hr, antisecretory effect is > 24 hr.
Drug: Optimal- take **esomeprazole**, **lansoprazole** or **omeprazole** 30-60 minutes before a meal- may
open cap & take c̄ acidic juice or sprinkle contents (beads) on 1 T cool applesauce. Do not chew beads.
Follow by cool water.
Take **dexlansoprazole**, **pantoprazole** or **rabeprazole** s̄ regard to food.
Swallow Tab or Cap whole- do not crush, chew, open or divide.
For **Prevacid cap**- may mix beads c̄ small amount Ensure pudding, yogurt, cottage cheese or strained
pears **or** 60 mL orange or tomato juice (rinse glass ≥ 2X c̄ juice & drink).
To administer through feeding tube- may open cap & mix contents c̄ 40 cc apple juice.
Flush tube c̄ additional apple juice to clear. Dissolve **Solu-Tab** on tongue s̄ liquid, swallow saliva.
Mix **Prevacid pkt** granules in 2T cool water **only**. Take immediately, do <u>not</u> chew or crush granules.
Diet: May ↓ abs of Fe. ↓ abs of Vit B_{12}. In one study, **omeprazole** ↓ Ca abs by 61%.[101]
Ca suppl may be advised. Ca citrate is better absorbed than Ca Carbonate c̄ PPI.
Avoid gingko or SJW c̄ **omeprazole**- ↓ drug level.
Oral/GI: ↓ *GASTRIC ACID SECRETION*, ↑ *GASTRIC pH*, nausea, abdominal pain, <u>diarrhea</u>.
S/Cond: Avoid alcohol. Not c̄ lactation. 95-98.8% serum pro bound. Caution c̄ severe ↓ hepatic func.
Other: Headache, dizziness, cough, rash, muscle/back pain. Rare- hepatitis, pancreatitis, pneumonia.[44]
Pregnancy: Category C- **omeprazole**. All others- Category B.
Blood/Serum: ↑ *GASTRIN*. Possible ↓ Vit B_{12}.
< 1%- ↑ AST, ↑ ALT, ↑ alk phos, ↑ LDH, ↑ GGT, ↑ chol, ↑ glucose, ↑ crea, dyscrasias.

esomeprazole	**Nexium/Nexium I.V.**	Cap (DR)- sugar spheres (sucrose & starch) (s-isomer of **omeprazole**)
		Granules for DR Oral Susp- sugar spheres
dexlansoprazole	**Kapidex**	Cap (DR) Dual action release- sugar spheres, sucrose
		(*R*-enantiomer of **lansoprazole**)
lansoprazole	**Prevacid/Prevacid I.V.**	Cap (DR)- starch, sucrose, sugar spheres (sucrose & starch)
	Prevacid 24HR	Cap (DR)- starch, sucrose, sugar spheres

	Prevacid Solu-Tab	ODT- lactose, mannitol, aspartame = 2.5 mg phenylalanine/15 mg
omeprazole	**Prilosec**	Cap (DR)- lactose
		Granules for DR Oral Susp- sugar sphres, xanthan gum
	Zegerid	Pwd for oral susp- sucrose, sucralose, xanthan gum, xylitol, Na BiCarb = 480 mg Na/dose
pantoprazole	**Protonix/Protonix I.V.**	Tab (DR)- mannitol, propylene glycol Parenteral (IV)- pwd
		Granules for DR Oral Susp
rabeprazole	**Aciphex**	Tab (DR)- mannitol, propylene glycol

Promacta	IDIOPATHIC THROMBOCYTOPENIC PURPURA TREATMENT (ITP)	
		See **eltrombopag p 122**

ProtonixProntonix I.V. **pantoprazole**	ANTIGERD, ANTISECRETORY	See **Proton Pump Inhibitors above**

Proventil HFA	BRONCHODILATOR	See **albuterol p 25**

Provera	HORMONE	See **progesterone p 265**

Prozac	ANTIDEPRESSANT, SSRI	See **fluoxetine p 148**

pseudoephedrine
  Sudafed
  Tab- cornstarch, lactose, sucrose
  Syrup- menthol, saccharin Na, sorbitol
  Sudafed 12 Hour (SR)
  Tab
  SR Cap- Canada only

DECONGESTANT, Sympathomimetic Amine
  Drug: Take last dose a few hr before bedtime. Swallow SR forms whole. SR cap contents may be mixed c̄ jam or jelly, do not chew.[13]
  Diet: Limit caffeine/xanthine- ↑ CNS stimulation, see p 379.
  Nutr: Anorexia.
  Oral/GI: Dry mouth/nose, N/V c̄ large dose.
  S/Cond: Not c̄ lactation. Caution c̄ diabetes- drug effects may be confused c̄ hypo or hyperglycemia.[2] Caution c̄ cardiac disease, HTN or hyperthyroidism. Syrup precipitates some TF.[8]
  Pregnancy: Category C.
  Other: <u>Nervousness</u>, <u>insomnia</u>, <u>restlessness</u>, <u>transient</u> <u>HTN</u>, tachycardia, dizziness, tremor, headache, drowsiness, weakness, nosebleed, ↑ sweating, tremor. **Urinary:** Painful or difficult urination.

psyllium   LAXATIVE, Bulk Forming   Also used as Antidiarrheal, Antihyperlipidemic

hydrophilic mucilloid   Tab, Pwd, Wafer

Metamucil-Pwd   **Drug:** Take 2 hr before or after other med. Do **not** swallow or inhale dry pwd.

Original or Smooth   Dissolve pwd in $\geq$ 8 oz water, milk or juice for laxative effect.

  3 g fiber, 3-5 mg Na,   Drink $\geq$ 8 oz cool fluid $\bar{c}$ wafer form for laxative effect.

  30 mg K, sucrose,   As antidiarrheal, use only 80 mL liquid.[6]

  25-45 cal/dose,   **Diet:** Appropriate for $\downarrow$ Na diet.

  7-12 g CHO/dose,   High fiber $\bar{c}$ 1500-2000 mL fluid/day to prevent constipation.

  gluten free   As antihyperlipidemic- $\downarrow$ fat, $\downarrow$ chol, ($\downarrow$ cal if needed) diet.

Sugar-Free Smooth   **Nutr:** $\downarrow$ appetite.

  20 cal/dose,   **Oral/GI:** N/V, abdominal cramps, bloating, diarrhea, flatulence.

  5 g CHO,   **S/Cond:** Not $\bar{c}$ dysphagia, bowel, esophageal or GI obstruction.

  aspartame =   Caution $\bar{c}$ diabetes- $\uparrow$ insulin needs, some forms contain significant CHO.

  25 mg phenylalanine,   **Pregnancy:** Category B.

  30 mg K, 3 mg Na   **Other:** Rare- allergic reactions to pwd.

                           Blood/Serum: $\downarrow$ *CHOL*, $\downarrow$ *LDL*.

Wafer- 6 g fiber, corn oil, cornstarch, fructose, molasses, oats, sucrose, wheat flour, 120 cal/dose, 17 g CHO, 0.5-0.7 g gluten

Pulmicort   ANTIASTHMA, Corticosteroid   See **budesonide p 64**

Pulmozyme   CYSTIC FIBROSIS MANAGEMENT   See **dornase alfa p 116**

Pylera   H.PYLORI TREATMENT (used in combination $\bar{c}$ **omeprazole**)

               Combination drug **biskalcitrate** (bismuth subcitrate potassium), **metronidazole**, **tetracycline**

               See listing for **bismuth subsalicylate p 58** See **metronidazole p 216**, See **Tetracyclines p 310**

pyrazinamide (PZA)   TUBERCULOSIS TREATMENT

Pyrazinamide   **Nutr:** Anorexia. **Oral/GI:** N/V.

Tab   **S/Cond:** Avoid alcohol. Not $\bar{c}$ lactation.

               Caution $\bar{c}$ diabetes or severe $\downarrow$ renal func.[58] Caution $\bar{c}$ geriatric.[12]

               Not $\bar{c}$ severe hepatic disease or acute gout. HIV patients may need

               a longer course of therapy.

               Pregnancy: Category C.

               Other: Hepatotoxicity, jaundice, muscle &/or joint pain, gout.

Rare- interstitial nephritis, photosensitivity c̄ reddish-brown skin discoloration, porphyria, fever, rash.
Blood/Serum: ↑ <u>URIC ACID</u>, ↑ <u>AST</u>, ↑ <u>ALT</u>.
Rare- dyscrasias, ↑ iron binding capacity, ↑ Fe.[6]
Urinary: ↓ <u>URIC ACID</u>. False ketone results. Rare- dysuria.
Monitor: Hepatic & renal func, uric acid. TB- sputum cultures, chest x-rays q 2-3 mo & at completion of therapy.

pyridoxine Some Parenteral brands- benzyl alcohol	B COMPLEX VITAMIN, VIT B_6	Oral or Parenteral (IM or IV)

Drug: 2.5-10 mg/day to treat Pyr def.[6] 50-100 mg/day to treat medication induced def. Swallow SR cap whole, do not chew or crush.
Nutr: AI (mg/day) Infants 0-6 mo = **0.1**. 7-12 mo = **0.3**.
RDA (mg/day) Children 1-3 yr = **0.5**. 4-8 = **0.6**. 9-13 = **1.0**.
Males 14-50 = **1.3**. 51-70+ = **1.7**.
Females 14-18 = **1.2**. 19-50 = **1.3**. 51-70+ = **1.5**. Lactation = **2.0**.
UL (mg/day) Children 1-3 yr = **30**. 4-8 = **40**. 9-13 = **60**. 14-18 = **80**.
Adult = **100**. Lactation = **80-100**. ↑ Pyr requirement c̄ ↑ pro intake.
Oral/GI: Nausea c̄ high dose.
S/Cond: Active form, pyridoxal phosphate is 100% serum pro bound.[13]
↑ need in HIV/AIDS, alcoholism, hepatic disease, cancer.
Def S/S:[47] Peripheral neuropathy, seborrhea, microcytic anemia, depression, confusion, EEG abnormalities, seizures.
Def ↓ conversion of tryptophan to Nia.
Pregnancy: Category A (oral & parenteral).
RDA = 1.9 mg/day. **UL = 80-100** mg/day.
Other: Headache, drowsiness, mild flushing, paresthesia.
LT use of megadose (≥ 2 g/day) causes chronic toxicity c̄ severe <u>sensory neuropathy</u>, <u>ataxia</u> & <u>skin lesions</u>.
Blood/Serum: High dose- ↑ AST, ↓ Fol, ↓ prolactin.

Pyridium	URINARY ANALGESIC, Azo Dye	See **phenazopyridine** p 251
Questran	ANTIHYPERLIPIDEMIC	See **cholestyramine** p 83

quetiapine
Seroquel[a,b]
 Tab- Na starch glycolate,
 lactose
Seroquel XR[a,c]
 Tab- lactose

ANTIPSYCHOTIC[a] (Second Generation), ANTIMANIC,[b]
 ADJUNCTIVE TREATMENT TO ANTIDEPRESSANTS[c]
Drug: Take regular tab $\bar{s}$ regard to meals, although food ↑ abs & bioavailability 15-25%. Take XR form $\bar{s}$ food or $\bar{c}$ a light meal (about 300 cal). Swallow XR tab whole- do not split, chew or crush.
Diet: Caution $\bar{c}$ grapefruit/related citrus, see p 390.
Nutr: ↑ APPETITE, ↑ WEIGHT, obesity, anorexia.
Oral/GI: DRY MOUTH, dyspepsia, abdominal pain, constipation.
S/Cond: Avoid alcohol. Not $\bar{c}$ lactation. Caution $\bar{c}$ geriatric or ↓ hepatic func. Caution $\bar{c}$ seizures/history of seizures.
↑ mortality in geriatrics $\bar{c}$ dementia-related psychosis.
Pregnancy: Category C.
Other: Drowsiness, dizziness, orthostatic hypotension, sedation (↑ risk $\bar{c}$ initial dose titration), diabetes,[17] headache, asthenia, ↑ HR, agitation, back pain, fever, rash, flu syndrome, cough, rhinitis, pharyngitis, tachycardia, palpitation, dyspnea, peripheral edema, sweating, double vision. Rare- hyper or hypothyroidism, seizures, TD, NMS, ↑ QT interval, suicidal thinking & behavior,
Blood/Serum: ↓ T_4, ↑ CHOL, ↑ TRIGLYCERIDES, transient ↑ AST, ↑ ALT, ↑ GGT, ↓ WBC, ↑ glucose. Rare- ↑ TSH, ↑ alk phos, ↓ glucose, ↑ prolactin, ↑ crea, ↓ K, ↓ platelets, anemia, ↑ WBC.
Monitor: Although in PI, eye exam for cataracts no longer advised.[15] Baseline wt then monthly.
Baseline BP, FBS, Hb A1$_c$ & lipids at 12 wk, then at least annually.[1]

quinapril
 Accupril/Accuretic

ANTIHYPERTENSIVE   See **Angiotensin Converting Enzyme Inhibitors p 36**
 Accuretic also contains **hydrochlorothiazide,** see p 166.

quinidine gluconate
Generic brand
Tab (SR)- sugar, cornstarch
IV

ANTIARRHYTHMIC　　　　　　　　　Oral or Parenteral (IM or IV)

Drug: May take c̄ food or milk to ↓ GI irritation.
Insure adequate fluid intake/hydration. Maintain urinary pH 6-7.
Swallow SR tab whole. May break Tab (SR) in 1/2, do not crush or chew.
Diet: Caution c̄ K suppl. Avoid high dose Ca suppl (↑ urinary pH).
Diet or medication resulting in alkaline urine (eg predominantly
milk/milk products, citrus fruit), ↑ drug blood levels due to ↓ excretion.
Not c̄ grapefruit/related citrus, see p 390. Dietary salt intake affects oral drug
abs- high salt intake ↓ serum drug levels.[104] Consistent salt intake stabilizes
drug levels.

quinidine sulfate
Generic brand
Tab (SR)- sucrose,
  guar gum, gelatin

Nutr: Anorexia. ↑ K may ↑ drug effects.[13]
Oral/GI: Bitter taste, esophagitis, N/V, CRAMPS, abdominal pain, DIARRHEA.
S/Cond: Not c̄ lactation.[6] Correct hypokalemia, hypocalcemia or
hypomagnesemia prior to drug use to ↓ risk of ECG changes.
80-90% serum pro bound. Caution c̄ geriatric.[26]
Hypoalbuminemia (< 3 g/dL)- may ↑ drug effects.[6] Caution c̄ ↓ hepatic func
or severe ↓ renal func. Caution c̄ CHF. Not c̄ G6PD def- risk of hemolysis.
Pregnancy: Category C.
Other: Cardiotoxicity (↑ QT interval, other ECG changes), headache,
dizziness, weakness, fatigue, rash, cinchonism (hearing loss, tinnitus),
flushing, hypotension, syncope, confusion, fever, visual disturbances.
Rare- hepatotoxicity, angioedema, SLE-like syndrome, photosensitivity.
Blood/Serum: ↑ AST, ↑ CPK (c̄ sulfate form). ↓ K (due to diarrhea).
Rare- ↓ platelets, hemolytic anemia, ↓ glucose.[18]
Monitor: BP. Drug level, CBC c̄ diff, hepatic & renal func.
Possibly electrolytes, Mg, ECG (continuously c̄ IV).

QVAR

ANTIASTHMA (Oral inhaler), Corticosteroid
See **beclomethasone p 51**

rabeprazole
  Aciphex

ANTIGERD　　　　　　　See **Proton Pump Inhibitors p 268**

raloxifene
Evista
Tab- lactose, propylene glycol

OSTEOPOROSIS TREATMENT & PREVENTION,
BREAST CANCER PREVENTION in Postmenopausal Women   SERM
Drug: Take s̄ regard to food.
Diet: Adequate Ca & Vit D intake or Ca-Vit D suppl essential. **Nutr:** ↑ wt.
S/Cond: For postmenopausal women only. Limit alcohol.
Not c̄ lactation. > 95% serum bound. Caution c̄ ↓ hepatic func.
Not c̄ immobilized or bedridden patient.
Not c̄ Hx of venous thromboembolism. **Pregnancy:** Category X.
Other: ↑ _BONE_ _MINERAL_ _DENSITY_, ↓ _BONE RESORPTION_, hot flashes, leg cramps, depression, migraine, peripheral edema, muscle pain, insomnia, rash, sinusitis. Rare- thromboembolism, hepatitis.
Blood/Serum: ↓ CHOL, ↓ LDL, ↓ LIPOPROTEINS (a) & b, ↓ FIBRINOGEN, ↑ total T_4. (Slightly ↓ Ca, ↓ P, ↓ TP, ↓ alb, ↓ platelets).

raltegravir
Isentress
Tab- lactose

ANTIRETROVIRAL (HIV/AIDS), Integrase Inhibitor for HIV-1
Drug: Take s̄ regard to food.
Oral/GI: N/V, gastritis, abdominal pain, diarrhea.
S/Cond: Not c̄ lactation. **Pregnancy:** Category C.
Other: Headache, pyrexia, asthenia, fatigue, dizziness, lipodystrophy.
Rare- myopathy, rhabdomyolysis, SJS.[5]
Blood/Serum: Anemia, ↑ CPK, ↑ FBS, ↑ bil, ↑ ALT, ↑ AST, ↑ alk phos, ↑ amylase, ↑ lipase.

ramelteon
Rozerem
Tab- lactose, starch

SLEEP AID, Melatonin Receptor Agonist
Drug: Take within 1/2 hr of bedtime.
Do not take c̄ or just after a ↑ fat meal- ↑ fat ↑ time to drug action & ↓ C_{max}.
Oral/GI: Taste changes, nausea.
S/Cond: Caution c̄ alcohol- ↑ CNS effects. Not c̄ lactation.
Caution c̄ COPD or sleep apnea. Geriatrics experience elevated drug levels. Caution c̄ moderate ↓ hepatic func. Not c̄ severe ↓ hepatic func.
Pregnancy: Category C. **Other:** Dizziness, fatigue, daytime drowsiness, depression, muscle/joint pain, flu, URTI, headache.
Rare- parasomnias c̄ amnesia (eg sleep walking).
Blood/Serum: ↓ cortisol, ↑ prolactin, ↓ testosterone.

ramipril
Altace

ANTIHYPERTENSIVE   See **Angiotensin Converting Enzyme Inhibitors p 36**

Raniclor

ANTIBIOTIC, Cephalosporin   See **cefaclor p 76**

ranitidine
Zantac

ANTIULCER, ANTIGERD, ANTISECRETORY   See **Histamine H$_2$ Receptor**
Oral or Parenteral (IM or IV)   **Antagonists p 162**

Rapaflo
silodosin

BPH treatment
Cap- starch   See **Alpha$_1$ Adrenergic Blockers p 28**

rasagiline
Azilect
Tab- mannitol, starch

PARKINSON'S TREATMENT, Irreversible MAO-B Inhibitor
Initial monotherapy or adjunct therapy to **levodopa**
Drug: take s̄ regard to food.
Diet: Avoid foods high in tyramine & other pressor amines during drug
use & for 2 wk after DC to prevent hypertensive crisis, see p 383.
Avoid tryptophan suppl.[93] Avoid SJW,[93] see p 286. Avoid ginseng.[93]
Nutr: Anorexia, ↓ wt.
Oral/GI: Dry mouth, gingivitis, N/V, dyspesia, abdominal pain,
hemorrhage, constipation, diarrhea.
S/Cond: Caution c̄ lactation. 88-94% serum pro bound.
Caution c̄ mild ↓ hepatic func. NOT with moderate-severe ↓ hepatic func.
Not c̄ pheochromocytoma. **Pregnancy:** Category C.
Other: Dyskinesia, accidental injury, fall, postural hypotension, ataxia,
joint/neck pain, muscle weakness/pain, paresthesia, dystonia,
tendon inflammation, ecchymosis, hernia, dyspnea, headache,
drowsiness, asthenia, anxiety, depression, abnormal dreams,
hallucinations, ↑ sweating, rash, ↑ cough, flu syndrome.
Blood/Serum: < 1%- ↓ Ca, anemia.
Urinary: Hematuria, incontinence.

Razadyne/Razadyne ER   ANTI-ALZHEIMER'S, Acetylcholinesterase Inhibitor
Trade name changed in USA- previously **Reminyl**   See **galantamine p 153**

R

Rebetol	ANTIVIRAL, HEPATITIS C TREATMENT, Nucleoside Analog	
		See **ribavirin p 278**
Rebif	MULTIPLE SCLEROSIS TREATMENT	See **interferon beta-1a p 178**
Reclast zoledronic acid	OSTEOPOROSIS TREATMENT, PAGET'S DISEASE TREATMENT Parenteral only (IV)	See **Bisphosphonates, Parenteral p 60**
Reglan	ANTIEMETIC, ANTIGERD	See **metoclopramide p 214**
Relistor	LAXATIVE Opioid Antagonist	See **methylnaltrexone p 214**
Relpax eletriptan	ANTIMIGRAINE Serotonin 5-HT$_1$ Receptor Agonist	See **Antimigraine p 39**
Remeron	ANTIDEPRESSANT	See **mirtazapine p 218**
Remicade infliximab	ANTIARTHRITIC (Rheumatoid Arthritis), CROHN'S DISEASE TREATMENT, TNF Inhibitor 500 mg sucrose/vial	See listing for **etanercept p 130**

Reminyl (Canada)   ANTI-ALZHEIMER'S, Acetylcholinesterase Inhibitor
Previous brand name in USA- now **Razadyne**   See **galantamine p 153**

Renagel	PHOSPHATE BINDER (for use in ESRD)	See **sevelamer HCl p 291**
Renvela	PHOSPHATE BINDER (for use in ESRD)	See **sevelamer carbonate p 291**

repaglinide
    Prandin
    Tab- maize starch

ORAL HYPOGLYCEMIC for Type 2 Diabetes, Meglitinide
Used alone or c̄ **metformin**, **rosiglitazone** or **pioglitazone**
Drug: Take 15-30 minutes before meals (do not take if meal is skipped).
Diet: Drug is adjunct to prescribed diabetic diet, exercise.
↓ cal if wt loss needed. **Nutr:** ↑ wt.[10] *STIMULATES INSULIN RELEASE*.
Oral/GI: Tooth disorder, N/V, diarrhea, constipation.
S/Cond: Limit alcohol. Not c̄ lactation. > 98% serum alb bound.
Caution c̄ malnutrition- ↑ risk of hypoglycemia.

Caution $\bar{c}$ ↓ hepatic func or severe ↓ renal func.
Not $\bar{c}$ type 1 diabetes or ketoacidosis. **Pregnancy:** Category C.
Other: URTI, hypoglycemia, joint, chest or back pain, headache, allergy.
Blood/Serum: ↑ *INSULIN*, ↓ *FASTING GLUCOSE*, ↓ *POSTPRANDIAL GLUCOSE*,
↓ *Hb A1$_C$*. Rare- ↑ AST, ↑ ALT.
Monitor: FBS periodically. Hb A1$_C$ q 3 mo.

Reprexain Tab	ANALGESIC Combination drug **hydrocodone** & **ibuprofen**	See listing for **codeine p 91** See **ibuprofen p 170**

Requip/Requip XL   ANTIPARKINSON, Dopamine Agonist   See **ropinirole p 285**

reserpine   ANTIHYPERTENSIVE, ANTIPSYCHOTIC   Rauwolfia alkaloid
  Generic brands   Also used to treat hyperthyroidism
  Tab- confectioner's sugar,   **Drug:** Take $\bar{c}$ food or milk to ↓ GI distress.
  cornstarch, lactose   **Diet:** ↓ Na, ↓ cal may be recommended. Avoid natural licorice, see p 374.
Avoid SJW, see p 286. **Nutr:** Anorexia, ↓ wt. ↑ appetite, ↑ wt.
Oral/GI: ↑ GI MOTILITY, dry mouth, N/V, stomach cramps, black tarry stools,
diarrhea, GI bleeding. **S/Cond:** Avoid alcohol. Not $\bar{c}$ lactation.
↑ risk of dental problems, see p 11 & 15.
Not $\bar{c}$ active peptic ulcer, colitis, gallstones or depression.
Caution $\bar{c}$ ↓ renal func, history of peptic ulcer, colitis, gallstones,
mental depression. 95% serum pro bound. **Pregnancy:** Category C.[7]
Other: ↓ *BP* $\bar{c}$ possible hypotension, dizziness, nasal congestion/bleeding,
drowsiness, headache, edema, rash, depression (may be severe),
nightmares, syncope, arrhythmias, bradycardia, anxiety, weakness,
blurred vision, muscle aches, gynecomastia, lactation, EPS $\bar{c}$ high dose.
Rare- Parkinsonian syndrome, hypersensitivity reaction.
Blood/Serum: ↑ prolactin. **Monitor:** BP.

Restoril temazepam	SLEEP AID	See **Benzodiazepines p 54**
retinol	VITAMIN	See **vitamin A p 336**
Retrovir	ANTIRETROVIRAL (HIV/AIDS), NRTI	See **zidovudine p 348**

Revatio	PULMONARY ARTERIAL HYPERTENSION TREATMENT	
		See **sildenafil p 292**
ReVia	ALCOHOL ABUSE DETERRENT, NARCOTIC ANTAGONIST	
		See **naltrexone p 224**
Reyataz	ANTIRETROVIRAL (HIV/AIDS), Protease Inhibitor	
		See **atazanavir p 45**
Rheumatrex	ANTIARTHRITIC	See **methotrexate p 212**
Rhinocort Aqua	ANTIASTHMA, Corticosteroid	See **budesonide p 64**

ribavirin

Rebetol
Cap- lactose
Soln- sucrose, sorbitol, propylene glycol
Copegus
Tab- starch, cornstarch

ANTIVIRAL, HEPATITIS C TREATMENT, Nucleoside Analog
(used c̄ **interferon alfa 2b, peginterferon alfa 2b** or **peginterferon alfa 2a**)
Drug: Take consistently c̄ or s̄ regard to food, high fat meal ↑ conc 70%.
(Test meal = 840 cal, 54 g fat, 32 g pro, 57 g CHO).
Dosage based on body wt.
Nutr: <u>Anorexia</u>.
Oral/GI: Taste changes, <u>N/V</u>, <u>dyspepsia</u>.
S/Cond: Not c̄ lactation. Caution c̄ ↓ renal func.
Not c̄ severe ↓ renal func, unstable cardiac disease, pancreatitis, hemoglobinopathies, autoimmune hepatitis, unstable thyroid disease.
Caution c̄ ↓ pulmonary func, diabetes, psychiatric disorder, geriatric.
Pregnancy: Category X.
Not to be used by male partners of pregnant women.
Other: <u>Insomnia</u>, <u>depression</u>, <u>rash</u>, <u>itching</u>, emotional lability, nervousness, dizziness, dyspnea, weakness, fatigue.
(See also i**nterferon alfa 2b**)
Blood/Serum: <u>Hemolytic</u> <u>anemia</u>, ↓ <u>WBC</u>, ↓ <u>platelets</u>, ↑ <u>bil</u>, ↑ uric acid.
Monitor: Baseline Hb, again at 2 & 4 wk.
CBC c̄ diff, platelets, hepatic func, TSH.[7]

Rifamate	ANTIBIOTIC, TUBERCULOSIS TREATMENT	See **isoniazid p 180**
Cap- Na starch glycolate	Combination drug	See **rifampin below**

rifampin
  Rifadin
  Cap- cornstarch
  IV- pwd

ANTIBIOTIC, TUBERCULOSIS TREATMENT, (also ANTI-MAC)
Oral or Parenteral (IV)

Drug: Take c̄ 8 oz water 1 hr before or 2 hr after food to ↑ abs.
May take c̄ food if GI upset, but food ↓ abs. May open cap & mix
contents c̄ applesauce or jelly.
Diet: May need Vit D suppl.
Nutr: Anorexia. May ↑ Vit D metabolism & ↓ BMD c̄ LT use.[93]
Oral/GI: Oral candidiasis, dyspepsia, N/V, <u>cramps</u>, <u>diarrhea</u>, flatulence.
Rare- pseudomembranous colitis.
S/Cond: Avoid alcohol. Not c̄ lactation. Caution c̄ ↓ hepatic func or geriatric.
Caution c̄ diabetics on sulfonylurea- ↑ glucose.
84-91% serum pro bound.[6] Potent CYP inducer- caution c̄ many other drugs.
Pregnancy: Category C.
Other: <u>Red/orange</u> <u>body</u> <u>fluids</u>, <u>rash</u>, flu-like syndrome, fever/chills,
fatigue, joint/muscle pain, allergic reaction, SJS, TEN, dizziness, ataxia,
drowsiness, confusion, visual changes, headache, flushing, itching,
facial & peripheral edema. Rare- jaundice & hepatitis, interstitial nephritis.
Rare- osteomalacia, anaphylaxis, acute renal failure c̄ high dose.
Blood/Serum: ↑ <u>AST</u>, ↑ <u>ALT</u>, ↑ <u>alk phos</u>, ↑ <u>bil</u> (<u>false</u> ↑ at start of drug use)[6],
↓ Vit D, ↑ PTH, ↑ BUN, ↑ crea, ↑ uric acid. Rare- dyscrasias.
Inaccurate microbiological Fol & Vit B$_{12}$ assays.
Urinary: <u>RED/ORANGE</u> <u>URINE</u>. False + opiates c̄ KIMS method.[6]
Monitor: Baseline & during treatment- CBC, platelets, hepatic func.

Rifater
  Tab- sucrose

ANTITUBERCULOSIS
Combination drug

See **rifampin above,** See **isoniazid p 180**
See **pyrazinamide p 270**

rifaxamin
  Xifaxan
  Tab- Na starch glycolate,
  propylene glycol

ANTIBIOTIC, Traveler's Diarrhea Treatment (diarrhea due to E. coli)
Drug: Take s̄ regard to food.
Oral/GI: All GI effects higher c̄ placebo than c̄ drug.
S/Cond: PI states not c̄ lactation, but little systemic abs.
Not c̄ fever or blood in stool.
Pregnancy: Category C.

R

rilpivirine
Edurant
Tab- lactose

ANTIRETROVIRAL (HIV/AIDS), NNRTI

Drug: Take tab once daily c̄ a meal.
Diet: Take Ca or Mg suppl or antacids 2 hr before or 4 hr after drug.
Not c̄ high protein nutrition drink- ↓ drug absorption.
Caution c̄ grapefruit/related citrus, see p 390. Not c̄ SJW, see p 286.
Nutr: ↓ appetite. **Oral/GI:** N/V, abdominal pain, diarrhea.
S/Cond: Not c̄ lactation. >99.7% serum pro bound- hypoalbuminemia
(< 3 g/dL) may ↑ drug effects. Not c̄ severe ↓ hepatic func.
Caution c̄ severe ↓ renal func. **Pregnancy:** Category B.
Other: Fatigue, headache, dizziness, insomnia, somnolence,
abnormal dreams, rash, body fat redistribution, depression, anxiety,
dysphoria, altered mood, suicidal thinking and behavior.
Rare- glomerulonephritis, cholecystitis, cholelithiasis,
immune reconstitution syndrome.
Blood/Serum: ↑ <u>ALT</u>, ↑ <u>AST</u>, ↑ <u>bil</u>, ↑ <u>chol</u>, ↑ <u>LDL</u>, ↑ TG, ↑ crea.
Monitor: Emergence or worsening of depressive disorders (eg depressed
mood, depression, suicide attempt, dysphoria).

Riomet

ANTIHYPERGLYCEMIC AGENT, Biguanide   See **metformin p 210**

risedronate
Actonel

OSTEOPOROSIS TREATMENT, PAGET'S DISEASE TREATMENT
                    See listing for **Bisphosphonates, Oral p 59**

risperidone
Risperdal
Tab- lactose, cornstarch,
 propylene glycol
Soln
Risperdal M-TAB (ODT)
aspartame = 0.28 mg
phenylalanine/mg,
mannitol, simethicone,
peppermint oil

ANTIPSYCHOTIC (Second Generation), ANTIMANIC, Oral or Parenteral (IM)
    TREATMENT OF IRRITABILITY IN AUTISM
    Also used to treat resistant depression or anxiety
Drug: Take s̄ regard to food.
Dissolve ODT on tongue c̄ or s̄ liquid, swallow saliva.
Nutr: ↑ <u>APPETITE</u>, ↑ <u>WEIGHT</u>, obesity.
Oral/GI: ↑ or ↓ salivation, dry mouth, dysphagia, N/V, dyspepsia,
abdominal pain, <u>constipation</u>, diarrhea.
S/Cond: Avoid alcohol. Not c̄ lactation. 90% serum pro bound.
Caution c̄ ↓ hepatic func or ↓ renal func, seizures/history of seizures, geriatric.

Risperdal Consta (IM/SR)
long acting microspheres
Risperdone Oral Soln-
sorbitol

Pregnancy: Category C.
Other: <u>DROWSINESS</u>, <u>insomnia</u>, <u>anxiety</u>, <u>weakness</u>, <u>akathisia</u>,
<u>EPS</u> at high dose, <u>rhinitis</u>, nose bleeds,[21] HTN, orthostatic hypotension,
diabetes, Parkinsonism, dizziness, rash, muscle pain, tachycardia,
↑ QT interval, sexual dysfunction, <u>AMENORRHEA</u>, <u>GALACTORRHEA</u>.
Rare- seizure, NMS, tardive dyskinesia, suicidal thinking & behavior.
↑ mortality in geriatric c̄ dementia-related psychosis.
Blood/Serum: ↑ <u>PROLACTIN</u> in <u>WOMEN</u> & <u>men</u>, ↑ <u>TG</u>, ↑ glucose.
< 1%- ↓ Na, ↓ K, ↑ CPK, ↑ AST, ↑ ALT, ↓ Hb & HCT,
↓ platelets, ↑ uric acid, ↑ P.
Monitor: Baseline ECG.[17] Baseline wt then monthly. Baseline BP, FBS,
Hb A1$_c$[21] & lipids at 12 wk, then at least annually.[1]

Ritalin PSYCHOSTIMULANT, ANTI-ADHD See **methylphenidate p 214**

ritonavir (RTV)
Norvir
Soln- ethanol, saccharin Na,
castor oil, propylene glycol,
peppermint oil &
caramel flavoring
Cap- castor oil,
ethanol

ANTIRETROVIRAL (HIV/AIDS), Protease Inhibitor
Drug: Take c̄ food. May mix soln c̄ chocolate milk or nutritional suppl.
Diet: Avoid SJW, see p 286. **Nutr:** Anorexia, ↓ wt.
Oral/GI: Taste changes, throat irritation, dyspepsia, <u>NAUSEA</u>, <u>vomiting</u>,
abdominal pain, <u>diarrhea</u>.
S/Cond: Avoid alcohol. Not c̄ lactation. 98% serum pro bound.
Caution c̄ ↓ hepatic func. Caution c̄ diabetes.
Strong CYP3A4 inhibitor- may affect many other drugs.
Pregnancy: Category B.
Other: <u>Hepatotoxicity</u>, <u>hepatitis</u>, <u>jaundice</u>, <u>circumoral</u> or peripheral
paresthesia, <u>weakness</u>, headache, dizziness, drowsiness, flushing,
muscle pain, fever, diabetes,[96] excessive menstrual bleeding.[74]
Rare- pancreatitis, gout, SJS, anaphylaxis.
May ↑ risk of lipodystrophy or nephrotoxicity.
Blood/Serum: ↑ <u>CPK</u>, ↑ <u>TG</u>, ↑ <u>VLDL</u>, ↑ <u>CHOL</u>, ↑ <u>AST</u>, ↑ <u>ALT</u>, ↑ GGT,
↑ alk phos, ↑ uric acid, ↑ amylase, ↑ BUN, ↑ glucose.[96]
Monitor: Baseline & periodically during therapy- hepatic func, GGT,
CPK, lipid panel, TG, glucose.

R

rituximab **Rituxan**	ANTINEOPLASTIC, Monoclonal Antibody for B-cell Non-Hodgkin's Lymphoma Parenteral only (IV)

Pretreatment antihistamine & acetaminophen usual

Diet: Insure adequate fluid intake/hydration to ↑ uric acid excretion.

Nutr: Anorexia.

Oral/GI: Taste changes, <u>throat irritation</u>, NAUSEA/V, dyspepsia, <u>abdominal pain</u>, <u>diarrhea</u>.

S/Cond: Not c̄ lactation. Caution c̄ cardiac disease, hepatitis B.

Pregnancy: Category C.

Other: <u>Fever</u>, <u>CHILLS</u>, <u>ALLERGIC INFUSION REACTION</u> (may be fatal), <u>WEAKNESS</u>, <u>INFECTION</u>, <u>hypotension</u> (may be severe), <u>HTN</u>, <u>headache</u>, <u>dizziness</u>, <u>angioedema</u>, <u>peripheral edema</u>, <u>muscle pain</u>, <u>rhinitis</u>, <u>bronchospasm</u>, <u>cough</u>, <u>dyspnea</u>, <u>rash</u>, <u>itching</u>, dry eyes, back pain, depression, anxiety, night sweats, fatigue, insomnia, flushing, paresthesia, tachycardia. Rare- anaphylaxis, SJS, TEN, tumor lysis syndrome & acute renal failure, arrhythmias (can be fatal).

Blood/Serum: ↓ <u>WBC</u>, ↓ <u>neutrophils</u>, ↓ <u>platelets</u>, anemia, ↑ LDH, ↑ <u>glucose</u>, ↓ Ca, ↑ uric acid.

Monitor: CBC & platelets, baseline & periodically. Heart rate, BP.

rivaroxaban **Xarelto** Tab- lactose	PREVENTION OF STROKE/SYSTEMIC EMBOLISM in NONVALVULAR ATRIAL FIBRILLATION, DVT PROHYLAXIS IN KNEE OR HIP REPLACEMENT SURGERY, Selective Factor Xa inhibitor

Drug: Take 10mg tab s̄ regard to food. Take 15 & 20 mg tab c̄ evening meal. Not for admin via J-tube.

Diet: Avoid herbal products c̄ antiplatlet/anticoagulent effects (ie ginger, garlic, ginseng & others). Avoid SJW, p 286. Caution c̄ grapefruit/related citrus, see p 390.

S/Cond: Avoid alcohol. Not c̄ lactation. 92-95% serum pro bound- hypoalbuminemia (< 3 g/dL) may ↑ drug effects.

Not c̄ severe ↓ renal func (CrCl < 30 mL/min).

Not c̄ moderate to severe ↓ hepatic func.

Not c̄ spinal/epidural anesthesia/puncture.

Do dental care cautiously, ↑ risk of bleeding.
Pregnancy: Category C.
Other: Bleeding (can be fatal), skin blister, itching, muscle spasm, extremity pain, syncope, hypersensitivity, jaundice, cytolytic hepatitis, subdural hematoma, epidural hematoma, retroperitoneal hemorrhage, SJS.
Blood/Serum: ↑ AST, ↑ ALT, ↑ <u>GGT</u>, ↓ platelets, ↑ bil, agranulocytosis.
Monitor: S/S of neurological impairment, S/S of bleeding/blood loss.

rivastigmine **Exelon** Cap Soln Transdermal Patch 24 hr Vit E	ALZHEIMER'S or PARKINSON'S DEMENTIA TREATMENT, Acetylcholinesterase Inhibitor Also used to treat vascular & mixed dementia **Drug:** Take BID c̄ food. Swallow soln directly or mix c̄ small glass water, cold fruit juice or soda. **Nutr:** <u>Anorexia</u>, ↓ wt, dehydration. **Oral/GI:** <u>NAUSEA/VOMITING</u> (<u>may be</u> severe), <u>dyspepsia</u>, abdominal pain, <u>diarrhea</u>, constipation, flatulence. Rare- esophageal rupture at high initial dose. **S/Cond:** Not c̄ lactation. Caution c̄ seizures, asthma, obstructive pulmonary disease. Caution c̄ peptic ulcer disease- drug may ↑ gastric acid secretion. Caution c̄ wt < 50 kg- ↑ risk of side effects. **Pregnancy:** Category B. **Other:** <u>Headache</u>, <u>dizziness</u>, insomnia, weakness, fatigue, drowsiness, syncope, tremor, ataxia, confusion, hallucinations, rhinitis, depression, ↑ BP. **Blood/Serum:** Anemia. **Urinary:** Hematuria.
rizatriptan **Maxalt**	ANTIMIGRAINE, Serotonin 5-HT$_1$ Receptor Agonist See **Antimigraine p 39**
Robaxin	SKELETAL MUSCLE RELAXANT See **methocarbamol p 211**
Robitussin Chest Congestion	EXPECTORANT See **guaifenesin p 159**
Rocaltrol	Ca REGULATOR, Active Vit D$_3$ See **calcitriol p 68**

Rocephin	ANTIBIOTIC, **ceftriaxone sodium** See **cephalosporins p 80**

roflumilast
  Daliresp
  Tab- lactose,
  corn starch

TO REDUCE COPD EXACERBATIONS IN PATIENTS c̄ SEVERE COPD,
Selective Phosphodiesterase 4 (PDE4) Inhibitor

> **Drug:** Take c̄ or s̄ food.
> **Diet:** Caution c̄ grapefruit/related citrus, see p 390. Not c̄ SJW, see p 286.
> **Nutr:** ↓ wt, ↓ appetite.
> **Oral/GI:** Diarrhea, N/V, abdominal pain, dyspepsia, gastritis.
> **S/Cond:** Not c̄ lactation. Not c̄ moderate - severe ↓ hepatic func.
> 99% serum pro bound- hypoalbuminemia (< 3 g/dL) may ↑ drug effects.
> Not for acute bronchodilation. **Pregnancy:** Category C.
> **Other:** Headache, back pain, muscle spasm, tremor, insomnia, dizziness,
> sinusitis, rhinitis, anxiety, depression, suicidal thinking & behavior.
> **Urinary:** UTI.
> **Monitor:** Wt regularly. Emergence or worsening of insomnia, anxiety,
> depression, suicidal thoughts or other mood changes.

romiplostim
  Nplate
  pwd- vial
  no preservatives
  mannitol, sucrose

IDIOPATHIC THROMBOCYTOPENIC PURPURA TREATMENT,

Parenteral only (SC)

Thrombopoietin Receptor Agonist Stimulates bone marrow to
produce ↑ platelets, ≥ 50 X 10^9/L to ↓ bleeding risk

> **Drug:** Given SC q wk.
> **Oral/ GI:** Dyspepsia, abdomonal pain.
> **S/Cond:** Not c̄ lactation. Caution c̄ ↓ hepatic func or ↓ renal func.
> Not c̄ blood cancer or myelodysplastic syndrome.
> Dose based on actual BW.
> **Pregnancy:** Category C.
> **Other:** Dizzines, muscle/joint pain, shoulder pain, extremity pain,
> insomnia, paresthesia, headache, bone marrow reticulin deposition,
> ST ↑ thrombocytopenia after DC of drug.
> Myelofibrosis, popliteal artery thrombosis, bleeding.[137]
> **Blood/Serum:** ↑ PLATELETS, ↓ RISK OF BLEEDING.
> **Monitor:** Prior to, during & ≥ 2wk after DC- CBC, platelets,
> peripheral blood smears.

ropinirole **Requip** Tab- lactose	ANTIPARKINSON, RESTLESS LEG SYNDROME TREATMENT Dopamine Receptor Agonist, Nonergot Derivative

Drug: Take s̄ regard to food, but food may ↓ nausea.
Nutr: Anorexia. ↑ or ↓ wt.
Oral/GI: Dry mouth, dysphagia, pharyngitis, <u>dyspepsia</u>, NAUSEA, <u>vomiting</u>, abdominal pain, diarrhea, constipation, flatulence.
S/Cond: Caution c̄ alcohol. Not c̄ lactation.
Caution c̄ ↓ hepatic func or severe ↓ renal func. **Pregnancy:** Category C.
Other: <u>DROWSINESS</u>, <u>fatigue</u>, <u>syncope</u>, weakness, dizziness, headache, peripheral edema, postural hypotension, ↑ BP, ↑ sweating, chest pain, tremor, palpitations, tachycardia, bradycardia, atrial fibrillation, confusion, amnesia, hallucinations, abnormal dreams, anxiety, hypokinesia, ↑ dyskinesia, yawning, flushing, visual changes, dry eyes, muscle pain/cramps. Rare- sleep attacks, compulsive behavior, melanoma.
Blood/Serum: ↑ alk phos, ↑ BUN, anemia.
< 1%- ↑ or ↓ glucose, ↑ LDH, ↑ CPK, ↑ P, ↑ or ↓ K, ↓ Na, ↑ chol.
Urinary: UTI, incontinence. **Monitor:** Possibly skin exams.

rosiglitazone **Avandia**	ANTIDIABETIC AGENT for Type 2 Diabetes	See **thiazolidinediones p 312**
rosuvastatin **Crestor**	ANTIHYPERLIPIDEMIC	See **HMG-CoA Reductase Inhibitors p 164**
Rowasa	ANTI-INFLAMMATORY (in ulcerative colitis)	See **mesalamine p 209**
Roxanol	ANALGESIC, Narcotic, Opioid	See **morphine p 221**
Roxicet Soln- 0.4% alcohol, sorbitol, fructose, saccharin Na, Tab- cornstarch	ANALGESIC, Narcotic, Opioid Combination drug	See **oxycodone p 241** See **acetaminophen p 22**
Roxicodone	ANALGESIC, Narcotic, Opioid	See **oxycodone p 241**
Rozerem	SLEEP AID	See **ramelteon p 274**

Safyral	ORAL CONTRACEPTIVE	See **Oral Contraceptives p 237**

St. John's wort (SJW)
  Hypericum perforatum
  Oral- pwd, liquid
  or solid forms
  Movana
  Tab- cornstarch

  Topical- liquid or
  semi-solid

  (note- many brands
  do not meet content
  claims)[75]

HERBAL PRODUCT (Not FDA approved)   Oral or Topical
  Used as Antidepressant, Antianxiety, topically to treat wounds, burns
  Drug: 4-8 wk minimum use for antidepressant effect. Take AM to ↓ insomnia.
  Diet: Weak MAOI- interaction theorized c̄ high SJW dose & ↑ intake of
  ↑ tyramine foods, see p 383.
  Oral/GI: Dry mouth, GI upset, abdominal pain, constipation.
  S/Cond: Not c̄ lactation. Not c̄ bipolar disorder- may induce mania.
  Not c̄ Alzheimer's or schizophrenia- may induce psychosis.
  Caution c̄ all other drugs- SJW induces CYP3A4, 2D6, 1A2 & p-glycoprotein,
  thus may ↑ metabolism of substrates of these systems & ↓ serum drug levels.[93]
  Caution c̄ drugs which ↑ serotonin, such as antidepressants- risk of
  serotonin syndrome.
  Pregnancy: Avoid use.
  Other: Insomnia, restlessness, headache, fatigue, sedation, anxiety,
  agitation, irritability, vivid dreams, paresthesias, dizziness, tremor.
  Photosensitivity at high dose. < 1%- confusion, allergic reaction/rash,
  serotonin syndrome. Withdrawal symptoms upon DC after LT use.
  Blood/Serum: ↓ glucose, ↑ TSH. ↓ PT/INR c̄ **warfarin** use.

Salagen   ANTIXEROSTOMIA, SJÖGREN'S SYNDROME TREATMENT, Cholinergic
         See **pilocarpine p 258**

salmeterol
  Serevent Diskus
  Pwd for inhalation-
  lactose

ANTIASTHMA (not for acute symptoms), COPD Treatment, EIB
  Also used to prevent Exercise Induced Bronchospasm (EIB)
  Long Acting Bronchodilator, Beta-2 agonist
  Drug: Do NOT exceed prescribed dose.
  Oral/GI: Dental pain, ↓ salivation, candidiasis, pharyngitis,
  throat irritation, N/V, stomachache, diarrhea.
  S/Cond: Not c̄ lactation. Caution c̄ ↓ hepatic func, cardiac disease,
  arrhythmias, diabetes, hyperthyroidism[7] or seizures.
  Caution c̄ milk allergy- rare allergic reaction.
  Pregnancy: Category C.

Other: <u>Headache</u>, tachycardia, palpitations, tremor, nervousness, rash, eczema, cough, rhinitis/congestion, keratitis, conjunctivitis, muscle/back pain, paresthesia, edema, paradoxical bronchospasm, HTN, dizziness, anxiety, allergic reaction, hypokalemia. ↑ QT interval, arrhythmias c̄ high dose.
Rare- asthma related deaths.
Blood/Serum: Rare- ↑ glucose, ↓ K.

Samsca	HYPONATREMIA TREATMENT	See **tolvaptan p 318**
Sanctura/Sanctura SR trospium	ANTIMUSCARINIC	See **Bladder Control Agents p 61**
Sandimmune	IMMUNOSUPPRESSANT	See **cyclosporine p 96**
Sandostatin	ANTIDIARRHEAL	See **octreotide p 232**
Saphris	ANTIPSYCHOTIC, Second Generation	See **asenapine p 43**

sapropterin
   Kuvan
   Tab- asorbic acid,
   mannitol, riboflavin

HYPERPHENYLALANEMIA TREATMENT, Enzyme Enhancer
in tetrahydrobiopterin (BH4-) responsive PKU   Synthetic BH4
Drug is only effective in pts c̄ sufficient residual
phenylalanine hydroxylase (PAH). BH4 stimulates PAH to metabolize Phe.
Drug: Take c̄ food to ↑ abs. Dissolve tab in 4-8 oz water or apple juice. May crush & stir, drink within 15 minutes. Dose based on BW.
Diet: Adjunct to restricted phenylalanine (Phe) diet.
Oral/GI: N/V, diarrhea.
S/Cond: Not c̄ lactation. Caution c̄ ↓ hepatic func.
Pregnancy: Category C.
Other: <u>Rhinorrhea/URTI</u>, <u>pharyngolaryngeal pain</u>, headache, cough, nasal congestion, confusion.
Blood/Serum: ↑ *PAH*, ↓ *PHENYLALANINE*, ↓ neutrophils.
Urinary: UTI.
Monitor: Phe level at 1 wk, then periodically, to prevent dangerously low Phe.

S

saquinavir (SQV)
  Invirase
  Cap- lactose 66.3 mg,
  Na starch glycolate
  Tab- lactose

ANTIRETROVIRAL (HIV/AIDS), Protease Inhibitor
  Drug: Take c̄ or within 2 hr of a full meal. (test meals were 54-57 g fat)
  Must be administered c̄ low dose **ritonavir**.
  Diet: Caution c̄ grapefruit/related citrus- see p 390.
  Avoid SJW or garlic suppl- ↓ drug level.
  Oral/GI: Mouth ulceration, taste changes, dysphagia, dyspepsia, <u>N/V</u>,
  <u>abdominal pain</u>, <u>diarrhea</u>, constipation, <u>flatulence</u>.
  S/Cond: Not c̄ lactation. 98% serum pro bound. Caution c̄ ↓ hepatic func.[5]
  Caution c̄ diabetes or geriatric.
  Pregnancy: Category B.
  Other: <u>Fatigue</u>, <u>pneumonia</u>, weakness, rash, itching, dry skin, eczema,
  photosensitivity, headache, insomnia, depression, fever, back pain,
  bronchitis, flu, sinusitis. Rare- SJS, seizures, diabetes.
  May ↑ risk of lipodystrophy.
  Blood/Serum: ↑ <u>glucose</u>, ↓ glucose, ↑ CPK, ↑ TG, anemia, ↓ platelets,
  ↓ neutrophils, ↑ K. <1%- ↓ K, ↑ TSH, ↑ AST, ↑ ALT, ↑ bil, ↑ amylase,
  ↑ GGT, ↑ LDH, ↑ or ↓ Ca, ↓ Na, ↓ P.
  Monitor: Baseline & periodic CBC, TG, blood chem,
  including hepatic func, glucose.

Sarafem

PMDD TREATMENT, SSRI   See **fluoxetine p 148**

sargramostim
  Leukine

COLONY STIMULATING FACTOR   See listing for **filgrastim p 142**
  Liquid- 1.1% benzyl alcohol Pwd- no preservatives Parenteral only (IV)

Savella

FIBROMYALGIA MANAGEMENT, SNRI   See **milnacipran p 217**

saxagliptin
  Onglyza
  Tab- lactose

ANTIDIABETIC AGENT, Incretin Enhancer
  DPP-4 (dipetidyl-peptidase-4) Inhibitor See listing for **sitagliptin p 293**

Seasonale/Seasonique

ORAL CONTRACEPTIVE, 91 day regimen   See **Oral Contraceptives p 237**

Sectral

ANTIHYPERTENSIVE, ANTIARRHYTHMIC See **acebutolol p 21**
Cardioselective Beta-Blocker

selegiline
Eldepryl
Cap- lactose

Generic brands
Tab- lactose,
maize starch

Emsam patch for
depression only
Zelapar ODT
gelatin, mannitol,
aspartame =
1.25 mg phenylalanine

ANTIPARKINSON (oral forms) (adjunct to carbidopa/levodopa),
ANTIDEPRESSANT (patch)   MAO-B Inhibitor
Drug: Take regular tab or cap c̄ breakfast & lunch-
bioavailability ↑ 3-4 X c̄ food.
Dissolve ODT on tongue c̄ or s̄ liquid once a day ≥ 5 minutes before food.
Swallow saliva
Diet: If oral dose of cap/tab > 10 mg/day or ODT > 2.5 mg, or c̄ 9 or
12 mg patch, avoid high tyramine foods, see p 383. Avoid SJW, see p 286.
Oral/GI: Dry mouth, dysphagia, <u>nausea</u>, abdominal pain.
S/Cond: Avoid alcohol. Not c̄ lactation.[10]
↑ risk of dental problems, see p 11 & 15. 85-90% serum pro bound.[6]
Caution c̄ geriatric
Pregnancy: Category C.
Other: <u>Dizziness</u>, <u>confusion</u>, hallucinations, headache, insomnia,
vivid dreams, depression, EPS, tardive dyskinesia, peripheral edema,
arrhythmias, syncope, HTN or postural hypotension,
suicidal thinking & behavior. <u>APPLICATION SITE REACTIONS</u> c̄ patch.
Blood/Serum: Transient ↑ AST, ↑ ALT.

Selzentry

ANTIRETROVIRAL (HIV/AIDS), CCR5 antagonist
See **maraviroc p 204**

senna — LAXATIVE, Stimulant
- **Ex-Lax**
- **Max** Tab- starch, sucrose, 25 mg sennosides/Tab
- **Reg** Chew Tab- cocoa, sugar, palm kernel oil, non-fat dry milk, lecithin, 15 mg sennosides/Tab
- **Senokot**
- Tab- mineral oil, lactose, 8.6 mg sennosides, 25 mg Ca
- **SenokotXTRA**
- Tab- lactose, cornstarch, 17.2 mg sennosides
- **Perdiem Overnight Relief**
- Tab- starch, sucrose, 15 mg sennosides, 55 mg Ca, propylene glycol

Drug: Take HS c̄ 8 oz water or juice.
Perdiem- Swallow tab whole, do not crush or chew. Do not use for > 1 wk.
Diet: High fiber c̄ 1500-2000 mL fluid/day to prevent constipation.
Nutr: Electrolyte imbalance c̄ excessive use.
Oral/GI: ↑ *INTESTINAL PERISTALSIS*, *BOWEL MOVEMENT IN 6-12 HR*. N/V, cramps, diarrhea, laxative dependence & loss of normal bowel func c̄ LT use/abuse.
S/Cond: Not c̄ rectal bleeding. Caution c̄ abdominal pain, N/V.
Pregnancy: Avoid stimulant laxatives in pregnancy.[2]
Urinary: Discolored urine.
Blood/Serum: LT or excess- ↑ glucose, ↓ K, ↓ Ca.

Senokot-S
Tab- 20 mg Ca, 4 mg Na

STIMULANT LAXATIVE, STOOL SOFTENER
Combination drug

See **senna above**
See **docusate sodium p 115**

Sensipar

HYPERPARATHYROIDISM TREATMENT

See **cinacalcet p 84**

Septra

ANTIBIOTIC

See **trimethoprim c̄ sulfamethoxazole p 324**

Serax (previous brand name)
oxazepam

ANTIANXIETY

See **Benzodiazepines p 54**

Serevent

ANTIASTHMA, COPD TREATMENT

See **salmeterol p 286**

Seroquel/Seroquel XR

ANTIPSYCHOTIC (Second Generation)

See **quetiapine p 272**

sertraline
 Zoloft
 Tab- Na starch glycolate
 Conc- alcohol 12%

ANTIDEPRESSANT, TREATMENT OF OCD, PANIC DISORDER, PTSD, PMDD or SOCIAL ANXIETY   SSRI
 Drug: Take consistently c̄ or s̄ food (food ↑ abs). Dilute conc in 4 oz water, ginger ale, lemon/lime soda, lemonade or orange juice (not c̄ any other liquids). Drink immediately.
 Diet: Avoid tryptophan suppl- may ↑ drug side effects.[3]
 Avoid SJW, see p 286.
 Caution c̄ grapefruit/related citrus, see p 390.
 Nutr: <u>Anorexia</u>, ↓ wt.
 Oral/GI: <u>Dry mouth</u>, <u>N</u>/V, <u>dyspepsia</u>, <u>diarrhea</u>, constipation.
 Rare- GI bleeding.
 S/Cond: Avoid alcohol. Caution c̄ lactation. 98% serum pro bound.
 Caution c̄ ↓ hepatic func. **Pregnancy:** Category C.
 Other: <u>Insomnia</u>, <u>dizziness</u>, <u>drowsiness</u>, ↑ <u>sweating</u>, <u>tremor</u>, twitching, headache, palpitations, agitation, anxiety, visual disturbances, sexual dysfunction, ↓ thyroid func.[21]
 Rare- SIADH, akathisia, serotonin syndrome, suicidal thinking & behavior.
 Blood/Serum: Slight ↑ chol & TG, ↓ uric acid, ↑ TSH.
 < 1%- ↑ AST, ↑ ALT, ↓ platelets, ↓ Na.

sevelamer HCl
 Renagel
 Tab

sevelamer carbonate
 Renvela
 Tab

PHOSPHATE BINDER (for use in ESRD)
 Drug: Take c̄ each meal. Swallow whole- do not crush, chew or divide. Take 1 hr after or 3 hr before other med.
 Diet: Low P diet.
 Oral/GI: No GI abs. <u>Nausea</u>, <u>dyspepsia</u>, diarrhea, constipation, flatulence.
 S/Cond: Caution c̄ lactation. Caution c̄ dysphagia, severe ↓ GI motility, GI surgery. Not c̄ hypophosphatemia or bowel obstruction.
 Pregnancy: Category C.
 Other: Acidosis- ↓ risk c̄ carbonate form.
 Blood/Serum: ↓ <u>*PHOSPHORUS*</u>, ↑ <u>Ca</u>, ↓ <u>LDL</u>, ↓ <u>CHOL</u>, ↓ <u>PTH</u>.
 Monitor: P, Ca, Cl, bicarb.

sildenafil
  Revatio[a]
  Tab- lactose
  Viagra[b]
  Tab- lactose

PULMONARY ARTERIAL HYPERTENSION TREATMENT[a]
  ERECTILE DYSFUNCTION TREATMENT[b]
  Also used to treat severe Raynaud's syndrome[1]
  Phosphodiesterase type 5 (PDE5) inhibitor
Drug: Take s̄ regard to food, but high fat meal ↓ rate & extent of abs.
Diet: Caution c̄ grapefruit/related citrus, see p 390. Avoid **sildenafil** containing dietary supplements eg **Shangai**/related products.
Oral/GI: <u>Dyspepsia</u>, gastritis, diarrhea.
S/Cond: Limit alcohol. Caution c̄ lactation. 96% serum pro bound. Caution c̄ geriatric, HTN, cardiac disease/MI history, sleep apnea,[21] retinitis pigmentosa, severe ↓ renal func or severe ↓ hepatic func. Not c̄ pulmpnary venoocclusive disease.
Pregnancy: Category B.
Other: <u>Nose bleed</u>, <u>nasal congestion</u>, <u>headache</u>, <u>flushing</u>, <u>insomnia</u>, erythema, dyspnea, rhinitis, sinusitis, ↓ sense of smell, muscle pain, fever, paresthesia, sleep apnea, dizziness, hypotension, visual changes. Rare- HTN, cardiac events, permanent vision loss, hearing loss[1] (usually in one ear).
Urinary: UTI. **Monitor:** Possibly BP, vision, hearing.

sildosin
  Rapaflo Cap- starch

BPH TREATMENT

                            See **Alpha₁ Adrenergic Blockers p 28**

simethicone
  GasAid Maximum Strength
  Softgel- peppermint oil
  Mylanta Gas
  Chew Tab- dextrose
  Softgel- peppermint oil
  Mylicon Drops
  Drops- maltitol, xanthan gum

ANTIFLATULENT
Drug: Take after meals &/or HS. Chew chewable tab well. May mix drops c̄ 1 oz cool water, infant formula or other liquid.
Diet: Proper diet & exercise important.[13] Avoid carbonated beverages & gas-forming foods to prevent flatulence.
Oral/GI: <u>Belching</u>. Not absorbed from GI tract.
Pregnancy: Category C.[2]

Phazyme Chew Tab- aspartame = 0.4 mg phenylalanine/tab, mannitol, maltodextrin, starch, Na 8 mg/tab
SoftgelCap

| **Simponi** | ANTIARTHRITIC, ANKYLOSING SPONDYLITIS TREATMENT |
| | See **golimumab p 158** |

| **simvastatin**
   Zocor | ANTIHYPERLIPIDEMIC | See **HMG-CoA Reductase Inhibitors p 164** |

| **Sinemet/Sinemet-CR** | ANTIPARKINSON | See **levodopa & carbidopa p 193** |

| **Sinequan** previous brand name ANTIDEPRESSANT | See **Tricyclic Antidepressants p 323** |
| **doxepin** | |

| **Singulair** | ASTHMA Prophylaxis & Chronic Treatment See **montelukast p 220** |

sitagliptin
   Januvia
   Tab

ANTIDIABETIC AGENT, DPP-4 (dipeptidyl-peptidase-4) Inhibitor
for adult Type 2 DM. Drug ↑ & prolongs incretin hormone level.
Drug: Take s̄ regard to food.
Diet: Adjunct to diabetic diet & exercise.
S/Cond: Caution c̄ lactation. Caution c̄ moderte to severe ↓ renal func.
Not c̄ Type 1 DM or ketoacidosis.
Does not cause hypoglycemia when used as single agent.
Pregnancy: Category B.
Other: Nasopharyngitis, URTI, headache. Rare- anaphylaxis,
angioedema, rash, urticaria, exfoliative skin, SJS, acute pancreatitis.
Blood/Serum: ↑ *INSULIN RELEASE* after meals, ↓ *GLUCAGON*.
Monitor: Baseline & periodic renal func. Glucose, $HbA1_C$.

| **Skelaxin** | SKELETAL MUSCLE RELAXANT, Sedative | See **metaxalone p 209** |

| **Slow Fe** | HEMATINIC, ANTIANEMIC, Mineral | See **ferrous salts p 140** |

| **Slow-Mag** | MINERAL SUPPLEMENT | See **magnesium p 202** |

sodium bicarbonate
  Sodium Bicarbonate
  ($NaHCO_3$)
  baking soda
  27% Na = 12 mEq Na/g

  90 mg (3.92 mEq)
  Na/325 mg Tab

  Parenteral- multiple conc
  972 mg (42.28 mEq)
  Na/tsp Pwd

ANTACID, ALKALINIZING AGENT   Oral or Parenteral (IV)
  Drug: As antacid- take after meals c̄ 8 oz water.
  Diet: Consider the Na content c̄ ↓ Na diet. Take Fe suppl separately, 1 hr before or 2 hr after drug. Caution c̄ Ca suppl or high milk intake c̄ LT use- may cause milk alkali syndrome.
  Nutr: ↑ thirst, ↑ wt (edema).
  Oral/GI: <u>Belching</u>, gastric distention, cramps, flatulence.
  S/Cond: Caution c̄ severe ↓ renal func, CHF, HTN. Caution c̄ ↓ hepatic func c̄ IV.[26]
  Pregnancy: Category C.[13] Not recommended due to Na content & danger of systemic alkalosis.
  Other: Peripheral edema. Rare- alkalosis, fluid overload.
  Blood/Serum: ↑ Na, ↓ K, ↓ Ca, ↑ *pH* c̄ IV. **Urinary:** ↑ *pH*.
  Monitor: Electrolytes, acid-base balance, serum pH c̄ IV.

sodium polystyrene
 sulfonate
  Kayexalate
  Pwd- 100 mg (4.1 mEq) Na/g

  Sodium Polystyrene
  Sulfonate
  (multiple brands)
  Susp- 1500 mg (65 mEq)
  Na/60 mL,
  0.1- 0.3% alcohol,
  saccharin Na
  Rectal suppository
  sorbitol, alcohol

ANTIHYPERKALEMIA, Cation Exchange Resin   Oral or Rectal
  Drug: Mix pwd c̄ 20-100 mL cool water or syrup. May mix pwd or susp c̄ cool food. DO NOT HEAT, DO NOT INHALE PWD.
  Diet: ↓ K, see p 387. Avoid K suppl. Consider Na content c̄ ↓ Na diet. Take Ca or Mg suppl or antacids separately by several hr. Not c̄ salt sub or sorbitol.
  Nutr: <u>Anorexia</u>. 33% of Na is abs = 33 mg (1.44 mEq) Na/g drug; 500 mg (21.75 mEq) Na/15 g dose.
  Oral/GI: N/V, gastric irritation, <u>CONSTIPATION</u>, fecal impaction, especially in pediatric or geriatric, diarrhea, bezoars, GI ulceration/necrosis.
  S/Cond: Caution c̄ lactation. Caution c̄ CHF, HTN, significant edema. Not c̄ obstructive bowel disease, severe constipation or hypokalemia.
  Pregnancy: Category C.
  Other: Edema, Na retention, hypokalemia, hypocalcemia, confusion, weakness, irritability, arrhythmia.
  Blood/Serum: ↓ <u>POTASSIUM</u>, ↓ <u>Mg</u>, ↓ <u>Ca</u>, ↑ Na.
  Monitor: Electrolytes, Mg, Ca.

solifenacin **Vesicare**	ANTIMUSCARINIC	See **Bladder Control Agents p 61**
Solodyn	ANTIBIOTIC, **minocycline**	See **Tetracyclines p 310**
Solu-Cortef	CORTICOSTEROID, **hydrocortisone**	See **corticosteroids p 94**
Solu-Medrol	CORTICOSTEROID, **methylprednisolone**	See **corticosteroids p 94**

Sorafenib
  Nexavar
  Tab

ANTINEOPLASTIC, Multikinase Inhibitor (Renal cell/Hepatocellular cancer)
> **Drug:** Take twice a day 1 hr before or 2 hr after food.
> **Diet:** Avoid SJW, see p 286.
> **Nutr:** <u>Anorexia</u>, WEIGHT <u>LOSS</u>.
> **Oral/GI:** N/V, <u>abdominal</u> <u>pain</u>, constipation, <u>DIARRHEA</u>.
> Rare- GI perforation.
> **S/Cond:** Not $\bar{c}$ lactation. Caution $\bar{c}$ ↓ hepatic func.
> Not $\bar{c}$ cardiac ischemia/infarction.
> **Pregnancy:** Category D.
> **Other:** <u>RASH</u>, HAND-FOOT <u>SYNDROME</u>, HAIR <u>LOSS</u>, <u>dry</u> <u>skin</u>, <u>itching</u>, <u>HTN</u>,
> <u>fatigue</u>, <u>hemorrhage</u>, <u>neuropathy</u>, <u>asthenia</u>, joint/musle pain,
> hepatic dysfunction, headache, dyspnea, hoarseness, depression,
> cardiac ischmia/infarction, erectile dysfunction.
> **Blood/Serum:** <u>HYPOPHOSPHATEMIA</u>, (↓ <u>P</u>), ↓ <u>alb</u>, ↑ <u>lipase</u>, ↑ <u>amylase</u>,
> ↑ <u>PT/INR</u>, ↓ <u>WBC</u>, ↓ <u>platelets</u>.
> **Monitor:** BP. PT/INR $\bar{c}$ concomitant use of **warfarin**.

sorbitol

LAXATIVE, Hyperosmotic
> **Drug:** Take HS.
> **Diet:** High fiber $\bar{c}$ 1500-2000 mL fluid/day to prevent constipation.
> Low CHO or diabetic food/candy may contain sorbitol or
> maltitol & ↑ drug GI effects.
> **Oral/GI:** <u>SWEET</u> <u>TASTE</u>, <u>bloating</u>, <u>cramps</u>, <u>flatulence</u>, diarrhea.
> **Pregnancy:** Consult physician.

sotalol
  Betapace
  Tab- lactose, starch
  Betapace AF
  Tab- lactose, starch

ANTIARRHYTHMIC, Non-selective Beta-Blocker
Drug: Food ↓ abs 20%. Take consistently c̄ or s̄ food.
Diet: Avoid natural licorice, see p 374. Take separately from Al or Ca, Mg antacids or Ca^9b or Mg suppl by at least 2 hr.
Nutr: Wt changes.
Oral/GI: N/V, dyspepsia, abdominal pain, diarrhea, flatulence.
S/Cond: Avoid alcohol. Not c̄ lactation. Caution c̄ diabetes- may mask symptoms of & prolong hypoglycemia. May reduce insulin release in response to hyperglycemia. Not c̄ hypokalemia or hypomagnesemia. Caution c̄ ↓ renal func or CHF. Extreme caution c̄ dialysis.[58]
Not c̄ severe ↓ renal func, ↑ QT interval or asthma/bronchospasm.
Pregnancy: Category B.
Other: ↓ BP c̄ possible hypotension, DIZZINESS, FATIGUE, weakness, headache, dyspnea, edema, rash, bradycardia, syncope, palpitations, proarrhythmia, ↑ QT interval, depression, peripheral vascular insufficiency, visual changes, paresthesia, bleeding.
Blood/Serum: Rare- ↑ AST, ↑ ALT, dyscrasias.
Monitor: BP. Heartrate. Baseline & periodic CBC, hepatic & renal func.

Spectracef

ANTIBIOTIC, Cephalosporin, 3rd generation   See **cefditoren p 77**

Spiriva Handihaler

BRONCHODILATOR   See **tiotropium p 315**

spironolactone
Aldactone
Tab- cornstarch

ANTIHYPERTENSIVE, DIURETIC, PRIMARY HYPERALDOSTERONISM TREATMENT
To treat Hypokalemia, Cirrhosis c̄ Ascites, PCOS, PMS, Hirsutism
Nephrotic Syndrome, K-Sparing Adjunct CHF Treatment
Drug: Take c̄ meals or milk to ↓ GI irritation & ↑ abs.
Diet: Avoid excessive K intake, K suppl, salt subs.
↓ Na, ↓ cal may be recommended. Discontinue Na restriction if
hyponatremia occurs. Avoid natural licorice, see p 374.

Aldactazide
Tab- cornstarch
also contains
hydrochlorothiazide,
see **p 166_**

Nutr: Anorexia, ↓ wt, ↑ thirst, dehydration.
Oral/GI: Dry mouth, <u>N/V</u>, gastritis, rare gastric bleeding, <u>cramps</u>, <u>diarrhea</u>.
S/Cond: Caution c̄ alcohol. Not c̄ lactation.
Caution c̄ mild to moderate ↓ renal func. Not c̄ severe ↓ renal func.[58]
98% serum pro bound. Not c̄ hypokalemia.
Pregnancy: Category C.
Other: ↓ *BP* c̄ possible hypotension, <u>HYPERKALEMIA</u>, <u>ARRHYTHMIA</u>,
headache, dizziness, ataxia, drowsiness, confusion.
Gynecomastia, endocrine effects, hyponatremia c̄ LT high dose.
Blood/Serum: ↑ <u>POTASSIUM</u>, ↓ Na, ↓ Cl, ↑ BUN, ↑ crea, ↑ Mg, ↑ <u>LDL</u>, ↓ <u>HDL</u>.[20]
Urinary: ↑ *Na*, ↑ Cl, ↑ *WATER*, ↓ K, ↑ Ca.
Monitor: BP, electrolytes, renal func. Possibly lipids.

Sporanox/Sporanox IV	ANTIFUNGAL, ANTICANDIDIASIS	See **itraconazole p 182**
Sprintec	ORAL CONTRACEPTIVE	See **Oral Contraceptives p 237**
St. John's wort	HERBAL PRODUCT	See **St. John's wort p 286**
Stalevo Tab- cornstarch, sucrose, mannitol	ANTIPARKINSON Combination drug	See **levodopa & carbidopa p 193** See **entacapone p 124**
Starlix	ORAL HYPOGLYCEMIC for TYPE 2 diabetes	See **nateglinide p 225**
statin	ANTIHYPERLIPIDEMIC	See **HMG-CoA Reductase Inhibitors p 164**

S

stavudine (d4T)
Zerit
Cap- lactose,
 Na starch glycolate
Pwd for Soln- sucrose
 (reconsituted by pharmacist)
Zerit XR (SR)
Cap- lactose

ANTIRETROVIRAL (HIV/AIDS), NRTI
Drug: Take s̄ regard to meals. **Nutr:** Anorexia, ↓ wt.
Oral/GI: Stomatitis, <u>N/V</u>, abdominal pain, <u>diarrhea</u>.
S/Cond: Limit alcohol. Not c̄ lactation.
Caution c̄ geriatric or ↓ renal func. **Pregnancy:** Category C.
Other: Peripheral <u>neuropathy</u>, <u>chills/fever</u>, headache, weakness,
muscle pain, dementia, insomnia, rash, bone marrow suppression,
pancreatitis (can be fatal), lipodystrophy, lactic acidosis.
Rare- hepatomegaly c̄ steatosis (can be fatal).
Highest incidence of lipodystrophy, hyperlipidemia &
lactic acidosis of all NRTI.[5]
Blood/Serum: ↑ <u>AST</u>, ↑ <u>ALT</u>, ↑ alk phos, ↑ bil, ↑ GGT, ↑ <u>amylase</u>,
↑ lipase, anemia, ↓ platelets, ↓ <u>neutrophils</u>, ↑ <u>chol</u>, ↑ <u>TG</u>.
Monitor: Hepatic func, amylase, lipase, lipid panel.

Stelara

PLAQUE PSORIASIS, Interleukin 12 & 23 Antagonist   Parenteral (SC)
See **ustekinumab p 327**

Strattera

ANTI-ADHD   See **atomoxetine p 46**

sucralfate (Al complex)
Carafate
Tab- starch
Susp- sorbitol,
 simethicone

ANTIULCER, Gastric Mucosa Protectant
Drug: Take c̄ water on empty stomach 1 hr before meals & HS.
May suspend tab in flavored syrup or other liquid.
Diet: Bland diet may be recommended.
Take Ca or Mg suppl or antacids separately by ≥ 30 minutes.
Oral/GI: ↓ <u>PEPSIN ACTIVITY</u> by 32%, constipation, cramps.
S/Cond: Avoid or limit alcohol. Caution c̄ lactation.
Caution c̄ ↓ renal func- high Al content.
Caution c̄ dysphagia, delayed gastric emptying or TF- possible bezoar
formation due to protein-binding properties of drug.[13] **Pregnancy:** Category B.
Monitor: Possibly renal func, especially in geriatric.

Sudafed

DECONGESTANT   See **pseudoephedrine p 269**

Sudafed PE
  phenylephrine   DECONGESTANT   See listing for **pseudoephedrine p 269**

Sular
  nisoldipine   ANTIHYPERTENSIVE, Ca Channel Blocker
  Tab (SR)- lactose   **Drug:** Do not take c̄ high fat meal- affects drug kinetics.
                                     Take on empty stomach 1 hr before or 2 hr after meal.
                                                    See listing for **nifedipine p 229**

sulfamethoxazole
  c̄ trimethoprim   ANTIBIOTIC, Sulfonamide   See **trimethoprim**
  Bactrim/Bactrim DS   **c̄ sulfasmethoxazole p 324**

sulfonylureas   ORAL HYPOGLYCEMIC, Sulfonylurea- 2nd generation
  Drug: Take **Glucotrol** 30 minutes before first meal of the day.[10] Food delays abs, but does not ↓ total abs.
  Take **glimepiride**, **glyburide** or **Glucotrol XL** c̄ first meal of the day.
  Swallow **Glucotrol XL** whole- do not chew, cut or crush.
  Diet: Adjunct to prescribed diabetic diet & exercise.
  Caution c̄ high dose (> 3 g) nicotinic acid- ↑ glucose.[6, 47]
  Nutr: ↑ or ↓ appetite, ↑ wt. **Oral/GI:** Dyspepsia, nausea, diarrhea, constipation.
  S/Cond: Avoid alcohol. Not c̄ lactation. 95-99% serum pro bound.
  Hypoalbuminemia (< 3 g/dL) may ↑ drug effects. Caution c̄ ↓ hepatic func or ↓ renal func.
  Caution c̄ geriatric or malnourished patient- ↑ risk of hypoglycemia.
  Caution c̄ G6PD def- ↑ risk of hemolytic anemia.
  Pregnancy: Category C, except **Glynase** & **Micronase**- Category B.
  Other: HYPOGLYCEMIA. Dizziness, headache, drowsiness, blurred vision, skin reactions.
  Rare- SIADH c̄ **glipizide**.
  Blood/Serum: ↓ _GLUCOSE_, ↓ _Hb A1_$_C$. Rare- ↑ AST, ↑ ALT, ↑ LDH, ↑ alk phos, ↑ BUN, ↑ crea, ↓ Na,
  dyscrasias.
  Urinary: ↓ _GLUCOSE_. ↑ volume c̄ **glipizide** or **glyburide**. **Monitor:** Glucose, Hb A1$_C$.

glimepiride	**Amaryl**	Tab- lactose, Na starch glycolate (May be used c̄ **insulin** or **metformin**)
glipizide	**Glucotrol** Tab- lactose, starch	**Glucotrol XL** Tab
glyburide	**DiaBeta** Tab	**Glynase PresTab**- lactose, cornstarch

S

sumatriptan
  Imitrex
  Sumavel DosePro

ANTIMIGRAINE, Serotonin 5-HT$_1$ Receptor Agonist
or CLUSTER HEADACHE TREATMENT

See **Antimigraine p 39**

sunitinib
  Sutent
  Cap- mannitol

ANTINEOPLASTIC, Tyrosine Kinase Inhibitor (Gastrointestinal Stromal Tumor or Advanced Renal Cancer)
  Drug: Take s̄ regard to food.
  Diet: Avoid SJW, see p 286. Avoid grapefruit/related citrus, see p 390.
  Nutr: Dehydration, anorexia, ↓ wt.
  Oral/GI: <u>Dry mouth</u>, <u>oral pain</u>, <u>TASTE CHANGES</u>, <u>STOMATITIS/MUCOSITIS</u>, GERD, <u>N/V</u>, dyspepsia, <u>abdominal pain</u>, <u>constipation</u>, <u>flatulence</u>, <u>DIARRHEA</u>.
  S/Cond: Not c̄ lactation. Not c̄ CHF. 95% serum pro bound. Caution c̄ hypothyroidism, heart disease or hx of ↑ QT interval.
  Pregnancy: Category D.
  Other: <u>SKIN DISCOLORATION (YELLOW)</u>, <u>HYPERTENSION</u>, <u>HAND-FOOT SYNDROME</u>, <u>graying of hair</u>, rash, <u>dry skin</u>, edema, asthenia, <u>back pain</u>, <u>muscle/limb/joint pain</u>, <u>cough</u>, hair loss, fatigue, insomnia, headache, hypothyroidism, pancreatitis, embolism, bleeding, ↑ QT interval.
  Blood/Serum: ↑ <u>CREATININE PHOSPHOKINASE</u>, ↑ <u>ALT</u>, ↑ <u>AST</u>, ↑ <u>alk phos</u>, ↑ <u>bil</u>, ↑ <u>amylase</u>, ↑ <u>lipase</u>, ↓ <u>LVEF</u>, ↑ <u>crea</u>, ↑ <u>uric acid</u>, ↓ <u>K</u>, ↑ <u>Na</u>, ↓ Na, ↓ P, ↑ or ↓ glucose. ↓ <u>PLATELETS</u>, ↓ <u>WHITE BLOOD CELLS</u>, ↓ <u>Hb/anemia</u>, ↓ <u>TSH</u>.
  Monitor: Baseline & periodic BP, ECG, CBC c̄ diff, platelets, P, blood chem, thyroid func.

Sustiva

ANTIRETROVIRAL (HIV/AIDS), NNRTI   See **efavirenz p 121**

Sutent

ANTINEOPLASTIC, Tyrosine Kinase Inhibitor   See **sunitinib above**

Symbicort
  budesonide & **formoterol**

ANTIASTHMA
  Combination drug

See **budesonide p 64**
See listing for **salmeterol p 286**

Symbyax
  Cap- starch

ANTIDEPRESSANT for Depression of Bipolar Disorder
  Combination drug

See **olanzapine p 233**
See **fluoxetine p 148**

Symlin	ANTIHYPERGLYCEMIC, Type 1 or 2 Diabetes	
		See **pramlintide p 262**
Symmetrel	ANTIPARKINSON, ANTIVIRAL	See **amantadine p 30**
Synthroid levothyroxine	THYROID HORMONE (T_4)	See **thyroid p 313**

tacrolimus
  Prograf
  Cap- lactose
  IV- 80% dehydrated
    alcohol, castor oil

IMMUNOSUPPRESSANT (To prevent organ transplant rejection)
  Adjunct to **corticosteroids**, some effects may be due to steroids, see p 94.
  Drug: Take consistently c̄ or s̄ food. High fat or high CHO meals ↓ abs of drug.
  Diet: Avoid K suppl or salt subs.
  Avoid grapefruit/related citrus,[123] see p 390. Avoid SJW, see p 286.
  Nutr: ANOREXIA. ↑ appetite. ↓ Fe.
  Oral/GI: Oral candidiasis, stomatitis, dysphagia, DYSPEPSIA,
  NAUSEA/VOMITING, gastritis, hemorrhage, GI perforation, ABDOMINAL PAIN,
  DIARRHEA, CONSTIPATION, flatulence.
  S/Cond: Avoid alcohol- to prevent flushing. Not c̄ lactation.
  Caution c̄ ↓ renal func or ↓ hepatic func. 99% serum pro bound.
  IV- not c̄ castor oil allergy. Limit sun exposure.
  Pregnancy: Category C.
  Other: DIABETES, NEUROTOXICITY, NEPHROTOXICITY, HEADACHE, TREMOR,
  PARESTHESIA, INSOMNIA, PLEURAL EFFUSION, DYSPNEA, EDEMA, ASCITES,
  HYPERTENSION, BACK OR MUSCLE PAIN, rash, dizziness, confusion, weakness,
  photosensitivity. Rare- myocardial hypertrophy. Anaphylaxis c̄ IV.
  Blood/Serum: ↑ or ↓ POTASSIUM, ↓ MAGNESIUM, ↓ PHOSPHORUS, ↑ GLUCOSE,
  ANEMIA, ↑ or ↓ WBC, ↓ platelets, ↑ BUN, ↑ CREA, ↑ AST, ↑ ALT,
  ↑ alk phos, ↑ LDH, ↑ bil, ↑ chol, ↓ glucose, ↓ Na, ↑ or ↓ Ca, ↑ P, ↓ CO_2,
  ↑ uric acid, ↓ alb.
  Urinary: ↑ frequency, incontinence, pro, hematuria, UTI, retention, alb.
  Monitor: Baseline & periodic- BP, electrolytes, Mg, P,
  renal func, hepatic func, CBC c̄ diff, platelets, drug level.

tadalafil
  Adcirca PULMONARY ARTERIAL HYPERTENSION TREATMENT
    Tab- lactose

  Cialis ERECTILE DYSFUNCTION TREATMENT, BPH TREATMENT
    Tab- lactose See listing for **sildenafil p 292**

Tagamet ANTIULCER, ANTIGERD, ANTISECRETORY
  cimetidine See **Histamine H$_2$ Receptor Antagonists p 162**

Tamiflu INFLUENZA TREATMENT OR PROPHYLAXIS See **oseltamivir p 239**

tamoxifen ANTINEOPLASTIC (Breast Cancer), BREAST CANCER PREVENTION
  generic Tab- lactose,   Estrogen Antagonist
    cornstarch **Drug:** Swallow EC tab whole. Take s̄ regard to food.
  Nolvadex-D (EC) **Diet:** Take Ca or Mg suppl separately from EC tab by 2 hr.
  (Canada only) Caution c̄ grapefruit/related citrus, see p 390.
  Tab- cornstarch, Avoid soy & other suppl with estrogenic effect.[93]
    gelatin, lactose **Nutr:** Anorexia, ↓ wt.
    Oral/GI: N/V.
    S/Cond: Not c̄ lactation. Not c̄ DVT or pulmonary embolus.
    Pregnancy: Category D.
    Other: HOT FLASHES, menstrual changes, peripheral edema, cough,
    headache, fatigue, rash, muscle/bone pain.
    Rare- ocular toxicity/cataracts, retinopathy, SJS, pancreatitis,
    endometrial changes, uterine sarcoma, hepatotoxicity,
    thrombotic event (can be fatal).
    Blood/Serum: ↑ Ca, ↑ AST, ↑ ALT, ↑ bil, ↑ alk phos, ↓ chol,[6] ↓ LDL,[6]
    ↑ BUN, ↑ crea, ↓ WBC, ↓ platelets. Rare- ↑ chol, ↑ TG, ↑ T$_4$.
    Monitor: CBC c̄ diff, platelets, hepatic func, lipid panel.
    Gyn exam, possibly ophthalmic exams.

tamsulosin BPH TREATMENT See **Alpha$_1$ Adrenergic Blockers p 28**
  Flomax

Tapazole
  methimazole
  Tab- lactose, cornstarch,
  starch
	ANTIHYPERTHYROID
	  Drug: Food may affect bioavailablity, take
	  consistently c̄ or s̄ food each day.[13]
		See listing for **propylthiouricil p 267**

tapentadol
  Nucynta
  Tab- lactose
  Nucynta ER
  Tab- polyethylene
  glycol, alpha tocopheral
  (Vit E)
	ANALGESIC, Opiod & Norepinephrine Reuptake Inhibitor
	  Drug: Take s̄ regard to food. Swallow ER tab whole.
	  Do not crush, split, divide, chew or dissolve.
	  Nutr: ↓ appetite.
	  Oral/GI: Dry mouth, dyspepsia, <u>nausea/vomiting</u>.
	  S/Cond: Avoid alcohol. Not c̄ lactation. Caution c̄ ↓ renal func, seizures,
	  geriatric, moderate ↓ hepatic func. Not c̄ severe ↓ hepatic func
	  or severe ↓ renal func. Not c̄ paralytic ileus. Not c̄ respiratory depression.
	  Not for patient < 18 yrs. May be habit forming c̄ LT use.
	  Pregnancy: Category C.
	  Other: <u>DIZZINESS</u>, headache,[9a] sweating, itching, rash,confusion, ataxia,
	  insomnia. Rare- seizures.	

Tarceva	ANTINEOPLASTIC	See **erlotinib p 127**

Tarka
  Tab- cornstarch, lactose, ethanol   Combination drug
    trandolapril (IR) **& verapamil** (SR)
	ANTIHYPERTENSIVE	See **Angiotensin Converting
		    Enzyme Inhibitors p 36**
		  See **verapamil p 332**

Taxol	ANTINEOPLASTIC, Antimitotic Agent	See **paclitaxel p 242**
Taxotere **docetaxel**	ANTINEOPLASTIC, Antimitotic Agent	See listing for **paclitaxel p 242**
Tazicef	ANTIBIOTIC, **ceftazidime**	See **cephalosporins p 80**
Taztia XT	ANTIANGINA, ANTIHYPERTENSIVE, Ca Channel Blocker See **diltiazem p 111**	
Teflero **ceftaroline**	ANTIBIOTIC	See **cephalosporins** (parenteral) **p 80**

| **Tegretol/Tegretol XR** | ANTIEPILEPTIC | See **carbamazepine p 72** |

| **Tekturna** | ANTIHYPERTENSIVE, Direct Renin Inhibitor | See **aliskiren p 26** |

telaprevir
Incivek
Tab- propylene glycol

TREATMENT FOR CHRONIC HEPATITIS C, Protease inhibitor
Drug: Take witin 30 min of a high fat ($\geq$ 20g fat) meal or snack.
Diet: Not c̄ low fat meal or snack.
Caution c̄ grapefruit/related citrus, see p 390. Not c̄ SJW, see p 286.
Oral/GI: <u>Dysgeusia</u>, <u>N/V</u>, <u>diarrhea</u>, <u>anal pruritis</u>, <u>anorectal discomfort</u>, <u>hemorrhoids</u>.
S/Cond: Not as monotherapy. Not c̄ lactation. Not c̄ moderate to severe ↓ hepatic func. Not in solid organ transplant recipients
Not c̄ concurrent HIV or HBV infection.
Pregnancy: Category X (when combined c̄ peginterferon alfa and ribavirin).
Contraindicated in men whose female partners are pregnant.
Negative pregnancy test required before starting treatment
Other: <u>RASH</u>, <u>PRURITIS</u>, <u>fatigue</u>. Rare- drug rash c̄ eosinophilia
and systemic symptoms (DRESS), SJS.
Blood/Serum: ↓ <u>HCT</u>, ↑ <u>Hgb</u>, ↓ WBC, ↓ <u>platelets</u>, ↑ <u>bil</u>, ↑ <u>URIC ACID</u>.
Monitor: HCV-RNA levels at weeks 4 & 12 & as clinically indicated.
CBC c̄ diff at weeks 2, 4, 8, 12 & as clinically indicated. Hgb prior to &
at least q 4 wks during therapy. Electrolytes, crea, uric acid, AST, ALT, bil,
TSH at wks 2, 4, 8, 12 & as clinically indicated.
Females- routine monthly pregnancy test during treatment & for 6 mos
after DC of treatment.

telbivudine
Tyzeka
Tab- Na starch glycolate
Soln- saccharin Na,
47 mg Na/30 mL

HEPATITIS B TREATMENT, Thymidine Nucleoside Analog
Drug: Take s̄ regard to food.
Oral/GI: <u>N/V</u>, dyspepsia, <u>abdominal pain</u>, diarrhea.
S/Cond: Not c̄ lactation. Caution c̄ ↓ renal func or geriatric.
Pregnancy: Category B.
Other: <u>URTI</u>, <u>fatigue</u>, <u>nasopharyngitis</u>, <u>pharyngolaryngeal pain</u>, <u>flu-like symptoms</u>, <u>dizziness</u>, <u>cough</u>, <u>headache</u>, rash, fever,

muscle/joint/back pain, rhinorrhea, insomnia, peripheral neuropathy.
Rare- lactic acidosis & hepatomegaly c̄ steatosis (can be fatal) reported c̄
other nucleoside analogs. Exacerbation of hepatitis B upon DC of drug.
Blood/Serum: ↑ CPK, ↑ ALT, ↑ AST, ↑ lipase, ↓ neutrophils.
Monitor: Baseline renal & hepatic func, then hepatic func periodically.

---

telmisartan
Micardis/Micardis HCT

ANTIHYPERTENSIVE   See **Angiotensin II Receptor Antagonists p 38**
Micardis HCT also contains **hydrochlorothiazide**, see **p 166**

---

temazepam
Restoril

SLEEP AID   See **Benzodiazepines p 54**

---

temozolomide
Temodar
Cap- lactose,
Na starch gycolate
IV Vial- mannitol 600 mg

ANTINEOPLASTIC, (Brain/Spinal Cord Cancer)   Oral or Parenteral (IV)
Imidazotetrazine Derivative
Drug: Oral- Swallow cap whole c̄ full glass of water- do not open or chew.
Dose based on body surface area, neutrophil & platelet counts.
Food ↓ rate & extent of abs of oral form slightly.
Nutr: Anorexia. ↑ wt (edema).
Oral/GI: Taste changes, stomatitis, dysphagia, NAUSEA/VOMITING,
abdominal pain, CONSTIPATION, diarrhea.
S/Cond: Not c̄ lactation.
Caution c̄ severe ↓ hepatic func or severe ↓ renal func.
Geriatrics & women have ↑ risk of bone marrow suppression.
Pregnancy: Category D.
Other: BONE MARROW SUPPRESSION, HAIR LOSS, FATIGUE, HEADACHE, rash,
convulsions, blurred vision, memory loss, weakness, confusion,
coughing, dyspnea, muscle pain, edema, paresthesia, ataxia, insomnia,
allergic reaction, visual changes.
IV- Infusion site reactions, hematoma, petechiae.
Rare- SJS/TEN, aplastic anemia (may be fatal).
Blood/Serum: ↓ WBC, ↓ platelets, ↓ neutrophils, ↓ LYMPHOCYTES, ↓ Hb.
Urinary: Incontinence, UTI, ↑ frequency.
Monitor: Weekly CBC, platelets.

temsirolimus **Torisel** Vial- 32.5% alcohol, 50.3% propylene glycol	ANTINEOPLASTIC (Renal Cell Carcinoma), mTOR Kinase Inhibitor Pretreatment antihistamine/diphenhydramine usual Parenteral only (IV) **Diet:** Avoid SJW, see p 286. Avoid grapefruit/related citrus, see p 390. **Nutr:** ANOREXIA, ↓ wt. **Oral/GI:** DYSGEUSIA, MUCOSITIS, NAUSEA/vomiting, ABDOMINAL PAIN, CONSTIPATION, DIARRHEA, fatal bowel perforation. **S/Cond:** Not c̄ lacataion. Not c̄ ANC < 1,000/mm³ or platelet count < 75,000/mm³. **Pregnancy:** Category D. **Other:** ASTHENIA, EDEMA, FEVER, INFECTIONS, BACK PAIN, DYSPNEA, COUGH, headache, chest pain, chills, pharyngitis, rhinitis, joint/muscle pain, nose bleed, nail disorder, dry skin, itching, acne, insomnia, conjunctivitis, allergic reaction, pneumonia, URTI, HTN, depression, ↓ wound healing, interstitial lung disease, thromboembolism. **Blood/Serum:** ANEMIA, ↓ PLATELETS, ↑ GLUCOSE, ↑ CHOL, ↑ LDL, ↑ TRIGLYCERIDES, ↑ ALK PHOS, ↑ CREA, ↓ P, ↑ AST, ↓ WHITE BLOOD CELLS, ↓ LYMPHOCYTES, ↓ POTASSIUM, ↓ neutrophils, ↑ bil. **Urinary:** UTI. **Monitor:** Baseline & periodic glucose, lipids, renal func, CBC c̄ diff, blood chem.
Tenex	ANTIHYPERTENSIVE See **guanfacine p 159**
tenofovir (TDF) **Viread** Tab- lactose, starch	ANTIRETROVIRAL (HIV/AIDS), CHRONIC HEPATITIS B TREATMENT, NRTI **Drug:** Take s̄ regard to food, but high fat meal ↑ AUC & bioavailability. **Diet:** Ca & Vit D suppl may help ↓ bone loss. **Nutr:** Anorexia, ↓ wt. **Oral/GI:** N/V, dyspepsia, abdominal pain, diarrhea, flatulence. **S/Cond:** Not c̄ lactation. Caution c̄ ↓ renal func or ↓ hepatic func or geriatric. Caution in pt c̄ both hepatitis B & HIV infection. **Pregnancy:** Category B. **Other:** Headache, weakness, dizziness, rash, muscle pain, sweating, peripheral neuropathy, depression, insomnia, pneumonia, ↓ bone mineral density. Rare- lactic acidosis, hepatomegaly c̄ steatosis,

pancreatitis, lipodystrophy, Fanconi syndrome, renal toxicity.
Blood/Serum: ↑ <u>ALT</u>, ↑ <u>AST</u>, ↑ amylase, ↓ neutrophils, ↓ P.
Monitor: Hepatic func, body wt, temp, serum P, urinalysis, renal func/CrCl, possibly bone density c̄ LT use.[5]

Tenoretic Tab- Na starch glycolate	ANTIHYPERTENSIVE, DIURETIC Combination drug	See **atenolol p 45** See **chlorthalidone p 82**
Tenormin	ANTIHYPERTENSIVE	See **atenolol p 45**
terazosin Hytrin Terazosin	ANTIHYPERTENSIVE, BPH TREATMENT	See **Alpha₁ Adrenergic Blockers p 28**

terbinafine
  Lamisil
  Tab[a]- Na starch glycolate
  Oral granules[b]-
   Na starch glycolate

ANTIFUNGAL[a], toenail or fingernail onychomycosis treatment,
  SCALP RINGWORM TREATMENT (Tinea capitis)[b]
Diet: Sprinkle granules on a spoonful of non-acidic food (eg pudding), swallow immediately, do not chew. Not c̄ applesauce or fruit based food. Limit caffeine- drug ↓ caffeine clearance 20%.
Nutr: ↓ wt due to taste changes.
Oral/GI: Taste changes/loss, dyspepsia, abdominal pain, diarrhea.
S/Cond: Limit alcohol- ↑ risk of hepatotoxicity.[13] Not c̄ lactation. Not c̄ hepatic disease or ↓ renal func. Not c̄ lupus erythematosus. > 99% serum pro bound. Not c̄ ANC ≤ 1000 cells/mm³.
Pregnancy: Category B.
Other: Headache, rash, itching, URTI, cough, nasopharyngitis, visual changes, fever.
Rare- anaphylaxis, SJS, TEN, hepatotoxicity (can be fatal).
Rare- induction or exacerbation of lupus erythematosus.
Blood/Serum: ↑ AST, ↑ ALT. Rare- ↓ WBC, ↓ neutrophils, ↓ platelets.
Monitor: Baseline hepatic func & for S/S of hepatotoxicity. CBC c̄ diff, platelets c̄ use > 6 wk.

teriparatide
Forteo
Prefilled 3 mL syringe-
45.4 mg mannitol
once daily

OSTEOPOROSIS TREATMENT for postmenopausal woman or man at high
   risk for fracture including Glucocorticoid-Induced Osteoporosis
   Recombinant Human Parathyroid Hormone   Parenteral only (SC)
Diet: Adequate (not excessive) Ca & Vit D intake essential.
Oral/GI: Nausea.
S/Cond: Indicated for men & postmenopausal women only (ie: not c̄
lactation or for children). Caution c̄ severe ↓ renal func- drug level ↑ 73%.
Not c̄ hypercalcemia, Paget's or ↑ alk phos.
Pregnancy: Category C.
Other: ↑ _BONE_ _FORMATION/DENSITY_. ↓ _BACK_ _PAIN_. Hypotension c̄ first doses,
dizziness, syncope, joint pain, leg cramps, depression, dyspnea.
Blood/Serum: ↑ Vit D, ↑ uric acid. Transient ↑ Ca, ↑ P.
Urinary: Transient ↑ Ca, ↑ P.
Monitor: Baseline & periodic Ca, P, bone density.

testosterone
(transdermal)
Androderm
Patch- alcohol
Axiron
Sol- ethanol,
 isopropol alcohol
AndroGel
Gel- ethanol
Fortesta
Gel- ethanol

MALE HORMONE REPLACEMENT, PRIMARY HYPOGONADISM,
HYPOGONADOTROPIC HYPOGONADISM, Androgen
Drug: Apply patch to a dry, clean hairless area of back, abdomen,
upper arm or thigh. Apply sol to axilla. Apply gel to upper arm and
shoulder.Cover application area c̄ shirt or t-shirt to avoid secondary
exposure of testosterone to women or children. Apply **Fortesta** gel to thigh.
Cover c̄ clothing to avoid secondary exposure. Do not apply to genital area.
Wash hands after application.
Nutr: ↑ appetite.
Oral/GI: N/V, diarrhea, GI bleeding.
S/Cond: Not c̄ lacatation (not indicated for women). Avoid if suspected
or confirmed breast cancer or prostate cancer. Caution c̄ BPH.
Caution c̄ diabetes- may ↓ insulin requirements.
Caution c̄ cancer patients at risk for hypercalcemia.
Pregnancy: Category X (not indicated for women)
Other: APPLICATION SITE- PRURITIS, irritation, erythema. Headache, back pain,
depression, hypertension, anxiety, confusion, acne, prostate carcinoma,
edema, gynecomastia, azoospermia.

Blood/Serum: ↑ Hb, ↑ HCT, ↑ <u>PSA</u>, hyperlipidemia, ↑ Ca. ↓ glucose.
Urinary: Nocturia, frequency, urgency, infection.
Monitor: Testosterone level 2 wk after initial dose or change in dose.
Baseline HCT & Hb. 3-6 mo after initial dose, then yearly. PSA, LFTs,
lipids periodically. Serum Ca in cancer pts.

tetrabenazine (TBZ)
  Xenazine
  Tab- lactose,
   maize starch
  Nitoman (Canada)

HUNTINGTON'S DISEASE CHOREA TREATMENT
    Also to treat Tourette Syndrome or Tardive Dyskinesia
    monamine-depleting agent for involuntary movements
    Drug: Take s̄ regard to food.
    Nutr: ↓ appetite.
    Oral/GI: <u>Nausea</u>, vomiting, dysphagia.
    S/Cond: Avoid alcohol. Not c̄ ↓ hepatic func. Not c̄ lactation.
    Caution c̄ CYP2D6 poor metabolizer;
    CYP2D6 genetic testing if dose ≥ 50 mg.
    Not c̄ suicidal state or active depression; caution c̄ a history of such.
    Pregnancy: Category C.
    Other: <u>INSOMNIA</u>, <u>SEDATION</u>, <u>akathisia</u>, <u>depression</u>, <u>anxiety</u>, <u>Parkinsonism</u>,
    <u>EPS</u>, <u>irritability</u>, <u>fatigue</u>, <u>instability</u>, unsteady gait, dizziness, headache,
    obsessiveness, bronchitis, SOB, URTI, ecchymosis, falls, ↑ QT interval.
    Rare- NMS, induction or worsening of tardive dyskinesia,
    suicidal thinking & behavior.
    Blood/Serum: Slightly ↑ AST, ↑ ALT.
    Urinary: Dysuria.
    Monitor: For akathisia, restlessness, agitation, depression.

Tetracyclines　　　　　　ANTIBIOTIC, Adjunct to periodontitis treatment (**Periostat**)
　　　　　　　　　　　　　　Also used as ANTIARTHRITIC (Rheumatoid) (**minocycline**), ANTI-ACNE (**minocycline**)

Drug: Take **Tetracycline** c̄ 8 oz water 1 hr before or 2 hr after food/milk, divalent/trivalent minerals/mineral fortified foods. (Food ↓ blood levels 50-80%).[7]
minocycline or **doxycycline** may be taken c̄ food or milk, but not minerals/mineral fortified foods.
Diet: Take Ca, Fe, Mg, Zn or MVI c̄ minerals, antacids or fortified foods (eg OJ c̄ Ca or breakfast cereals) separately by 3 hr before or 1 hr after drug. Avoid SJW- ↑ photosensitivity.
Nutr: Anorexia. Chelate formation c̄ Ca, Fe, Mg or Zn- ↓ both drug & mineral abs. In theory, may also chelate c̄ Mn.[93] Possible ↓ Vit K due to ↓ bacterial synthesis in intestine. Possible B Vit def c̄ LT use.[6] Caution c̄ Vit A suppl- ↑ risk of benign intracranial HTN.[13] ↓ skeletal growth in children ≤ 8.
Oral/GI: Stomatitis, black & hairy tongue, oral candidiasis, esophagitis,[6] dysphagia, <u>N/V</u>, <u>cramps</u>, <u>diarrhea</u>, flatulence, anogenital lesions/candidiasis. Lower GI effects, eg diarrhea, are less common c̄ **doxycycline** or **minocycline**. Discoloration of teeth in children ≤ 8. Rare- pseudomembranous colitis.
S/Cond: Not c̄ lactation. Caution c̄ diabetes- ↓ glucose.[18] Caution c̄ ↓ hepatic func. Caution c̄ ↓ renal func c̄ **Tetracycline**. (**Doxycycline** is drug of choice c̄ ↓ renal func[58]). Caution c̄ TF- chelation c̄ minerals may ↓ both drug & mineral abs.[8] **Doxycycline** is > 90% serum pro bound.
Pregnancy: Category D.[13] Permanent infant tooth discoloration if used in 2nd half of pregnancy.
Other: <u>Ataxia</u>, <u>dizziness</u>, <u>photosensitivity</u>, headache, rash. **minocycline**- <u>DIZZINESS</u>, <u>ATAXIA</u>, <u>headache</u>, <u>drowsiness</u>. Rare- hepatotoxicity, pancreatitis, benign intracranial HTN, anaphylaxis, SJS, TEN, lupus-like syndrome.
Blood/Serum: ↑ alk phos, ↑ bil, ↑ AST, ↑ ALT, ↑ amylase. ↓ Pyr, ↓ Vit B_{12}, ↓ pantothenic acid, ↓ conc of Vit C in WBC.[6]　　**Tetracycline**- ↑ BUN.　　**minocycline**- Rare- + ANA.
Urinary: ↑ Rib, ↑ N, ↑ Vit C.[6] **Monitor:** CBC, renal & hepatic func c̄ LT use.

doxycycline	minocycline	Tetracycline
Vibramycin	**Dynacin**	Cap- lactose
Cap, Tab- propylene glycol	Cap- cornstarch, lactose	
Pwd for Oral Susp- sucrose	**Minocin**	
Syrup- CaCl, propylene glycol,	Cap	
simethicone, Na metabisulfite, sorbitol	**Solodyn** (SR)	
	Tab- lactose	

Oracea Cap (30 mg IR & 10 mg DR beads)- sugar sphere
Periostat (low dose) Tab- lactose
Doryx (SR) Tab- lactose, cornstarch,
　75 mg Tab- 4.5 mg (0.196 mEq) Na
　100 mg Tab- 6 mg (0.261 mEq) Na
　150 mg Tab- 9.0 (0.392 mEq) Na

Teveten/Teveten HCT
  eprosartan

ANTIHYPERTENSIVE   See **Angiotensin II Receptor Antagonists p 38**
        Teveten HCT also contains **hydrochlorothiazide**, see **p 166**.

theophylline
  Elixophyllin
  Elixir- 20% alcohol
  Theo-24
  Cap (SR)-
   starch, sucrose
  Theolair
  Tab- lactose, starch
  Uniphyl
  Tab (SR)

  Check generic brand
  for- lactose,
  sucrose, starch,
  sorbitol, sulfites
  &/or benzyl alcohol

BRONCHODILATOR, Methylxanthine   Oral or Parenteral (IV)
        Also used for apnea & bradycardia of prematurity
        Drug: Follow PI about taking c̄ food.
        Food affects abs in some SR forms. Swallow enteric-coated & SR forms
        whole, do not crush or chew. Dosage based on IBW.
        Diet: Consistent intake of pro & CHO for consistent drug levels.
        Avoid drastic changes in caffeine intake,[3] see p 379.
        10 mg Pyr/day ↓ CNS effects (eg tremor).[38]
        Nutr: <u>Anorexia</u>. ↑ pro, ↓ CHO- ↑ metabolism of drug & ↓ blood level.
        Drug is pyridoxal kinase antagonist, therefore ↑ Pyr requirement.
        Oral/GI: Bitter aftertaste, GERD, <u>N</u>/V, epigastric pain.
        S/Cond: Caution c̄ alcohol- single large dose ↓ drug clearance.[10]
        Not c̄ lactation. Caution c̄ diabetes- ↑ glucose c̄ high dose.
        Caution c̄ ↓ hepatic func, seizures, cardiac disease.
        Pregnancy: Category C.
        Other: <u>Nervousness</u>, <u>insomnia</u>, dizziness, headache, tachycardia,
        palpitations, tremor, hypotension, rash, seizures, SIADH.
        Blood/Serum: ↑ glucose, ↑ AST,[6] ↑ uric acid, ↓ <u>Pyr</u>, ↓ <u>Thi</u>.[11]
        Urinary: Pro, diuresis (↑ Na, ↑ output), ↑ frequency.
        Monitor: Serum drug level.

Theraflu
  Acesulfame K,
  maltitol syrup,
  propylene glycol, benzyl alcohol

COLD & COUGH CONGESTION TREATMENT   See **acetaminophen p 22**
Combination drug   See **phenylephrine p 255**
                  See **guaifenesin p 159**

thiamine
thiamin

B COMPLEX VITAMIN, ANTIBERIBERI, VIT B$_1$ Oral or Parenteral (IM or IV)
Used to prevent Wernicke/Korsakoff syndrome due to chronic alcohol abuse
Drug: Oral antiberiberi dose is 5-10 mg 3X/day.[1, 13]
Nutr: ↑ <u>Thi</u> requirement c̄ ↑ CHO intake or gastric bypass.
AI (mg/day) Infants 0-6 mo = **0.2**, 7-12 mo = **0.3**.
RDA (mg/day) Children 1-3 yr = **0.5**. 4-8 = **0.6**. 9-13 = **0.9**.
Males 14-70+ = **1.2**. Females 14-18 = **1.0**. 19-70+ = **1.1**.
Lactation = **1.4**. No documented toxicity- no **UL** set.[47]
Oral/GI: IV- Nausea.
S/Cond: Alcohol inhibits abs.[13] Gastric bypass ↑ risk of def.
Alcoholism ↑ risk of def & optic neuropathy.
Def S/S (beriberi)- anorexia, ↓ wt, confusion, irritability, ↓ short term
memory, apathy, weakness, enlarged heart, edema, muscle wasting,
peripheral neuropathy.[52]
Pregnancy: Category A, oral & parenteral. **RDA** = **1.4** mg/day.
Other: IV- feeling of warmth, weakness, allergic reaction, rash.[26]

thiazolidinediones

ANTIDIABETIC AGENT for Type 2 diabetes
Monotherapy or c̄ **metformin** and/or **sulfonylurea**

Drug: Take s̄ regard to food. If once a day, take in the morning.
Diet: Prescribed diabetic diet. ↓ cal if wt loss needed. Avoid SJW, see p 286.
Nutr: ↑ <u>WEIGHT</u>. ↑ <u>INSULIN SENSITIVITY IN MUSCLE & FAT TISSUE</u>. ↓ <u>GLUCONEOGENESIS</u>.
Oral/GI: Tooth disorder, pharyngitis.
S/Cond: Not c̄ lactation. > 99% serum pro bound. Not c̄ active hepatic disease or
↑ hepatic enzymes > 2.5 X normal. Caution c̄ CVD, stable CHF, edema. Not c̄ severe or symptomatic CHF.
Pregnancy: Category C.
Other: URTI, injury, edema, headache, fatigue, muscle pain, sinusitis. ↑ risk of fractures in women,
Rare- new onset CHF, possible ↑ risk of MI.
Blood/Serum: ↓ <u>INSULIN</u>, ↓ <u>FASTING GLUCOSE</u>, ↓ <u>POSTPRANDIAL GLUCOSE</u>, ↓ *Hb A1$_C$*, ↑ <u>PLASMA VOLUME</u>,
anemia, ↓ WBC. Rare- hypoglycemia. **rosiglitazone**- ↑ <u>CHOL</u>, ↑ <u>LDL</u>, ↓ <u>HDL</u>, ↑ <u>TG</u>.
pioglitazone- ↓ <u>CHOL</u> ↓ <u>LDL</u> ↑ <u>HDL</u> ↓ <u>TG</u>.
Monitor: FBS & Hb A1$_C$ q 3-6 mo. Hepatic func- baseline, then q 2 mo for 12 mo, then periodically.
Possibly lipids.

pioglitazone	**Actos**	Tab- lactose
rosiglitazone	**Avandia**	Tab- lactose, Na starch glycolate

Thorazine previous brand name   ANTIPSYCHOTIC   See **Phenothiazines p 254**
  chlorpromazine

thyroid   THYROID HORMONE   Oral or Parenteral (IV or IM)
  levothyroxine   **Drug:** Take c̄ full glass water on empty stomach before breakfast to ↑ abs.
    many generic brands-   Pediatric dose based on body weight.
    check ingredients   May crush tab, suspend in water, drink immediately.
    Synthroid (T_4)   **Diet:** Take Fe, Ca[12] or Mg[3] suppl separately from drug by ≥ 4 hr[7] (may ↓ abs).
    Tab- lactose, sugar,   ↓ abs also reported c̄ soy, soy milk, soy infant formula, walnuts,
      cornstarch   cottonseed meal[87] & high fiber foods.[92] Caution c̄ grapefruit/related
                                     citrus, see p 390. Take drug 2-3 hr before soy.[4]
    Generic Brand   **Nutr:** Appetite changes, ↓ wt. **Oral/GI:** Rare- nausea, diarrhea.
    Inj- 10 mg mannitol/5 mL   **S/Cond:** Caution c̄ lactation- adjust dose. Caution c̄ diabetics on
    Levothroid   medication- ↑ glucose. Caution c̄ CVD, HTN or geriatric.
    Tab   > 99% serum pro bound. **Pregnancy:** Category A. ↑ dose required.
    Levoxyl   **Other:** Rare- headache, tremor, nervousness, insomnia, ↑ BP, ↑ pulse,
    Tab   palpitations. Overdose in postmenopausal women- ↑ bone resorption,
    Unithroid   ↓ bone density. **Blood/Serum:** ↑ T_4, ↑ T_3, ↓ TSH, ↑ glucose, ↓ CHOL,
    Tab- lactose, cornstarch,   ↓ LDL. Overdose in postmenopausal women- ↑ Ca, ↑ P, ↑ alk phos, ↓ PTH.
      Na starch glycolate   **Monitor:** Thyroid func, TSH.

tiagabine   ANTIEPILEPTIC, Adjunct Therapy for ≥ 12 yr old
  Gabitril   **Drug:** Take c̄ food. **Nutr:** ↑ appetite.
    Tab- ascorbic acid,   **Oral/GI:** Mouth ulcers, pharyngitis, N/V, abdominal pain, diarrhea.
      lactose, starch   **S/Cond:** Caution c̄ alcohol. Caution c̄ lactation. 96% serum pro bound.
                                     Hypoalbuminemia (< 3 g/dL)- may ↑ drug effects.
                                     Caution c̄ ↓ hepatic func. **Pregnancy:** Category C.
                                     Other: Dizziness, weakness, nervousness, tremor, vasodilation,
                                     drowsiness, insomnia, ataxia, confusion, agititation, hostility,
                                     memory/concentration difficulties, depression, speech disorder,
                                     paresthesia, cough, flu syndrome, muscle pain, rash.
                                     Rare- suicidal thoughts & behavior.
                                     Rare- seizures c̄ off-label use in pt c̄ no previous epilepsy diagnosis.[124]

Tiazac	ANTIANGINA, ANTIHYPERTENSIVE, Ca Channel Blocker See **diltiazem p 111**

ticagrelor
  Brilinta
  Tab- mannitol, starch

ACUTE CORONARY SYNDROME TREATMENT, REDUCTION OF MI, CVA, CV DEATH, platelet aggregation inhibitor

Drug: Take s̄ regard to food. Take c̄ low dose aspirin 75-100 mg daily. Doses of aspirin > 100 mg ↓ effectiveness of drug.
Diet: Caution c̄ grapefruit/related citrus- ↑ drug effect see p 390. Avoid SJW- ↓ drug effect see p 286.
Oral/GI: Nausea, diarrhea.
S/Cond: Not c̄ lactation. Not c̄ Hx of intracranial hemorrhage. Not c̄ cond that ↑ bleeding eg peptic ulcer. Caution c̄ moderate ↓ hepatic func. Not c̄ severe↓ hepatic func. Do dental care cautiously- ↑ risk of bleeding. 99% serum pro bound- hypoalbuminemia (< 3 g/dL) may ↑ drug effects. Caution c̄ dysphagia.
Pregnancy: Category C.
Other: <u>Dyspnea</u>, <u>headche</u>, bleeding (can be fatal), bradycardia, cough, dizziness, atrial fibrillation, hypertension, hypotension, chest pain, fatigue, back pain. < 1% gynecomastia.
Blood/Serum: ↑ uric acid, ↑ <u>crea</u>.
Monitor: S/S of bleeding/blood loss, dyspnea.

Tigan	ANTINAUSEANT, ANTIEMETIC See **trimethobenzamide p 324**

tigecycline
  Tygacil
  pwd- preservative free, lactose

ANTIBIOTIC, Glycylcycline Parenteral only (IV)
  derivative of **minocyline**, designed to overcome resistance to **tetracyclines**
Drug: Given IV every 12 hr for 5-14 days.
Diet: Avoid SJW,[93] see p 286.
Oral/GI: Dyspepsia, <u>N/V</u>, abdominal pain, diarrhea. Discoloration of teeth in children ≤ 8. Rare- pseudomembranous colitis.
S/Cond: Caution c̄ lactation. Caution c̄ severe ↓ hepatic func.
Pregnancy: Category D.
Permanent infant tooth discoloration if used in the 2nd half of pregnancy.
Blood/Serum: ↑ amylase, ↑ BUN, ↑ alk phos, ↑ bil, ↑ AST, ↑ ALT, ↓ alb, ↓ P, ↑ PT/INR.

Tikosyn   ANTIARRHYTHMIC, Selective Potassium Channel Blocker See **dofetilide p 115**

Timentin   ANTIBIOTIC, penicillin   See listing for **penicillin p 249**
  ticarcillin disodium   Pwd- 104 mg (4.5 mEq) Na/g,   Parenteral (IV only)
  & **clavulanate potassium**   6 mg (0.15 mEq) K/g

timolol   ANTIHYPERTYENSIVE, ANTIMIGRAINE, POST MI TREATMENT
  Blocadren (previous brand name) Tab (IR)- starch Nonselective Beta-Blocker   See listing for **propranolol p 267**

tinidazole   ANTIBIOTIC, AMEBICIDE, ANTITRICHOMONAL
  Tindamax   Longer duration of action than **metronidazole**   See listing for
  Tab- cornstarch   **metronidazole p 216**

tiotropium   BRONCHODILATOR, Anticholinergic for COPD TREATMENT Oral Inhalant
  Spiriva Handihaler   **Drug:** DO NOT SWALLOW CAP.
  Cap   Must be administered once a day c̄ inhalation device <u>only</u>.
  Pwd- lactose   **Oral/GI:** <u>Dry mouth</u>, stomatitis, GERD, dyspepsia, abdominal pain, constipation.
  Long Acting   **S/Cond:** Caution c̄ lactation. Caution c̄ moderate to severe ↓ renal func.
                                    Caution c̄ glaucoma. Not c̄ milk allergy. Caution c̄ preexisting urinary retention.
                                    Pregnancy: Category C.
                                    Other: <u>URTI</u>, sinusitis, pharyngitis, rhinitis,
                                    chest pain, edema, nosebleed, rash, fungal growth, blurred vision,
                                    ↑ heart rate, cough, flu-like symptoms. Rare- paradoxical bronchospasm.
                                    Urinary: UTI, retention.

tipranavir (TPV)
  Aptivus
  Cap- dehydrated
  alcohol 0.1 g/cap,
  castor oil,
  propylene glycol
  Soln- propylene glycol
  Vit E derivative =
  116 IU/mL

ANTIRETROVIRAL (HIV/AIDS), Non-peptidic Protease Inhibitor
  Must be taken c̄ **ritonavir**, see also p 281. (Effects may be due to **ritonavir**)
  Drug: Swallow cap whole c̄ high fat meal to ↑ bioavailability.
  Diet: Avoid SJW, see p 286. Avoid Vit E suppl > RDI, see p 341.
  Nutr: Anorexia, ↓ wt.
  Oral/GI: Dyspepsia, GERD, N/V, abdominal pain, <u>diarrhea</u>, flatulence.
  S/Cond: Not c̄ lactation. Not in treatment naive pt.
  Caution c̄ mild ↓ hepatic func, geriatric or diabetes. Not c̄ moderate-
  severe ↓ hepatic func. Caution c̄ sulfonamide allergy.
  Caution c̄ hepatitis B or C co-infection. **Pregnancy:** Category C.
  Other: <u>Rash</u>, fatigue, insomnia, headache, bronchitis, peripheral neuropathy,
  pancreatitis, hepatotoxicity. May ↑ risk of lipodystrophy or diabetes.
  Very rare- intracranial hemorrhage (may be fatal), new onset diabetes.
  Blood/Serum: ↑ amylase, ↑ <u>chol</u>, ↑ <u>TG</u>, ↑ glucose, anemia, ↓ WBC,
  ↓ platelets, ↑ <u>AST</u>, ↑ <u>ALT</u>.
  Monitor: Baseline & periodic- hepatic func, lipid panel, glucose.

tizanidine
  Zanaflex
  Tab- lactose
  Cap- sugar spheres
  (sucrose, starch)

SKELETAL MUSCLE RELAXANT, ANTISPASMODIC
  alpha-2 agonist- similar to **clonidine**
  Drug: Food ↑ abs & conc of drug, more ↑ c̄ tab than cap. May ↑ drug effects.
  Oral/GI: <u>DRY MOUTH</u>, pharyngitis, dyspepsia, N/V, constipation, diarrhea.
  S/Cond: Avoid alcohol- ↑ CNS effects.
  Caution c̄ lactation- drug expected to pass into milk.
  Caution c̄ moderate to severe ↓ renal func, ↓ hepatic func, geriatric.
  Pregnancy: Category C.
  Other: ↓ <u>BP</u> c̄ POSSIBLE <u>HYPOTENSION</u>, <u>ASTHENIA</u>, <u>DROWSINESS</u>, <u>DIZZINESS</u>,
  <u>bradycardia</u>, dyskinesia, nervousness, anxiety, depression, paresthesia,
  blurred vision, flu syndrome, fever, sweating, infection, rhinitis, rash,
  skin ulcer, speech disorder, back pain, muscle weakness, hepatotoxicity.
  Blood/Serum: ↑ ALT, ↑ AST. **Urinary:** UTI, ↑ frequency.
  Monitor: BP. Hepatic func- baseline, at 1, 3 & 6 mo, then periodically.

TMP-SMZ

ANTIBIOTIC, Sulfonamide   See **trimethoprim c sulfamethoxazole p 324**

tobramycin
ANTIBIOTIC, Aminoglycoside   Parenteral only (IM or IV) or Inhalation Soln
generic (Parenteral)
multiple dose vial contains 3.2 mg Na metabisulfite
TOBI (Inhalation Soln)- preservative free Fewer systemic effects. Rare- ototoxicity, voice changes, SJS.
See listing for **gentamicin p 156**

tocilizumab
Actemra
vial- sucrose- 50mg/mL,
polysorbate 80- 0.5mg/mL

ANTIARTHRITIC, Rheumatoid Arthritis (Adult or Juvenile) Parenteral only (IV)
Interleukin-6 (IL-6) inhibitor

Drug: Dosage based on body weight.
Nutr: ↑ wt.
Oral/GI: mouth ulceration, upper abdominal pain, gastritis, oral herpes simplex, stomatitis, gastric ulcer.
S/Cond: Not c̄ lacation. Caution c̄ geriatric- ↑ infection.
Not c̄ moderate to severe ↓ renal func. Not c̄ active hepatic disease or ↓ hepatic func. Not c̄ live vaccines. Not c̄ active infection.
Not c̄ ANC < 1000 or platelets < 100,000.
Pregnancy: Category C.
Other: URTI, nasopharyngitis, HTN, headache, dizziness, bronchitis, rash, hives, pruritis, dyspnea, cough, peripheral edema, conjunctivitis, nephrolithiasis, hypothyroidism, hypersensitivity reaction.
Rare- gastrointestinal perforation, anaphylaxis (can be fatal).
Urinary: UTI.
Blood/Serum:↑ AST, ↑ ALT, ↓ platelets, ↓ neutrophils, leukopenia, ↑ LDL, ↑ HDL, ↑ TG, ↑ bil, ↓ CRP.
Monitor: Neutrophils, platelets, AST, ALT, bil q 4-8 wks.
Lipids at 4-8 wks, then q 24 wks.

tocopherol
VITAMIN, Fat Soluble, Antioxidant
See **vitamin E p 341**

Tofranil/Tofranil PM
imipramine HCl or pamoate
ANTIDEPRESSANT
See **Tricyclic Antidepressants p 323**

tolterodine
Detrol/Detrol LA
ANTIMUSCARINIC
See **Bladder Control Agents p 61**

tolvaptan
 Samsca
 Tab- cornstarch,
  lactose

HYPONATREMIA TREATMENT (in CHF, SIADH, Cirrhosis),
 Vasopression Antagonist For Na < 125 mEq/L & resistant to fluid restriction.
 Drug: Take s̄ regard to meals.
 Diet: Drink to thirst only. Avoid grapefruit/related citrus, see p 390.
 Avoid SJW, see p 286. **Nutr:** <u>Thirst</u>, anorexia.
 Oral/GI: <u>Dry mouth</u>, <u>nausea</u>, <u>constipation</u>, ischemic colitis.
 S/Cond: Not c̄ lactation. 99% serum pro bound. Caution c̄ cirrhosis.
 Not c̄ anuric pt or pt unable to sense thirst.
 Limit serum Na increase to < 12 mEq/L in 24 hr.[1] **Pregnancy:** Category C.
 Other: <u>Asthenia</u>, fever, DVT, rhabdomyolysis, CVA, pulmonary embolism,
 respiratory failure, ventricular fibrillation, diabetes/ketoacidosis,
 hypotension, vaginal hemorrhage. Rare- cardiogenic shock, gout,
 disseminated intravascular coagulation.
 Blood/Serum: ↑ <u>glucose</u>, ↑ PT/INR, ↑ <u>Na</u>. Rare- ↑ uric acid.
 Urinary: <u>Polyuria</u>, ↑ urgency, urethral hemorrhage.
 Monitor: Na, K, neurologic & volume status.

topiramate
 Topamax
 Tab- lactose,
  Na starch glycolate
 Sprinkle Cap-
  sugar spheres,
  (sucrose, starch)

ANTIEPILEPTIC, MIGRAINE PROPHYLAXIS Also used to treat Bipolar Disorder[21]
 Drug: Take s̄ regard to meals. Swallow Tab whole- do not break (bitter taste).
 Swallow Cap whole or open & sprinkle on one tsp soft food.
 Swallow immediately, do NOT chew.
 Diet: Insure adequate fluid intake/hydration to ↓ risk of kidney stones.
 Nutr: ↓ <u>WEIGHT</u>,[21] <u>anorexia</u>. ↑ appetite, ↑ wt.
 Oral/GI: Dry mouth, gingivitis, taste changes, GERD, <u>nausea</u>, dyspepsia,
 <u>abdominal pain</u>, constipation, diarrhea.
 S/Cond: Avoid alcohol. Caution c̄ lactation.
 Caution c̄ ↓ hepatic func or ↓ renal func. **Pregnancy:** Category C.
 Other: <u>DROWSINESS</u>, <u>PSYCHOMOTOR SLOWING</u>, <u>FATIGUE</u>, <u>dizziness</u>, <u>ataxia</u>,
 <u>tremor</u>, <u>confusion</u>, <u>nervousness</u>, <u>mood problems</u>, <u>speech/language
 problems</u>, <u>memory</u> impairment, <u>concentration/attention</u> <u>difficulty</u>,
 <u>depression</u>, <u>paresthesia</u>, <u>back pain</u>, visual abnormalities including acute
 myopia/glaucoma, ↓ sweating, ↑ body temp, hair loss, apathy, weakness,
 muscle pain, breast pain, kidney stones, edema, menstrual changes,

metabolic acidosis. Rare- suicidal thoughts & behavior.
Blood/Serum: ↓ BICARB, anemia, ↓ WBC. < 1%- ↑ AST, ↑ ALT,
↑ GGT, ↓ platelets. **Urinary:** Hematuria, incontinence, UTI, ↑ frequency.
Monitor: Baseline & periodic bicarb levels.

Toprol-XL	ANTIHYPERTENSIVE, ANTIANGINA	See **metoprolol p 215**

toremifene
  Fareston
ANTINEOPLASTIC (Breast Cancer), Estrogen Antagonist
  Tab- starch, lactose   See listing for **tamoxifen p 302**

Torisel
ANTINEOPLASTIC, mTOR Kinase Inhibitor   See **temsirolimus p 306**

torsemide
  Demadex
ANTIHYPERTENSIVE, DIURETIC   See **Diuretics, Loop p 114**

Toviaz (SR)
  fesoterodine
ANTIMUSCARINIC   See **Bladder Control Agents p 61**
  Tab- lactose

Tradjenta
  linagliptin
ANTIDIABETIC AGENT, Incretin Enhancer
DPP-4 (dipeptidyl-peptidase-4) Inhibitor
Tab- mannitol, pregelatinized starch, corn starch   See listing for **sitagliptin p 293**

tramadol
  Ultram
  Tab- lactose,
   cornstarch,
   Na starch glycolate
  Ultram ER
  Tab
ANALGESIC, Opioid
  Drug: Take s̄ regard to food. Do not chew, crush or split ER tab.
  Diet: Caution c̄ SJW, theoretical interaction.⁹³ **Nutr:** Anorexia.
  Oral/GI: Dry mouth, dyspepsia, NAUSEA/vomiting, abdominal pain,
  CONSTIPATION, diarrhea, flatulence.
  S/Cond: Avoid alcohol. Not c̄ lactation. **Ultram-** caution c̄ ↓ renal func,
  seizures, geriatric or hepatic cirrhosis. **Ultram ER-** not c̄ severe ↓ hepatic
  func or severe ↓ renal func (CrCl < 30 mL/minute).
  May be habit forming c̄ LT use. ↑ risk of dental problems, see p 11 & 15.
  Pregnancy: Category C. **Other:** DIZZINESS, HEADACHE, DROWSINESS, itching,
  weakness, sweating, rash, visual changes, anxiety, confusion, ataxia,
  vasodilation. Rare- seizures, SJS, TEN.
  Blood/Serum: < 1%- ↑ crea, ↑ AST, ↑ ALT, ↓ Hb.
  Urinary: Pro. Retention, ↑ frequency.

| **Trandate** | ANTIHYPERTENSIVE | See **labetalol p 185** |

trandolapril
 Mavik

ANTIHYPERTENSIVE   See **Angiotensin Converting Enzyme Inhibitors p 36**

Tranxene
 clorazepate

ANTIANXIETY, ANTIEPILEPTIC   See **Benzodiazepines p 54**

tranylcypromine
 Parnate
 Tab- lactose

ANTIDEPRESSANT, MAOI   See listing for **phenelzine p 252**
Other: Lower incidence of insomnia & more rapid onset of action, but more severe HTN than other MAOI.[23]

trastuzumab
 Herceptin
 Pwd- preservative free
 Diluent- 1.1% benzyl
  alcohol

ANTINEOPLASTIC, Monoclonal Antibody (Breast Cancer c̄ HER2 Overexpression)
In combination c̄ **paclitaxel** for first treatment of metastatic disease
Single agent after previous treatment   Parenteral only (IV infusion)
Diet: Insure adequate fluid intake/hydration.
Nutr: Anorexia.
Oral/GI: NAUSEA/VOMITING, dyspepsia, ABDOMINAL PAIN, DIARRHEA, CONSTIPATION.
S/Cond: Not c̄ lactation. Caution c̄ cardiac disease or ↓ pulmonary func.
Pregnancy: Category B, but use not advised.
Other: FEVER, CHILLS, INFUSION REACTION, WEAKNESS, PAIN, HEADACHE, BACK PAIN, INFECTION, ↑ COUGH, DYSPNEA, pulmonary toxicity, insomnia, dizziness, bone/joint pain, flu syndrome, paresthesia, depression, rhinitis, pharyngitis, sinusitis, rash, acne, CHF, edema, tachycardia, peripheral neuritis, neuropathy, nail disorder, nose bleed, URTI, allergic reaction, ↓ LVEF.
Rare- fatal anaphylactic reaction or cardiomyopathy.
Blood/Serum: ↓ WBC, anemia.
Urinary: UTI.
Monitor: CBC c̄ diff & platelets, baseline & periodically.
Baseline cardiac & pulmonary func & periodic LVEF.

trazodone
  Desyrel
  (previous brand name)
  Tab- lactose,
  Na starch glycolate in
   some brands
  Oleptro (ER)
  Tab- polyethylene glycol

ANTIDEPRESSANT, Heterocyclic
Also used to treat insomnia,[17] aggression, panic attacks.[7]
Drug: Take c̄ meals/snack to ↓ GI effects & ↓ risk of postural hypotension. ER tab should be swallowed whole or broken along scored line. Do not crush or chew.
Diet: Avoid SJW, see p 286, ginkgo, ginseng, or valerian.
Caution c̄ grapefruit/related citrus, see p 390. **Nutr:** ↑ appetite, ↑ or ↓ wt.
Oral/GI: Unpleasant taste, DRY MOUTH, N/V, constipation.
Rare, but serious, upper GI bleeding.[68]
S/Cond: Avoid alcohol. Caution c̄ lactation. ↑ risk of dental problems, see p 11 & 15. 89-95% serum pro bound. Caution c̄ cardiac disease, ↓ hepatic func or ↓ renal func.[13] **Pregnancy:** Category C.
Other: DROWSINESS, dizziness, blurred vision, ataxia, headache, HTN or hypotension, fatigue, syncope, tremor, edema, paresthesia, allergic reaction.
Rare- suicidal thinking & behavior, priapism, SIADH, arrhythmia.
Blood/Serum: Mildly ↑ AST, ↑ ALT, ↑ alk phos. < 1%- ↓ WBC, ↓ neutrophils.
Monitor: WBC, ANC.[13]

Trental

ANTIPERIPHERAL VASCULAR DISEASE   See **pentoxifylline p 250**

treprostinil
  Tyvaso
  Inhalation Soln
treprostinil Na
  Remodulin
  Parenteral (IV or SC)
  5.3 mg Na/20 mL
   in 1, 2, & 5 mg/mL forms
  4 mg Na/20 ml
   in 20 mg/mL form

PULMONARY ARTERIAL HYPERTENSION TREATMENT, Vasodilator
Drug: Do not ingest. **Diet:** Avoid ginkgo.
Oral/GI: Nausea, diarrhea. GI hemorrhage.[9a]
S/Cond: Caution c̄ lactation. Caution c̄ hepatic func or ↓ renal func.
Caution c̄ geriatric. Caution c̄ low BP= ↑ risk of hypotension.
91% serum pro bound. Dosage based on BW.**Pregnancy:** Category B.
Other: Hypotension, bleeding. **Inhaler:** COUGH, throat irritation, headache, flushing, syncope, dizziness. **SC:** INFUSION SITE REACTIONS, SITE PAIN, jaw pain, edema, vasodilatation, dizziness, headache, rash, itching.
Blood/Serum: ↓ PLATELET AGGREGATION.

Treximet
  Tab

ACUTE TREATMENT OF MIGRAINE ATTACKS
Combination drug   See **antimigraine p 39**
  sumatriptan & **naproxen**   See **naproxen p 224**

triamcinolone
  Kenalog 10 & Kenalog 40-
  (Parenteral- benzyl alcohol)

CORTICOSTEROID   See **corticosteroids p 94**

Drug: IM, intra-articular (joint), intravitreal (eye)
Nutr: <u>Anorexia</u>, unlike other corticosteroids, which may ↑ appetite.[13]

triamcinolone
  Azmacort[a]- Aerosol Inhalant
  1% dehydrated alcohol

  Nasacort AQ[b]- Nasal Spray
  dextrose

ANTIASTHMA[a], ALLERGIC RHINITIS TREATMENT[b]   Corticosteroid
Not for acute asthma attack
Drug: Rinse mouth after using inhaled form. Do not swallow rinse water.
Nutr: ↑ wt. **Oral/GI:** <u>Oral</u> <u>candidiasis</u>,[7] <u>dry mouth</u>, toothache, <u>sore throat</u>,
<u>PHARYNGITIS</u> (↑ c̄ aerosol), N/V, dyspepsia, abdominal pain, diarrhea.
S/Cond: Caution c̄ lactation. Good oral hygiene essential.
Pregnancy: Category C. **Other:** <u>Headache</u>, cough, facial edema, otitis,
photosensitivity, rash, sinusitis. Nosebleed c̄ nasal forms.

triamterene
  Dyrenium
  Cap- lactose
  Tab- Canada only

  Dyazide Cap- lactose,
  Na starch glycolate,
  benzyl alcohol

  Maxzide Tab

  Dyazide & **Maxzide**
  also contain
  hydrochlorothiazide
  see **p 166**

DIURETIC, K sparing   (adjunct to antihypertensive therapy)
Chemically related to Fol (weak dihydro-folate reductase antagonist)
Drug: Take after meals or c̄ milk to ↓ GI irritation.
Diet: Avoid excessive K intake. Avoid K suppl or salt subs.
↓ Na, ↓ cal may be recommended. Discontinue Na restriction if
hyponatremia occurs. Avoid natural licorice, see p 374.
Nutr: ↓ utilization of Fol. **Oral/GI:** < 1%- taste changes, N/V, diarrhea.
S/Cond: Not c̄ lactation. Caution c̄ geriatric, diabetes, moderately ↓ hepatic
func or ↓ renal func. Not c̄ severe ↓ hepatic func or severe ↓ renal func.
Pregnancy: Category C.
Other: Dizziness, headache, photosensitivity, hyperkalemia.
Rare- hyponatremia, hypomagnesemia, metabolic acidosis.[6]
Blood/Serum: ↑ <u>K</u>, ↓ <u>Mg</u>, ↓ bicarb, ↑ uric acid, ↓ Fol.
Rare- ↓ platelets, anemia, ↑ BUN, ↑ crea, ↓ Na, ↑ Cl.
Urinary: ↑ <u>Na</u>, ↑ Cl, ↑ <u>WATER</u>, slight ↓ K, ↑ Ca, ↑ Mg, ↑ bicarb, ↑ pH.
Monitor: Electrolytes, Mg, renal func, BP, CBC c̄ diff, platelets.

triazolam
  Halcion

SLEEP AID   See **Benzodiazepines p 54**

TriCor

ANTIHYPERLIPIDEMIC, Fibrate   See **fenofibrate p 138**

Tricyclic Antidepressants (TCA) ANTIDEPRESSANT,[a] ANTIANXIETY,[b] To Treat ENURESIS,[c] OCD,[d] ITCHING[e]
Also used to treat ADHD, Panic Disorder, Migraine, Bulimia Nervosa, Insomnia, Neuropathies
Drug: May take c̄ food to ↓ GI distress. Dilute **doxepin** conc in 4 oz water, milk or juice.
Conc is incompatible c̄ carbonated beverages or grape juice.[13]
Diet: ↑ fiber may ↓ drug effect.[3] Limit caffeine, see p 379. Avoid SJW, see p 286.
Caution c̄ grapefruit/related citrus c̄ **clomipramine**, see p 390.
Nutr: ↑ WT, ↑ APPETITE, especially for sweets, CHO. ↑ need for Rib.[41] Anorexia.
Oral/GI: DRY MOUTH, taste changes, black tongue, stomatitis, dysphagia, esophagitis, N/V, CONSTIPATION, diarrhea, flatulence. Rare- paralytic ileus.
S/Cond: Avoid alcohol. Not c̄ lactation. ↑ risk of dental problems, see p 11 & 15. 90-97% serum pro bound. Not c̄ glaucoma.[17] Caution c̄ cardiac disease, ↓ hepatic func, geriatric[84], seizures, thyroid dysfunction, BPH, urinary retention. **desipramine-** Not c̄ family Hx of sudden death, cardiac dysrhythmias/conduction disturbances.[22]
Pregnancy: Category C. **imipramine-** Category D.[23] Topical **doxepin-** Category B.
Other: SEDATION, DROWSINESS, BLURRED VISION, delirium, dizziness, fine tremor, headache, weakness, orthostatic hypotension, ataxia, confusion, hallucinations, agitation, nightmares, gynecomastia, galactorrhea, edema, ↑ sweating, rash, mania/hypomania.
Rare- cardiotoxicity/arrhythmias, SIADH, jaundice, hepatitis, tinnitus, seizures, paresthesias, EPS (↑ in geriatric), NMS c̄ **amitriptyline**,[6] photosensitivity c̄ **clomipramine** or **imipramine**.[6] Suicidal thinking & behavior.
Blood/Serum: Dyscrasias, ↑ or ↓ glucose, ↑ prolactin, ↑ ALT, ↑ AST, ↑ alk phos, ↑ bil.
Rare- ↑ amylase, ↑ lipase, ↓ Na.
Urinary: Retention, ↑ Rib. **Monitor:** CBC c̄ diff, hepatic func c̄ LT use. BP, heart rate. Possibly ECG.

amitriptyline[a]	**Elavil** (previous brand name) Tab- lactose, starch
clomipramine[d]	**Anafranil** Cap- cornstarch
desipramine[a]	**Norpramin** Tab- sucrose, cornstarch, soy oil, mineral oil, mannitol
	Active metabolite of **imipramine**, less sedating, lower anticholinergic effects.
doxepin	**Sinequan**[a, b] (previous brand name) Cap- starch. Conc- peppermint oil.
	Zonalon Cream[e] (topical)
imipramine HCl[a, c]	**Tofranil**- Tab- sucrose, Na starch glycolate.
imipramine pamoate[a]	**Tofranil-PM** Cap- starch
nortriptyline[a]	**Pamelor** Cap- starch. Soln- 4% alcohol, 2 mg/mL sorbitol.
	nortriptyline- active metabolite of **amitriptyline**, less sedating, lower anticholinergic effects.

See "Guide to the Use of This Book" inside front cover.

| **Triglide** | ANTIHYPERLIPIDEMIC, Fibrate | See **fenofibrate p 138** |

trihexyphenidyl
   Artane (previous brand name)
   Generic brands
   Elixir- 5% alcohol,
    NaCl, sorbitol
   Tab- cornstarch,
    starch

ANTIPARKINSON, ANTI-EPS, Anticholinergic
Drug: Take c̄ meals to ↓ GI distress.
Oral/GI: <u>DRY MOUTH</u>, <u>MILD NAUSEA</u>/vomiting, <u>constipation</u>.
S/Cond: Avoid alcohol. May inhibit lactation. ↑ risk of dental problems, see p 11 & 15. Will not improve & may aggravate tardive dyskinesia. Caution in hot weather. Caution c̄ ↓ hepatic func or ↓ renal func, geriatric, BPH, glaucoma.
Pregnancy: Category C.
Other: <u>DIZZINESS</u>, <u>BLURRED VISION</u>, <u>DEPRESSION</u>,[17] <u>drowsiness</u>, <u>weakness</u>, <u>nervousness</u>, ↓ sweating, <u>confusion</u>, agitation, headache, tachycardia.
Urinary: <u>Retention</u>.

| **Trilafon** (previous brand name)
  perphenazine | ANTIPSYCHOTIC | See **Phenothiazines p 254** |

| **Trileptal** | ANTIEPILEPTIC | See **oxcarbazepine p 72** |

trimethobenzamide
   Tigan
   IM-
    0.45% phenol preservative
   Cap- lactose,
    starch

ANTIEMETIC, ANTINAUSEANT   Oral or Parenteral (IM only)
Diet: Insure adequate fluid intake/hydration.
Oral/GI: Diarrhea. **S/Cond:** Avoid alcohol. Not c̄ lactation.
Caution c̄ geriatric[84] or pediatric pt.
Pregnancy: Category C.
Other: <u>Drowsiness</u>, dizziness, blurred vision, depression, hypotension, headache, muscle cramps/spasm, rash.
Rare- hepatotoxicity (jaundice), seizures, EPS.
Blood/Serum: Rare- dyscrasias.

trimethoprim with
sulfamethoxazole (TMP-SMZ)
   Bactrim/Bactrim DS
   Tab- starch,
    Na starch glycolate,

ANTIBIOTIC, Sulfonamide   Oral or Parenteral (IV)
Drug: Take c̄ food & ≥ 8 oz water.
Diet: Insure adequate fluid intake/hydration to insure output of ≥ 1500 cc/day.[1]
May need Fol suppl. Avoid SJW,[12] see p 286.
Nutr: <u>Anorexia</u>. Interferes c̄ Fol metabolism.

docusate Na,
Na benzoate
Parenteral- 1% benzyl
alcohol,
0.1% Na metabisulfite

Septra/Septra DS
Tab- Na starch glycolate,
docusate Na
Septra Susp & Grape Susp
Susp- 0.26% alcohol,
0.1% Na benzoate,
saccharin Na, sorbitol

Oral/GI: Stomatitis, glossitis, <u>N/V</u>, diarrhea.
Rare- pseudomembranous colitis.
S/Cond: Avoid alcohol- possible disulfiram-like reaction.[9b]
Not c̄ lactation. Caution c̄ diabetics on sulfonylurea- ↓ glucose.
Do dental care cautiously, see p 11 & 15.
Caution c̄ G6PD def- risk of hemolytic anemia. Not c̄ sulfa allergy.
Not c̄ megaloblastic anemia due to Fol def.
Caution c̄ ↓ hepatic func or ↓ renal func, geriatric, HIV/AIDS (↑ side effects).
Pregnancy: Category C.
Other: <u>Allergic reaction</u>, <u>rash</u>, <u>photosensitivity</u>, <u>fatigue</u>, <u>dizziness</u>,
<u>headache</u>, ataxia, depression, edema, insomnia, peripheral neuritis.
Rare- hepatitis, jaundice, SJS, TEN, pancreatitis (can be fatal).
Blood/Serum: ↑ AST, ↑ ALT, ↑ bil, ↑ BUN, ↑ crea, ↓ Fol, ↑ K, ↓ Na.
Rare- megaloblastic anemia, dyscrasias, ↓ platelets c̄ LT IV.
False ↑ crea c̄ Jaffe method.
Urinary: Crystalluria, stones.
Monitor: CBC, urinalysis, renal func c̄ LT use.

Trimox	ANTIBIOTIC	See **amoxicillin p 32**
TriNessa	ORAL CONTRACEPTIVE	See **Oral Contraceptives p 237**
Tri-Norinyl	ORAL CONTRACEPTIVE	See **Oral Contraceptives p 237**
triptans	ANTIMIGRAINE	See **Antimigraine p 39**
Tri-Sprintec	ORAL CONTRACEPTIVE	See **Oral Contraceptives p 237**
Trivora-28	ORAL CONTRACEPTIVE	See **Oral Contraceptives p 237**
Trizivir (TZV) Tab- Na starch glycolate	ANTIRETROVIRAL (HIV/AIDS), NRTI Three drug combination **S/Cond:** Not c̄ pediatric pts, hepatic or renal failure, body wt < 40 kg.[6]	See **abacavir p 19** See **lamivudine p 187** See **zidovudine p 348**

trospium **Sanctura/Sanctura SR**	ANTIMUSCARINIC	See **Bladder Control Agents** p 61
Truvada Tab- lactose, pre-gelatinized starch Gluten Free Combination drug	ANTIRETROVIRAL (HIV/AIDS), NRTI	See **emtricitabine** p 123 See **tenofovir** p 306
Tums	ANTACID, Mineral Supplement	See **calcium carbonate** p 70
Tussionex **hydrocodone** & **chlorpheniramine** SR Susp- alcohol free, ascorbic acid, sucrose, corn syrup, starch, vegetable oil, xanthan gum	ANTITUSSIVE	See listing for **codeine** p 91 See **chlorpheniramine** p 82
Tygacil	ANTIBIOTIC, Glycylcycline	See **tigecycline** p 314
Tykerb	ANTINEOPLASTIC	See **lapatinib** p 189
Tylenol	ANALGESIC	See **acetaminophen** p 22
Tylox Cap- Na metabisulfite, cornstarch Combination drug	ANALGESIC, Narcotic, Opioid	See **oxycodone** p 241 See **acetaminophen** p 22
Tyvaso	PULMONARY ARTERIAL HYPERTENSION TREATMENT (Inhalation Form) See **treprostinil** p 321	
Tyzeka	HEPATITIS B TREATMENT, Thymidine Nucleoside Analog See **telbivudine** p 304	
ubiquinone	ANTIOXIDANT	See **coenzyme Q-10** p 91
Uloric	ANTIGOUT, Xanthine Oxidase Inhibitor	See **febuxostat** p 136
Ultracet Tab- cornstarch, Na starch glycolate Combination drug	ANALGESIC	See **tramadol** p 319 See **acetaminophen** p 22
Ultram/Ultram ER	ANALGESIC	See **tramadol** p 319
Ultrase/Ultrase MT	PANCREATIC ENZYMES	See **pancrelipase** p 244
Unasyn	ANTIBIOTIC	See **ampicillin & sulbactam** p 35

Uniphyl	BRONCHODILATOR	See **theophylline p 311**
Uniretic Tab- lactose	ANTIHYPERTENSIVE, DIURETIC	
	Combination drug	See **Angiotensin Converting Enzyme Inhibitors p 36**
		See **hydrochlorothiazide p 166**
Unithroid	THYROID HORMONE	See **thyroid p 313**
Univasc moexipril	ANTIHYPERTENSIVE	See **Angiotensin Converting Enzyme Inhibitors p 36**
Urocit-K	URINARY ALKALINIZER	See **potassium citrate p 260**
UroPhos K	URINARY ALKALINIZER	See **phospates p 257**
Uroxatral alfuzosin	BPH TREATMENT	See **Alpha₁-Adrenergic Blockers p 28**

ustekinumab
Stelara
Sucrose-
38 mg/45mg vial
76 mg/90 mg vial

PLAQUE PSORIASIS, Interleukin 12 & 23 Antagonist   Parenteral (SC)
Drug: Given SC initially then 4 wk later, then q 12 wk
S/Cond: Caution c̄ lactation. Pt wt $\geq$ 220 lb requires higher dose.
Not for < 18 yr old.
Pregnancy: Category B.
Other: Headache, fatigue, dizziness, back pain, itching, infection,
nasopharyngitis. Rare- serious infection, malignancy.
Monitor: For active TB prior to & during treatment.
Urinary: UTI

valacyclovir
Valtrex Tab

ANTIVIRAL (Herpes Zoster & Genital Herpes)   Oral only
Pro drug of **acyclovir**   See listing for **acyclovir p 23**

valganciclovir
Valcyte Tab

ANTI-CMV, also to ↓ risk of heterosexual transmission of genital herpes
Pro drug of **ganciclovir**   See listing for **ganciclovir p 154**

Valium
diazepam

ANTIANXIETY, SKELETAL MUSCLE RELAXANT, ANTIEPILEPTIC
See **Benzodiazepines p 54**

T/U/V

valproic acid
  Depakene[a]
  Cap- corn oil
  Syrup- sorbitol,
   sucrose
divalproex sodium
  Depakote
  Sprinkle Cap[a]
  Tab (DR)[a,b,c]- cornstarch
  Depakote ER[a,b,c]
  Tab (DR)-
   lactose, propylene glycol
valproate sodium
  Depacon (IV)[a]

ANTIEPILEPTIC[a], ANTIMANIC[b], MIGRAINE PROPHYLAXIS[c]

Oral or Parenteral (IV)

Drug: Take c̄ meals to ↓ GI irritation. Swallow cap/tab whole c̄ water- do not crush or chew. Do not take syrup in carbonated beverages- will liberate drug & may cause mouth/throat irritation or unpleasant taste.[6] May mix contents of sprinkle cap c̄ 5 mL (1 tsp) semi-solid food (eg applesauce, pudding) (do not chew). Swallow immediately.

Diet: ↑ Ca & Vit D intake or suppl. Possibly carnitine suppl c̄ poor diet.[1, 93]

Nutr: ↑ appetite, ↑ wt. Anorexia, ↓ wt. ↑ Vit D metabolism.

Oral/GI: Periodontal abscess, NAUSEA/VOMITING, dyspepsia, cramps, gastroenteritis, diarrhea, constipation, fecal incontinence, flatulence.

S/Cond: Avoid alcohol. Not c̄ lactation. Not c̄ ↓ hepatic func or hepatic disease or urea cycle disorder. 82-90% serum pro bound. (↑ free fraction of drug c̄ ↓ hepatic func, ↓ renal func or geriatric[7]). Hypoalbuminemia (< 3.0 g/dL) may ↑ drug effects.[13] ↑ risk of osteoporosis c̄ LT use.[21]

Pregnancy: Category D.

Other: ↓ BONE DENSITY,[21] TREMOR, WEAKNESS, drowsiness, sedation, dizziness, peripheral edema, headache, rash, hair loss, nystagmus, fever/chills, chest pain, neck or muscle pain, ataxia, confusion, depression, amnesia, HTN or hypotension, hallucinations, emotional lability, photosensitivity, paresthesia, blurred vision, hearing abnormality, dyspnea. Rare- tardive dyskinesia, SIADH, suicidal thinking & behavior, pancreatitis, hepatotoxicity (either can be fatal).

Blood/Serum: ↓ VITAMIN D, ↑ alk phos, ↑ AST, ↑ ALT, ↑ LDH, ↑ bil, ↑ NH_3, ↓ WHITE BLOOD CELLS, ↓ NEUTROPHILS, ↓ PLATELETS, ↑ T_3, ↓ T_4, ↑ coagulation time, ↓ alb, ↓ prealbumin. Rare- ↑ glycine, ↑ amylase, ↓ carnitine, ↓ Na.

Urinary: False + ketones. Incontinence.

Monitor: Baseline hepatic func, CBC c̄ diff, platelets, electrolytes, then q mo x 6 mo, then q 3 mo for a year. Baseline PT/INR then at 2 wk, then q 3 mo.[21] Drug level, BW, renal func, amylase/lipase, NH_3, Vit D.

valsartan
  Diovan/Diovan HCT

ANTIHYPERTENSIVE   See **Angiotensin II Receptor Antagonists p 38**
    Diovan HCT also contains **hydrochlorothiazide,** see **p 166**

Valtrex
  valacyclovir

ANTIVIRAL, (Herpes Zoster & Genital Herpes)   Oral only- Tab
    Pro drug of **acyclovir**   See listing for **acyclovir p 23**

Valturna
  Tab

ANTIHYPERTTENSIVE   See **aliskiren p 26**
    Combination drug **aliskiren** & **valsartan** See **Angiotensin II Receptor Antagonists p 38**

vancomycin
  IV Vial generic
  Vancocin-
  Cap

ANTIBIOTIC   Oral or Parenteral (IV)
    Oral form indicated to treat Staph aureus enterocolitis or C. difficile
    (pseudomembranous colitis) only.
    IV form to treat/prevent MRSA or endocarditis.
    Drug: Pediatric dose based on body wt.
    Oral/GI: Little GI abs. Bitter taste, nausea.
    IV- Rare- pseudomembranous colitis.
    S/Cond: Not c̄ lactation. Caution c̄ ↓ renal func.
    Pregnancy: Cap- Category B. Soln & IV- Category C.
    Other: <u>Allergic reaction</u>, <u>rash.</u>
    IV- "<u>red man syndrome</u>", nephrotoxicity, ototoxicity, SJS, TEN.
    Blood/Serum: ↓ <u>WBC</u>, eosinophilia, ↑ BUN, ↑ crea. Rare- ↓ platelets.
    Monitor: Renal func, urinalysis, drug level. WBC c̄ LT use.

varenicline
Chantix
Tab

SMOKING CESSATION AID, Nicotinic Receptor Agonist
  Drug: Take after eating c̄ a full glass of water to ↓ nausea.
  Nutr: ↑ appetite, ↑ wt. Anorexia, ↓ wt.
  Oral/GI: Dry mouth, taste changes, gingivitis, dyspepsia, GERD, nausea/vomiting, abdominal pain, constipation, flatulence.
  S/Cond: Caution c̄ alcohol- may exacerbate psychological effects. Not c̄ lactation. Caution c̄ ↓ renal func.
  May cause mild physical dependence.
  Pregnancy: Category C.
  Other: Insomnia, abnormal dreams, headache, sleep disorder, drowsiness, lethargy, fatigue, URTI, rhinorrhea, ↑ sweating, dyspnea, rash, edema, joint/muscle/back pain, menstrual disorder, hot flush, HTN. Depression, anxiety, emotional disorder, irritability, restlessness, aggression. Rare, but may be serious- psychosis, suicidal thinking & behavior, hallucinations, euphoria.
  Blood/Serum: Abnormal hepatic func tests, anemia.
  Urinary: Polyuria.

Vaseretic
Tab- lactose, starch

ANTIHYPERTENSIVE, DIURETIC See **Angiotensin Converting Enzymes p 36**
  Combination drug **enalapril** & **hydrochlorothiazide**
                                          See **hydrochlorothiazide p 166**

Vasotec
  enalapril

ANTIHYPERTENSIVE   See **Angiotensin Converting Enzymes p 36**

Vectibix

ANTINEOPLASTIC (Colorectal Cancer)   See **panitumumab p 245**

Vectical

PLAQUE PSORIASIS TREATMENT   See **calcitriol** ointment **p 69**

Velban (generics only)

ANTINEOPLASTIC, Vinca Alkaloid   See **vinblastine p 334**

Velcade

ANTINEOPLASTIC (Multiple Myeloma), Proteasome Inhibitor
                                          See **bortezomib p 63**

venlafaxine	ANTIDEPRESSANT[a], ANTIANXIETY[b], TREATMENT of PANIC ATTACKS[b],

venlafaxine
  Effexor[a]
  Tab- lactose,
  Na starch glycolate

  Effexor XR[a,b] (SR)
  Cap

ANTIDEPRESSANT[a], ANTIANXIETY[b], TREATMENT of PANIC ATTACKS[b], SOCIAL ANXIETY[b] SNRI (Serotonin-Norepinephrine Reuptake Inhibitor)
    Also used to treat PMDD, hot flashes
    Drug: Take c̄ food to ↓ GI upset. Swallow XR cap whole c̄ liquid, do not divide, crush or chew.
    Diet: Avoid SJW, see p 286.
    Nutr: <u>Anorexia</u>, ↓ wt. ↑ appetite, ↑ wt. ↓ <u>growth</u> <u>in</u> <u>children</u>.
    Oral/GI: <u>Dry</u> <u>mouth</u>, taste changes, <u>N</u>/V, dyspepsia, <u>constipation</u>, diarrhea, flatulence, bleeding.
    S/Cond: Avoid alcohol. Not c̄ lactation.
    Caution c̄ ↓ hepatic func or ↓ renal func.
    Pregnancy: Category C.
    Other: <u>Drowsiness</u>, dizziness, <u>weakness</u>, insomnia, <u>nervousness</u>, <u>sweating</u>, <u>sexual</u> <u>dysfunction</u>, anxiety, confusion, tremor, headache, ↑ BP, blurred vision, flushing, edema, tachycardia, chills, rash, bruising, suicidal thinking & behavior. Withdrawal symptoms upon DC of drug. < 1%- seizures, SIADH.
    Blood/Serum: ↑ <u>chol</u>. < 1%- ↓ Na, dyscrasias, ↑ or ↓ glucose, ↑ uric acid, ↑ AST, ↑ alk phos, ↓ K.
    Monitor: BP.

Venofer	HEMATINIC, ANTIANEMIC	See **ferrous salts, parenteral p 141**
Ventolin HFA	BRONCHODILATOR	See **albuterol p 25**
VePesid (VP-16)	ANTINEOPLASTIC, Mitotic Inhibitor	See **etoposide p 132**
Veramyst fluticasone	ANTI-ALLERGIC RHINITIS	See listing for **beclomethasone p 51**

verapamil	ANTIARRHYTHMIC[a], ANTIANGINA[b], ANTIHYPERTENSIVE[c]	
Calan[a, b, c]	Ca Channel Blocker, Diphenylalkylamine Oral or Parenteral (IV)	
Tab- cornstarch, lactose	**Drug:** Swallow SR form whole c̄ food or milk.	
Calan SR[a]	May open **Verelan** Cap & sprinkle granules on 1 spoon cool applesauce.	
Tab- cornstarch	Swallow immediately- do not chew granules. Follow c a glass of cool water.	
Covera-HS (SR)[b, c]	Take other forms s̄ regard to food. Take PM/HS form at bedtime.	
Tab	**Diet:** ↓ Na, ↓ cal may be recommended. Avoid SJW,[125] see p 286.	
Isoptin SR Tab[c]	Caution c̄ grapefruit/related citrus, see p 390. Avoid natural licorice, see p 374.	
Verelan (SR)[c]	Limit caffeine (drug ↓ caffeine clearance), see p 379.	
Cap- sugar spheres (sucrose & starch)	Caution c̄ very high dose Ca &/or Vit D suppl (above UL)[93]- hypercalcemia ↓ effect of drug.	
Verelan PM (SR)[c]	**Oral/GI:** Gingival hyperplasia (rare), dyspepsia, nausea, <u>constipation</u>.	
Cap- starch, sugar spheres (sucrose & starch)	**S/Cond:** Avoid or limit alcohol- drug ↑ alcohol effect. Not c̄ lactation. 90% serum pro bound. Hypoalbuminemia (< 3 g/dL)- may ↑ drug effects. Caution c̄ ↓ hepatic func, ↓ renal func or CHF. **Pregnancy:** Category C. **Other:** ↓ <u>*BP*</u> c̄ possible hypotension, headache, dizziness, fatigue, weakness, rash, peripheral &/or pulmonary edema, bradycardia, tachycardia. Rare- hepatitis. **Blood/Serum:** ↑ AST, ↑ ALT. **Monitor:** BP, pulse. Hepatic func c̄ LT use.	
Versed midazolam	ANESTHESIA ADJUNCT, Sedative	See **Benzodiazepines p 54**
Vesicare solifenacin	ANTIMUSCARINIC	See **Bladder Control Agents p 61**
Vfend	ANTIFUNGAL	See **voriconazole p 342**
Viactiv	CALCIUM SUPPLEMENT	See **calcium carbonate p 70**
Candy Chew	500 mg Ca, 100 IU Vit D, 40 μg Vit K	See **vitamin D p 340**
20 cal/candy,	10 mg Na, 4 g CHO, 0.5 g fat	
corn syrup, sugar, non-fat milk, cocoa butter, soy lecithin		
Viagra	ERECTILE DYSFUNCTION TREATMENT	See **sildenafil p 292**

| **Vibramycin** | ANTIBIOTIC | See **Tetracyclines p 310** |
| doxycycline | | |

V-Cillin K previous brand name ANTIBIOTIC See **penicillin p 249**

Vicodin	ANALGESIC, Narcotic, Opioid	See listing for **oxycodone p 241**
Tab- starch	**hydrocodone bitartrate &**	See **acetaminophen p 22**
	acetaminophen	

| **Vicoprofen** | ANALGESIC, Narcotic, Opioid | See listing for **oxycodone p 241** |
| Tab- cornstarch | **hydrocodone bitartrate & ibuprofen** | See **ibuprofen p 170** |

Victoza ANTIHYPERGLYCEMIC, ADJUNCT TO DIET AND EXERCISE
IN ADULTS WITH TYPE 2 DIABETES MELLITUS, Glucagon like Peptide
Receptor Agonist, Incretin Mimetic See **liraglutide p 196**

Vidaza ANTINEOPLASTIC, Pyrimidine Nucleoside See **azacitidine p 48**

Videx ANTIRETROVIRAL (HIV/AIDS), NRTI See **didanosine (ddI) p 108**

vilazodone ANTIDEPRESSANT, SSRI
 Viibryd
 Tab- lactose,
 polyethylene glycol

   Drug: Take c̄ food to ↑ absorption of drug.
   Diet: Caution c̄ grapefruit/related citrus, see p 390. Not c̄ SJW, see p 286
   Nutr: ↑ appetite, ↓ appetite.
   Oral/GI: <u>Diarrhea</u>, <u>N</u>/V, <u>dry mouth</u>, dyspepsia, flatulence, gastroenteritis.
   S/Cond: Avoid alcohol. Caution c̄ lactation. 96-99% serum pro bound.
   Caution c̄ seizures. Not c̄ severe ↓ hepatic func. Caution c̄ bleeding risk.
   Pregnancy: Category C.
   Other: Dizziness, somnolence, paresthesia, tremor, insomnia,
   abnormal dreams, fatigue, feeling jittery, palpitations, restlessness, joint pain,
   sweating, migraine, withdrawal symptoms upon DC of drug.
   Rare- serotonin syndrome, NMS, mania/hypomania hyponatremia,
   suicidal thinking or behavior

V

Vimpat	ANTIEPILEPTIC	See **lacosamide p 186**

vinblastine
Velban
(previous brand name)
Generic Brand-
preservative free

ANTINEOPLASTIC, Vinca Alkaloid   Parenteral only (IV)
Multiple Indications   (not for intrathecal use- can be fatal)
Diet: Insure adequate fluid intake/hydration.
Nutr: <u>Anorexia</u>, ↓ wt.
Oral/GI: <u>Stomatitis</u>, pharyngitis, sore throat, <u>NAUSEA/VOMITING</u>, abdominal pain, ileus, <u>CONSTIPATION</u>, diarrhea. Rare- GI bleeding.
S/Cond: Not c̄ lactation. Do dental care cautiously, see p 11 & 15. Caution c̄ ↓ hepatic func, ↓ pulmonary func,[6] bone marrow suppression or gout.
Pregnancy: Category D.
Other: <u>BONE MARROW SUPPRESSION</u>, <u>HTN</u>, <u>HAIR LOSS</u>, <u>jaw & bone pain</u>, <u>neurotoxicity</u>, <u>peripheral neuritis</u>, <u>headache</u>, <u>depression</u>, <u>convulsions</u>, asthenia, bronchospasm, dizziness, skin lesions.
Blood/Serum: ↓ <u>WHITE BLOOD CELLS</u>, ↓ platelets, ↑ uric acid.[13] Rare- anemia.
Urinary: ↑ uric acid.[13]
Monitor: WBC before each dose. Weekly CBC c̄ diff, platelets, hepatic func.

vincristine
Oncovin (previous brand name)
Generic Brand
Parenteral
 mannitol 100 mg/mL
Vincasar PFS
Parenteral-
 mannitol 100 mg/mL
 preservative free

ANTINEOPLASTIC, Vinca Alkaloid   Parenteral only (IV)
Multiple Indications   (not for intrathecal use- can be fatal)
Diet: Insure adequate fluid intake/hydration.
Nutr: Anorexia, ↓ wt.
Oral/GI: Altered taste, rare stomatitis, <u>dysphagia</u>, mild N/V, bloating, <u>cramps</u>, ileus, <u>severe CONSTIPATION</u>, impaction.
Rare- intestinal necrosis &/or perforation, diarrhea.
S/Cond: Not c̄ lactation. Caution c̄ ↓ hepatic func, bone marrow suppression or gout.
Pregnancy: Category D.
Other: <u>NEUROTOXICITY</u> (<u>PERIPHERAL NEUROPATHY</u>, <u>PARESTHESIA</u>, <u>ATAXIA</u>, <u>NEURITIC PAIN</u>), <u>HAIR LOSS</u>, acute <u>uric acid nephropathy</u>, <u>jaw & bone pain</u>, <u>muscle pain</u>/wasting, HTN or hypotension, bronchospasm, headache, rash. Rare- SIADH.

Blood/Serum: ↑ <u>URIC</u> <u>ACID</u>, ↑ K. Rare- ↓ Na, ↓ WBC, anemia, ↓ platelets.
Urinary: ↑ <u>URIC</u> <u>ACID</u>, retention.
Monitor: Uric acid. Weekly CBC c̄ diff, platelets, hepatic func.

vinorelbine **Navelbine** preservative free	ANTINEOPLASTIC, Vinca Alkaloid, Lung Cancer	Parenteral only (IV) (not for intrathecal use- can be fatal)

Diet: Insure adequate fluid intake/hydration.
Nutr: <u>Anorexia</u>, possible ↓ wt.
Oral/GI: <u>Stomatitis</u>, <u>NAUSEA/VOMITING</u>, <u>severe</u> <u>CONSTIPATION</u>, <u>diarrhea</u>,
paralytic ileus, obstruction, intestinal necrosis &/or perforation.
S/Cond: Not c̄ lactation. Do dental care cautiously, see p 11 & 15.
Caution c̄ ↓ hepatic func, ↓ pulmonary func or bone marrow suppression.
Pregnancy: Category D.
Other: <u>BONE</u> <u>MARROW</u> <u>SUPPRESSION</u>, <u>PERIPHERAL</u> <u>NEUROPATHY</u>, <u>PARESTHESIA</u>,
<u>ASTHENIA</u>, <u>FATIGUE</u>, <u>HAIR</u> <u>LOSS</u>, jaw, muscle or bone pain, rash, cough,
pulmonary reactions/edema, dyspnea, bronchospasm,
HTN or hypotension, vasodilation, tachycardia. Rare- SIADH.
Blood/Serum: ↓ <u>WHITE</u> <u>BLOOD</u> <u>CELLS</u>, <u>MILD</u> <u>ANEMIA</u>, <u>severe</u> <u>anemia</u>, ↑ <u>AST</u>,
↑ <u>ALT</u>, ↑ <u>bil</u>, ↑ alk phos. Rare- ↓ platelets.
Monitor: CBC c̄ diff & bil before each dose, then 1-2x/wk.[26]
Hepatic func frequently.

Viokase	PANCREATIC ENZYMES	See **pancrelipase p 244**
Viracept	ANTIRETROVIRAL (HIV/AIDS), Protease Inhibitor	See **nelfinavir p 226**
Viramune	ANTIRETROVIRAL (HIV/AIDS), NNRTI	See **nevirapine p 226**
Viread	ANTIRETROVIRAL (HIV/AIDS), NRTI	See **tenofovir p 306**
Vistaril	ANTIANXIETY	See **hydroxyzine p 169**

V

vitamin A (retinol)
  Aquasol A (parenteral)
  50,000 IU/mL

  beta carotene
  (provitamin A)

VITAMIN, ANTIOXIDANT, Fat Soluble   Oral or Parenteral (IM)
  1 IU = 0.3 RAE (Retinol Activity Equivalent). 1 RAE = 1 µg retinol =
  12 µg beta carotene = 3.33 IU Vit A activity from retinol.
  eg: 5000 IU (half as beta carotene) = 1500 µg
  Drug: My mix soln $\bar{c}$ food or juice. Water miscible form ↑ abs.
  Diet: Adequate fat, pro, Vit E needed for proper abs.
  Vit E, Fe & Zn needed for proper utilization. Avoid MVI.
  Nutr: AI (µg/day) Infants 0-6 mo = **400**. 7-12 mo = **500**.
  RDA (µg/day) Children 1-3 yr = **300**. 4-8 = **400**. 9-13 = **600**.
  Males 14-70+ = **900**. Females 14-70+ = **700**.
  UL (µg/day preformed Vit A) Infants 0-12 mo = **600**. Children 1-3 yr = **600**.
  4-8 = **900**. 9-13 = **1700**. 14-18 = **2800**. Adults 19-70+ = **3000**.
  Lactation = **1200-1300**. **UL** = **2800-3000** µg/day preformed Vit A.
  Malnutrition ↑ Vit A requirements.
  Excessive Vit A ↓ Vit D effect on Ca abs.[93] Anorexia, ↓ wt $\bar{c}$ toxicity.
  Oral/GI: Toxicity causes stomatitis, N/V, abdominal discomfort.
  S/Cond: Excessive alcohol intake ↓ hepatic Vit A stores & ↑ toxicity of Vit A.
  Vit A abs is ↓ $\bar{c}$ chronic diarrhea, steatorrhea, parasites & infections,
  cystic fibrosis, hepatic &/or pancreatic disease, celiac disease.
  Avoid high dose $\bar{c}$ ↓ hepatic func or severe ↓ renal func.
  Def S/S- xerophthalmia (night blindness, dry corneas & conjunctiva,
  corneal lesions), anorexia, hyperkeratosis, ↑ infection, ↓ growth, diarrhea.
  Pregnancy: RDA = 750-770 µg/day.
  UL = (teratogenic potential) **2800-3000** µg/day preformed Vit A.
  Category X for parenteral.
  Other: Intakes ≥ 30,000 µg for months or years cause **hypervitaminosis A**
  (chronic toxicity). Acute toxicity $\bar{c}$ single dose of ≥ 150,000 µg in adults &
  proportionately less in children.[47]
  Signs of chronic toxicity (hypervitaminosis)- Ascites, ataxia, brittle
  nails, bone pain/fragility, conjunctivitis, depression, dizziness,
  dry skin, lips & mucous membranes, fatigue, fever, hair loss,
  headache, hepatotoxicity/hepatomegaly (can be fatal), irritability,
  itching, muscle pain, osteoporosis/↑ risk of hip fracture,

psychosis, visual changes.

Infants & young children- N/V, desquamation, skin lesions, hyperirritability, skeletal abnormalities, intracranial pressure (bulging fontanel).

Blood/Serum: Toxicity- ↑ Vit A, ↑ BUN, ↑ crea, ↑ chol, ↑ TG, ↑ Ca, ↑ AST, ↑ ALT, ↑ Alk Phos, ↓ WBC, ↓ RBC, ↓ platelets, ↓ prothrombin.

Urinary: ↑ frequency c̄ toxicity, ↑ Ca.

vitamin B$_1$	B COMPLEX VITAMIN	See **thiamine p 312**
vitamin B$_3$	B COMPLEX VITAMIN	See **niacin p 228**
vitamin B$_6$	B COMPLEX VITAMIN	See **pyridoxine p 271**

V

vitamin B$_{12}$
  cyanocobalamin
   CaloMist
   Nasal Spray-
   benzyl alcohol
   25 µg Vit B$_{12}$/spray

Nascobal
   Nasal Spray
   4.35% cobalt
   2.3 mL bottle = 8 sprays
   500 µg Vit B$_{12}$/spray

hydroxocobalamin
   Many Parenteral brands-
   benzyl alcohol

B COMPLEX VITAMIN, ANTIANEMIC, Water Soluble

Oral, Nasal or Parenteral (IM or SC)

Drug: Parenteral preferred to initially treat pernicious anemia, severe def or Vit B$_{12}$ malabs. Use **Nascobal** once a week in one nostril only. **CaloMist** 1-2x daily in both nostrils. Use spray $\geq$ one hr before or after hot food/liquid.

Diet: Caution $\bar{c}$ Fol suppl- may mask pernicious anemia & result in progressive nerve demyelination.

Nutr: AI (µg/day) Infants 0-6 mo = **0.4**. 7-12 mo = **0.5**.
RDA (µg/day) Children 1-3 yr = **0.9**. 4-8 = **1.2**. 9-13 = **1.8**.
14 & adult = **2.4**. Lactation = **2.8**.
IOM recommendation for adults $\geq$ 51- use Vit B$_{12}$ fortified foods or supplements to meet much of the RDA.[47] No documented toxicity- no **UL** set.[47]
Intrinsic factor & adequate Ca needed for proper abs of oral Vit B$_{12}$.

Oral/GI: Mild transient diarrhea. Nausea $\bar{c}$ spray.

S/Cond: Limit alcohol. $\downarrow$ abs of Vit B$_{12}$ $\bar{c}$ achlorhydria/atrophic gastritis (common in geriatric), gastrectomy, ileal resection, pancreatic insufficiency, small bowel disease, Crohn's, HIV/AIDS (especially $\bar{c}$ chronic diarrhea), antiulcer drugs, H. pylori gastritis.[103]
Vegan vegetarian or PKU diet may need suppl.
Not $\bar{c}$ Leber's disease- Vit B$_{12}$ causes optic atrophy.
Vit B$_{12}$ def- treat $\bar{c}$ IM form or oral form $\geq$ 500 µg/day.[126]

Def S/S- paresthesia, $\downarrow$ sense of vibration or position, unsteadiness, ataxia, neuropsychiatric disorders, dementia, visual changes, $\downarrow$ growth, $\uparrow$ MCV, $\uparrow$ MCH, $\downarrow$ Hb, $\downarrow$ HCT, pernicious anemia (macrocytic, megaloblastic), $\uparrow$ homocysteine, $\uparrow$ methylmalonic acid.
Neuropsychiatric damage due to subclinical def is not accompanied by anemia in 30% of cases.

Pregnancy: RDA = 2.6 µg/day. Category A for oral RDA dose.
Category C[7] for parenteral & nasal.

Other: Hypokalemia in first 48 hr of parenteral treatment (can be fatal), itching. Rare- anaphylactic shock. Nasal spray- rhinitis, headache.

Blood/Serum: ↓ K, ↑ platelets, ↓ <u>homocysteine</u>, ↑ *Vit B₁₂*.
Monitor: Baseline CBC, Vit B₁₂, Fe, Fol, then CBC, Vit B₁₂ after 1 mo, then q 3-6 mo. K & platelets (for first 48 hr of parenteral treatment & c̄ **Nascobal**).

vitamin C
  ascorbic acid
  Ca ascorbate
  94 mg Ca/g
  Na ascorbate
  115 mg Na/g
  Cap
  Chew Tab
  Crystals
  Liquid
  Lozenge
  Pwd
  Soln
  Tab
  Tab (SR)

  Parenteral
  250 mg/mL

VITAMIN, ANTISCURVY   Oral or Parenteral (IV, IM, SC)
  Water Soluble, Antioxidant
  Drug: 100-500 mg/day to treat scurvy.[6] Do <u>not</u> stop high dose abruptly-taper slowly.[7] May mix oral soln c̄ food or fruit juice.
  Diet: Take c̄ Fe suppl to ↑ Fe abs.
  Nutr: AI (mg/day) Infants 0-6 mo = **40**. 7-12 mo = **50**.
  RDA (mg/day) Children 1-3 yr = **15**. 4-8 = **25**. 9-13 = **45**.
  Males 14-18 = **75**. 19-70+ = **90**. Females 14-18 = **65**. 19-70+ = **75**.
  Lactation = **115-120**.
  UL (mg/day) Children 1-3 yr = **400**. 4-8 = **650**.
  9-13 = **1200**. 14-18 = **1800**. Adults 19-70+ = **2000**.
  Lactation = **1800-2000**. LT high dose (> 2 g/day)[13] may cause systemic conditioning, rebound scurvy if DC abruptly- but evidence is inconsistent.[47]
  Oral/GI: N/V, dyspepsia, gastric cramps, diarrhea c̄ > 1 g/day.[6]
  Excess use of chewable tabs breaks down tooth enamel & ↑ caries.
  S/Cond: Tobacco smoking & chewing ↑ Vit C requirements.[47]
  Caution c̄ G6PD def- risk of hemolytic anemia c̄ high dose Vit C.
  Caution c̄ ↓ renal func- risk of oxalate stones.
  Caution c̄ hemochromatosis- ↑ Fe abs ↑ Fe toxicity.[47]
  Def S/S: (scurvy)- Gum inflammation/bleeding, slow wound healing, joint pain, hyperkeratosis, petechiae & other hemorrhagic effects, edema, weakness, fatigue, depression, psychological changes.
  Pregnancy: RDA = **80-85** mg/day. UL = **1800-2000** mg/day.
  Category C[13] for parenteral.
  Blood/Serum: False ↓ bil.
  Urinary: ↑ <u>oxalate</u>, ↑ Ca,[6] ↓ Na,[6] ↑ or ↓ uric acid (dose dependent).
  <u>False values</u>- + Hb c̄ <u>dipstick</u>, ↑ <u>glucose</u> (CuSO₄), ↓ <u>glucose</u> (glucose oxidase).

V

vitamin D
  cholecalciferol (D$_3$)
  ergocalciferol (D$_2$)
  Cap
  Soln

VITAMIN, Ca REGULATOR, ANTIRICKETS
Fat Soluble 1µg = 40 IU   Oral or Parenteral (IM or IV)
Drug: Soln may be dropped directly in mouth or mixed c̄ soft food or juice.
Nutr: ↑ _CALCIUM ABS_. Vit D$_2$ is as effective as Vit D$_3$ in maintaining serum levels of active Vit D.[127] Anorexia, ↓ wt, ↑ thirst.
AI (µg/day) Birth-50 yr = **5** (200 IU). 51-70 = **10** (400 IU). 70+ = **15** (600 IU). Lactation = **5** (200 IU).
UL (µg/day) Infants = 0-12 mo = **25** (1,000 IU). 1-70+ yr = **50** (2,000 IU). Lactation = **50** (2,000 IU).
Sunshine (UV) causes skin production of Vit D3- metabolized by the liver & kidneys to the active form of 1,25 dihydroxy D3 (1,25 [OH]$_2$ - D$_3$)[127]. See **calcitriol p 68**.
Oral/GI: Dry mouth, metallic taste, N/V, constipation, diarrhea.
S/Cond: Not c̄ hypercalcemia or hyperphosphatemia. Caution c̄ ↓ renal func or ↓ cardiac func. ↑ risk of def c̄ low sun exposure, use of topical sun screen. Excessive Vit A ↓ Vit D effect on Ca abs.[93]
For geriatric- 1000 IU recommended to ↓ risk of fracture.[73, 78]
Def S/S- Rickets, poor bone growth in children, osteomalacia or osteoporosis in adults, bone pain, muscle cramps, palpitations, irritability, ↑ risk of Type 1 diabetes (risk ↑ 234%).[139]
To treat def in adult- 50,000 IU Vit D$_2$/wk X 8 wk.[127a]
Pregnancy: AI = 5 µg/day (200 IU). **UL = 50** µg/day (2,000 IU).
Other: 250-1500 µg/day in adults or ≥ 45 µg/day in children causes hypervitaminosis D.[13, 47]
Toxicity c̄ LT use- polydipsia, depression, headache, drowsiness, weakness, bone Ca loss/bone pain, hypercalcemia & metastatic calcification of soft tissues in kidney, heart, blood vessels, lungs. Poor growth in children. **Blood/Serum:** ↑ Ca, ↑ P, ↑ or ↓ alk phos, ↑ Mg. ↑ BUN, ↑ crea, ↑ AST, ↑ ALT, ↑ chol. ↓ PTH in hyperparathyroidism.
Urinary: ↑ Ca c̄ Vit D ≥ 60 µg (2,400 IU)/day, ↑ P, ↑ alb. Polyuria.
Monitor: Ca, P, renal func.

vitamin E
α-tocopherol

VITAMIN, Fat Soluble, Antioxidant

IU of natural Vit E X 0.67 = mg α-tocopherol (30 IU = 20 mg)
IU of synthetic Vit E X 0.45 = mg α-tocopherol (30 IU = 13.5 mg)
Drug: Water miscible form ↑ abs.
Swallow cap whole- do not crush or chew.[7] Mix soln c̄ food or juice.
Diet: High PUFA intake ↑ Vit E requirements.
High dose Vit E (> 10 IU/kg body wt) ↓ hematologic response to Fe in
children c̄ Fe def anemia.[6]
Nutr: AI (mg/day) Infants 0-6 mo = **4**. 7-12 mo = **5**.
RDA (mg/day) Children 1-3 yr = **6**. 4-8 = **7**. 9-13 = **11**.
14-adult 70+ = **15**. Lactation = **19**.
UL (mg/day) Children 1-3 yr = **200**. 4-8 = **300**. 9-13 = **600**. 14-18 = **800**.
Adults 19-70+ = **1,000**. Lactation = **800-1,000**.
Se antioxidant action is synergistic c̄ Vit E.[2]
Adequate Vit E essential for Vit A abs, storage, utilization,
but high Vit E (> 800 IU) ↓ beta carotene blood levels by 20%.[93]
Oral/GI: Toxicity- nausea, diarrhea, flatulence.
S/Cond: Steatorrhea, chronic diarrhea, parasites, cystic fibrosis,
or pancreatic disease- ↓ abs of Vit E. Caution c̄ Vit K def or
use of anticoagulants- high dose Vit E ↑ risk of hemorrhage.
Pregnancy: RDA = 15 mg/day. **UL = 800-1,000**.
Other: LT intakes ≥ 1,100 mg/day[47] can cause toxicity & fatigue,
emotional disturbances, thrombophlebitis, breast soreness,
thyroid effects.
Blood/Serum: Toxicity- ↑ CPK, ↑ chol, ↑ TG, ↓ thyroxine,
↓ triiodothyronine.[6]
Urinary: ↑ crea c̄ toxicity.

vitamin K
phytonadione (K₁)
  Parenteral
  0.9% benzyl alcohol
  Mephyton
  Tab- lactose,
  starch

VITAMIN, To Treat HYPOPROTHROMBINEMIA & ↑ Blood Clotting
  Fat Soluble   Oral or Parenteral (IM or SC preferred)
  Diet: See Vit K sources, p 388. Caution c̄ **coenzyme Q10**- ↑ risk of clotting.[93]
  Maintain consistent Vit K intake if taking anticoagulant (eg **warfarin**).
  Nutr: AI (µg/day) Infants 0-6 mo = **2** (infant AI assumes prophylactic
  Vit K given at birth). 7-12 mo = **2.5**.
  Children 1-3 yr = **30**. 4-8 = **55**. 9-13 = **60**. 14-18 = **75**.
  Males 19-70+ = **120**. Females 19-70+ = **90**. Lactation = **75-90**.
  No documented toxicity- no **UL** set.[47]
  S/Cond: Caution c̄ lactation c̄ pharmacologic dose. Caution c̄ use of
  anticoagulants- high dose Vit E suppl antagonizes Vit K action & ↑ risk of
  hemorrhage. Vit K ↓ anticoagulant activity & ↑ risk of clot formation.
  Caution c̄ ↓ hepatic func c̄ high dose Vit K.
  Pancreatic or intestinal disease may ↓ Vit K abs.
  Def S/S- Rare- ↑ PT/INR, bleeding, bruising.
  Pregnancy: AI = **75-90** µg/day. Category C for pharmacologic dose.
  Other: Parenteral- Rare anaphylactic reaction (especially c̄ IV), flushing,
  dizziness, sweating, ↓ BP, rash.
  Blood/Serum: ↓ PT/INR, ↑ clotting factors.
  Rare- hemolytic anemia, ↑ bil in neonate c̄ ↑ dose.[6]
  Urinary: ↓ Ca. **Monitor:** PT/INR.

Vivarin	STIMULANT	See **caffeine p 67**
Vivelle/Vivelle DOT	HORMONE	See **Hormone Therapy p 165**
Vivitrol	ALCOHOL DEPENDENCE TREATMENT Once a month Parenteral	See **naltrexone p 224**
Voltaren	ANTIARTHRITIC, NSAID	See **diclofenac sodium p 107**

voriconazole
  Vfend
  Tab- lactose,
  starch

ANTIFUNGAL for esophageal candidiasis, aspergillosis and other
  severe infections   Oral or Parenteral (IV)
  Drug: Take tab or susp one hr before or after food to ↑ abs.
  Diet: Avoid SJW,[3a] see p 286.

Pwd for Oral Susp-
sucrose, xanthan gum

Vfend I.V.
Pwd for IV

Oral/GI: Dry mouth, <u>N/V</u>, abdominal pain, diarrhea.
S/Cond: Not c̄ lactation. Correct hypokalemia, hypocalcemia or hypomagnesemia prior to drug use. Caution c̄ mild to moderate ↓ hepatic func. Not c̄ severe ↓ hepatic func.
IV- Not c̄ moderate to severe ↓ renal func.
Do not drive at night due to abnormal vision & photophobia.
Drug levels are ↑ in CYP2C19 poor metabolizers. **Pregnancy:** Category D.
Other: <u>VISUAL DISTURBANCES</u>, <u>rash</u>, <u>fever</u>, hallucinations, chills, dizziness, headache, peripheral edema, tachycardia, HTN, hypotension, photosensitivity, respiratory distress/disorder- eg dyspnea, pleural effusion, ↓ glucose tolerance.
Rare- hepatotoxicity, acute renal failure, anaphylaxis, SJS, TEN, ↑ QT interval, CHF, seizures.
Blood/Serum: ↑ <u>AST</u>, ↑ <u>ALT</u>, ↑ <u>alk phos</u>, ↑ bil, ↓ or ↑ K, ↓ or ↑ Mg, ↓ platelets, ↑ CPK, ↑ or ↓ Ca, ↑ chol, ↑ or ↓ Na, ↓ P, ↑ uric acid, ↑ glucose. Rare- dyscrasias, ↑ crea, ↑ BUN. **Urinary:** Alb.
Monitor: Vision. Baseline & periodic- hepatic func, renal func, electrolytes.

vorinostat
Zolinza
Cap

ANTINEOPLASTIC (cutaneous Tcell lymphoma- CTCL)
Histone Deacetylase (HDAC) Inhibitor
Drug: Take once a day c̄ food. Do not open or crush cap.
Diet: Insure adequate hydration/fluid intake c̄ ≥ 2 L/day.
Nutr: <u>ANOREXIA</u>, ↓ <u>wt</u>. Dehydration.
Oral/GI: <u>Dry</u> <u>mouth</u>, <small>TASTE CHANGES</small>, <small>NAUSEA</small>/vomiting, <small>DIARRHEA</small>, constipation.
S/Cond: Not c̄ lactation. Caution c̄ ↓ hepatic func. Not c̄ ↑ QT interval, hypokalemia, or hypomagnesemia. **Pregnancy:** Category D.
Other: <u>FATIGUE</u>, <u>muscle spasms</u>, <u>hair loss</u>, chills, dizziness, <u>edema</u>, <u>headache</u>, <u>itching</u>, <u>URTI</u>, <u>cough</u>, <u>fever</u>, pulmonary embolism.
Rare- ↑ QT interval.
Blood/Serum: ↓ <small>PLATELETS</small>, anemia, ↑ <small>CREA</small>, ↑ <small>GLUCOSE</small>, ↑ <u>PT/INR</u>, c̄ **warfarin** use. **Urinary:** <small>PROTEIN</small>.
Monitor: Baseline CBC, blood chem, electrolytes c̄ K, Mg, Ca, glucose, crea q 2 wk for the first 2 mo, then q mo. Baseline & periodic ECG.

VoSpire ER (SR)	BRONCHODILATOR	See **albuterol** p 25
Votrient	ANTINEOPLASTIC	See **pazopanib** p 246
VP-16 (VePesid)	ANTINEOPLASTIC, Mitotic Inhibitor	See **etoposide** p 132
Vytorin Tab- lactose	ANTIHYPERLIPIDEMIC Combination drug **simvastatin** & **ezetimibe**	See **ezetimibe** p 134 See **HMG-CoA Reductase Inhibitors** p 164
Vyvanse **lisdexamfetamine**	ADHD TREATMENT Cap	See listing for **amphetamines** p 33 pro-drug of **dextroamphetamine**

warfarin
Coumadin
Tab- lactose,
 starch
Parenteral-
 mannitol 38 mg/mL

ANTICOAGULANT Oral or Parenteral (IV)

Diet: Consistent intake of Vit K essential, see p 388. ↑ Vit K ↓ drug effect & ↓ Vit K ↑ drug effect. Caution c̄ Vit K or MVI suppl- changes in intake will ↑ or ↓ PT/INR. Caution c̄ Vit E > 400 IU- alters PT/INR.[3]
Do not exceed UL for Vit A- risk of bleeding, see p 336. ↑ pro/↓ CHO diet ↓ drug effect & ↓ PT/INR.[1] Caution c̄ ≥ 60 g raw, fried or boiled onions- ↓ platelet aggregation/↑ fibrinolytic activity/INR.[51, 85]
Avoid or limit natural products which affect coagulation (eg garlic, ginger, ginkgo, ginseng, saw palmetto, or horse chestnut).
Avoid Coenzyme Q10, SJW or avocado- counteract drug effect & ↓ PT/INR.[91] Case report of interaction c̄ fish oil- ↑ PT/INR.[3a]
Case reports of interaction c̄ soy milk or green tea- ↓ PT/INR.[93]
Quinine,[3] cranberry, papaya[93] or mango[3] reported to ↑ effect of drug & ↑ PT/INR. Multiple studies found NO interaction c̄ ≤ 250 mL cranberry juice- no effect on PT/INR.[128a]
Oral/GI: Taste changes, N/V, cramps, diarrhea.
S/Cond: Caution c̄ alcohol- chronic alcohol abuse ↑ metabolism of drug & ↓ PT/INR; acute intoxication ↓ metabolism of drug & ↑ PT/INR. Caution c̄ lactation, ↓ hepatic func, ↓ renal func, CHF, severe diabetes, pediatric or geriatric. Caution c̄ Asian pt- may need ↓ initial & maintainence dose. Genetic variations in CYP2C9 enzyme may affect **warfarin** metabolism. Genetic variation of VKORC1 may alter effect of

warfarin on Vit K. Either variation or both may require ↓ dose.
Genetic testing for these variations is available.
Do dental care cautiously, ↑ risk of bleeding. 99% serum pro bound.
Hypoalbuminemia (< 3 g/dL)- may ↑ drug effects.
Caution c̄ TF- monitor PT/INR after change in formula or rate.[25]
Pregnancy: Category X.
Other: Hemorrhage, fever, rash.
Rare- hepatitis or jaundice, systemic chol microembolization,
purple toes syndrome, priapism, hair loss.
Rare- skin necrosis, gangrene (may be fatal).
Blood/Serum: ↑ *PT/INR*, ↓ *CLOTTING FACTORS*.
Rare- ↓ WBC, ↑ AST, ↑ ALT, ↑ alk phos, ↑ bil.
Monitor: PT/INR frequently. CBC, hepatic func, fecal occult blood.

Welchol	ANTIHYPERLIPIDEMIC, Bile Acid Sequestrant	See **colesevelam p 92**

Wellbutrin/Wellbutrin SR   ANTIDEPRESSANT   See **bupropion p 65**
Wellbutrin XL

wheat dextrin   LAXATIVE, Bulk Forming Soluble Fiber
  Benefiber   **Drug:** Stir 2 t (3.5 g) pwd in ≥ 4 oz beverage or soft food.
  Gluten free   Not c̄ carbonated beverages. Follow c̄ 4-8 oz additional fluid.
  (< 20 ppm of gluten)   **Diet:** High fiber c̄ 1500-2000 mL fluid/day to prevent constipation.
  Pwd 2 t- 15 cal, 4 g CHO,   **Oral/GI:** Nausea, stomach pain, GI pain/discomfort, diarrhea, FLATULENCE.
  3 g fiber, Na free, sugar free   **Pregnancy:** Consult doctor about use in pregnancy.
  Chew Tab- 10 cal, 2.7 g CHO, sugar free, 1 g fiber/tab, sorbitol, cornstarch, sucralose, aspartame
  Tab- 5 cal, 1 g fiber, 1.3 g CHO

Xanax/Xanax XR   ANTIANXIETY   See **Benzodiazepines p 54**
  alprazolam

V/W/X

Xarelto	PREVENTION OF STROKE/SYSTEMIC EMBOLISM in NONVALVULAR ATRIAL FIBRILLATION, DVT PROPHYLAXIS IN KNEE OR HIP REPLACEMENT SURGERY, Selective Factor Xa inhibitor See **rivaroxaban p 282**	
Xeloda	ANTINEOPLASTIC, Antimetabolite See **capecitabine p 72**	
Xenazine	HUNTINGTON'S DISEASE CHOREA TREATMENT See **tetrabenazine p 309**	
Xenical	WEIGHT CONTROL AGENT, Lipase Inhibitor See **orlistat p 238**	
Xgeva	PREVENTION OF SKELETAL RELATED EVENTS IN PATIENTS WITH BONE METASTASES FROM SOLID TUMORS, RANK ligand inhibitor See **denosumab p 104**	
Xifaxan	ANTIBIOTIC See **rifaximin p 279**	
Xolair	ANTIASTHMA See **omalizumab p 234**	
Xopenex Inhalation Soln (nebulizer)	ANTIASTHMA, BRONCHODILATOR See listing for **albuterol p 25** Short acting R-isomer of **albuterol**	

Xopenex HFA Aerosol (inhaler/puffer)- dehydrated alcohol
  levalbuterol

Xyzal **levocetirizine** Tab- lactose	ANTIHISTAMINE for Allergic Rhinitis or Chronic Urticaria Active enantiomer of **cetirizine** See **cetirizine p 81**	
Yasmin-28	ORAL CONTRACEPTIVE See **Oral Contraceptives p 237**	
Yaz	ORAL CONTRACEPTIVE See **Oral Contraceptives p 237**	
Zanaflex	SKELETAL MUSCLE RELAXANT, ANTISPASMODIC See **tizanidine p 316**	
Zantac **ranitidine**	ANTIULCER, ANTIGERD, ANTISECRETORY See **Histamine H_2 Receptor Antagonists p 162**	

Zaroxolyn	DIURETIC	See **metolazone p 215**
Zebeta	ANTIHYPERTENSIVE	See **bisoprolol p 58**
Zegerid omeprazole	ANTIULCER, ANTIGERD, ANTISECRETORY	See **Proton Pump Inhibitors p 268**
Zelapar ODT	ANTIPARKINSON (adjunct to carbidopa/levodopa)	See **selegiline p 289**
Zemplar paricalcitol Cap- medium chain triglycerides, alcohol IV- propylene glycol 30%, alcohol 20%	TREATMENT OF SECONDARY HYPERPARATHYROIDISM in ESRD synthetic **Vitamin D**	Oral & Parenteral (IV) See listing for **calcitriol p 68**
Zenpep	PANCREATIC ENZYME	See **pancrelipase p 244**
Zerit/Zerit XR	ANTIRETROVIRAL (HIV/AIDS), NRTI	See **stavudine p 298**
Zestril/Zestoretic lisinopril	ANTIHYPERTENSIVE See **Angiotensin Converting Enzyme Inhibitors p 36** **Zestoretic** also contains **hydrochlorothiazide**, see **p 166**.	
Zetia	ANTIHYPERLIPDEMIC, Chol Abs Inhibitor See **ezetimibe p 134**	
Ziac Tab- starch, cornstarch	ANTIHYPERTENSIVE, DIURETIC Combination drug	See **bisoprolol p 58** See **hydrochlorothiazide p 166**
Ziagen	ANTIRETROVIRAL (HIV/AIDS), NRTI	See **abacavir p 19**

X/Y/Z

zidovudine
(AZT or ZDV)
Retrovir
Cap- cornstarch,
 starch
Tab- Na starch glycolate
Syrup- sucrose,
 Na benzoate 0.2%
IV- preservative free

ANTIRETROVIRAL (HIV/AIDS), PREVENTION OF MATERNAL-FETAL HIV TRANSMISSION, NRTI,　　　Also used as Anti-PML, dementia & to ↓ effects of cryptosporidiosis[61]　　　　　Oral or Parenteral (IV)
Drug: Take s̄ regard to food.
Diet: High fat meal (about 40 g) ↓ abs of drug.[3]
Nutr: ∧norexia.
Oral/GI: Taste changes, mouth ulcer, oral pigment changes, NAUSEA/vomiting, dyspepsia, dysphagia, pain, constipation, flatulence.
S/Cond: Avoid alcohol. Not c̄ lactation. Caution c̄ anemia, ↓ hepatic func, ↓ renal func, pediatric or geriatric. Extreme caution c̄ granulocytes < 1000 cells/mm³ or Hb < 9.5 g/dL.[7]
Pregnancy: Category C.
Prevention of HIV transmission to infant- Oral **zidovudine** wks 14-34, IV during labor, & syrup or IV to the neonate.
Other: BONE MARROW SUPPRESSION, headache, weakness, fatigue, confusion, dizziness, paresthesia, fever, muscle pain, insomnia, rash. Rare- lactic acidosis & hepatomegaly c̄ steatosis (↑ risk c̄ obesity) (can be fatal). Rare- SJS, TEN, rhabdomyolysis, neuropathy.
Blood/Serum: Severe ANEMIA, ↓ WHITE BLOOD CELLS, ↑ or ↓ platelets, other dyscrasias. Rare- ↑ AST, ↑ ALT, ↑ bil, ↑ LDH, ↑ CPK.
Monitor: Baseline CBC c̄ diff, then monthly x 3 months, then q 3 months, hepatic func.

Zinacef

ANTIBIOTIC, Cephalosporin　　　　　　See **cefuroxime sodium p 78**

zinc

Zn gluconate-
  14.3% zinc

Zn sulfate-
  23% zinc

Zn chloride-
  48% zinc

MINERAL SUPPLEMENT   Oral or Parenteral (IV as part of TPN)

Drug: Take 1 hr before or 2 hr after meals.[13]
If GI upset occurs take $\bar{c}$ food, but not ↑ fiber or ↑ phytate food.[47]
Diet: To avoid nonabsorbable complexes, take Zn ≥ 2 hr apart from Cu,
Fe, Ca suppl or food high in bran fiber, P rich pro (eg milk casein)
or phytate, see p 382. No interaction $\bar{c}$ Fol.
No interaction $\bar{c}$ P salts, Ca or Fe in food.[47]
↑ Zn requirement $\bar{c}$ vegan diet.
Nutr: ↑ bioavailability from animal protein sources.
LT excess suppl may cause Cu def, anorexia.
AI (mg/day) Infants 0-6 mo = **2**. **RDA** (mg/day) 7-12 mo = **3**.
Children 1-3 yr = **3**. 4-8 = **5**. 9-13 = **8**. Males 14-70+ = **11**.
Females 14-18 = **9**. 19-70+ = **8**. Lactation = **12-14**.
UL (mg/day) Infants 0-6 mo = **4**. 7-12 mo = **5**.
Children 1-3 yr = **7**. 4-8 = **12**. 9-13 = **23**. 14-18 = **34**.
Adults 19-70+ = **40**. Lactation = **34-40**.
Oral/GI: Intake > 50 mg/day- metallic taste, dyspepsia, N/V,
abdominal pain, diarrhea.
S/Cond: LT high alcohol intake ↑ risk of Zn def due to ↓ Zn abs &
↑ excretion. ↑ need in vegan diet, HIV, malabsorption syndromes, eg-
celiac, Crohn's. Avoid Zn suppl in Menkes' disease to avoid ↓ Cu.
Zn sulfate may precipitate TF,[8] see p 393.
Def S/S- ↓ growth, delayed wound healing, ↓ taste acuity, ↓ mental func,
↓ immune func, anorexia, diarrhea, hypogonadism, dermatitis,
eye lesions, night blindness, photosensitivity, hair loss, nail dystrophy,
↓ retinol binding pro, ↓ conversion of tryptophan to Nia,[47] ↓ alb, ↓ pre-alb.[47]
Pregnancy: RDA = 11-13 mg/day. **UL = 34-40**. Category C for parenteral.
Other: LT intake of 100-300 mg/day causes chronic toxicity- GI upset,
Cu def, CNS changes, headache, chills, fever, fatigue.
Acute toxicity occurs $\bar{c}$ single dose of ≥ 2 g.
Blood/Serum: ↑ Zn, ↑ alk phos.[13] Transient ↓ HDL $\bar{c}$ excessive intake.
Rare- ↓ Cu, dyscrasias- sideroblastic anemia (due to Cu def),
↓ neutrophils, ↓ WBC.

ziprasidone HCl
  Geodon
  Cap- lactose,
  starch
  Oral Susp-
  xylitol, xanthan gum
 	
ziprasidone mesylate
  Vial- single dose
	ANTIPSYCHOTIC, ANTIMANIC (Bipolar Disorder Treatment), Second
	    Generation Oral or Parenteral (IM for acute agitiation in psychosis)
	Drug: Take cap $\bar{c}$ meal containing $\geq$ 30% fat to $\uparrow$ abs approximately two-fold.
	Diet: Avoid grapefruit/related citrus $\bar{c}$ oral form, see p 390.
	Nutr: Anorexia. $\uparrow$ wt, primarily $\bar{c}$ baseline BMI < 23. $\downarrow$ wt $\bar{c}$ BMI > 27.
	Oral/GI: Dry mouth, $\uparrow$ salivation, tongue edema, dysphagia, N/V,
	dyspepsia, diarrhea, constipation.
	S/Cond: Avoid alcohol. Not $\bar{c}$ lactation. 99% serum pro bound.
	Hypoalbuminemia (< 3 g/dL) may $\uparrow$ drug effects.
	Not $\bar{c}$ hypokalemia, hypomagnesemia or cardiac arrhythmias.
	Caution $\bar{c}$ geriatric, Alzheimer's or seizures/history of seizures.
	IM- caution $\bar{c}$ $\downarrow$ renal func. **Pregnancy:** Category C.
	Other: <u>Drowsiness</u>, <u>respiratory disorders</u> (cold symptoms, URTI),
	orthostatic hypotension, <u>dizziness</u>, <u>EPS</u>, <u>akathisia</u>, $\uparrow$ QT interval,
	tachycardia, chest pain, dyspnea, nasal discharge,[17] weakness,
	muscle pain, vision changes, fungal dermatitis, rash, hypomania.[21]
	$\uparrow$ mortality in geriatrics $\bar{c}$ dementia-related psychosis.
	Blood/Serum: $\uparrow$ prolactin. Rare- $\uparrow$ glucose, $\uparrow$ Hb A1$_c$.
	Monitor: Baseline ECG. Serum K, Mg.[21] Baseline wt, then monthly.
	Baseline BP, Hb A1$_c$ & lipids at 12 wk, then at least annually.[1]

Zipsor	ANALGESIC	See **diclofenac potassium p 107**
Zirgan (ophthalmic gel)	ACUTE HERPETIC KERATITIS TREATMENT	See **ganciclovir p 154**
Zithromax	ANTIBIOTIC	See **azithromycin p 49**
Zmax	ANTIBIOTIC	See **azithromycin p 49**
Zocor simvastatin	ANTIHYPERLIPIDEMIC	See **HMG-CoA Reductase Inhibitors p 164**
Zofran/Zofran ODT	ANTIEMETIC, ANTINAUSEANT	See **ondansetron p 235**

Zoladex
  goserelin
	ENDOMETRIOSIS TREATMENT, ANTINEOPLASTIC, Hormone
	    SC Implant
		See listing for **leuprolide p 190**

zoledronic acid	HYPERCALCEMIA TREATMENT, ANTINEOPLASTIC[a]
Zometa[a]	OSTEOPOROSIS TREATMENT, PAGET'S DISEASE TREATMENT[b]
Reclast[b]	See **Bisphosphonates, Parenteral p 60**

Zolinza   ANTINEOPLASTIC, Skin Cancer   See **vorinostat p 343**

zolmitriptan   ANTIMIGRAINE, Serotonin 5-HT$_1$ Receptor Agonist   See **Antimigraine p 39**
  Zomig/Zomig-ZMT

Zoloft   ANTIDEPRESSANT, SSRI   See **sertraline p 291**

zolpidem   SLEEP AID, Non-Benzodiazepine, 8 hr duration
  Ambien   **Drug:** Take HS. Do not take immediately after a meal.
  Tab- lactose,   Food ↓ abs & delays onset of drug action.
  Na starch glycolate   Take **CR** tab whole, do not divide, crush or chew. Place sublingual tab
  Ambien CR   under tongue, do not swallow or take c̄ water. SL (**Intermezzo**) tab is
  Tab- lactose,   intended for middle of the night when return to sleep is difficult.
  Na starch glycolate   Tab should only be taken if at least 4 hr remain until wake up time.
  (2 layer- IR & SR)   **Oral/GI:** Dry mouth, pharyngitis, N/V, hiccups, diarrhea, constipation.
  Edluar sublingul tab   **S/Cond:** Avoid alcohol. Not c̄ lactation. 93% serum pro bound.
  mannitol, saccharin Na   Caution c̄ ↓ hepatic func, depression or geriatric.
  Intermezzo SL tab   **Pregnancy:** Category B. **Intermezzo** & **Edluar** SL tab, **CR** tab- Category C.
  mannitol, sorbitol,   **Other:** Daytime drowsiness, drugged feeling, dizziness, ataxia, headache,
  sucralose   rash, confusion, weakness, anxiety, depression, ↑ BP, hallucinations,
    memory problems, visual changes, tinnitus, muscle pain, tremor.
    Rare- parasomnias c̄ amnesia (eg sleep walking).

Zometa   HYPERCALCEMIA TREATMENT, ANTINEOPLASTIC
  zoledronic acid   See **Bisphosphonates, Parenteral p 60**

Zomig/Zomig-ZMT   ANTIMIGRAINE   See **Antimigraine p 39**
  zolmitriptan   Serotonin 5-HT$_1$ Receptor Agonist

Zonalon   ANTIPRURITIC   See **Tricyclic Antidepressants p 323**
  doxepin   topical cream

Z

zonisamide
  Zonegran
  Cap- vegetable oil

ANTIEPILEPTIC, Sulfonamide
  Drug: Swallow cap whole, do not open or chew.
  Diet: Insure adequate fluid intake/hydration to ↓ risk of kidney stones.
  Oral/GI: Dry mouth, taste changes, hiccups, <u>N</u>/V, dyspepsia, abdominal pain, diarrhea, constipation.
  Nutr: <u>Anorexia</u>, ↓ wt.
  S/Cond: Not c̄ lactation. Caution c̄ ↓ hepatic func, mild ↓ renal func or geriatric. Not c̄ moderate to severe ↓ renal func or sulfa allergy.
  Pregnancy: Category C.
  Other: <u>Drowsiness</u>, <u>dizziness</u>, ataxia, agitation, anxiety, confusion, insomnia, ↓ thought processes, speech abnormalities, paresthesias, headache, weakness, double vision, flu syndrome, rhinitis, cough, rash, kidney stone, status epilepticus, tinnitus, tremor, asthenia.
  Rare- SJS, TEN, heat stroke/hyperthermia (↑ in pediatrics).
  Rare- suicidal thinking & behavior; metabolic acidosis (may be more severe & frequent in younger pts).
  Blood/Serum: ↑ BUN, ↑ crea, ↑ alk phos.
  Monitor: Renal func. Baseline bicarbonate & periodically during treatment.

Zortess

IMMUNOSUPPRESSANT (To prevent organ transplant rejection)
                                        See **everolimus p 132**

Zosyn
  64 mg (2.79 mEq) Na/g

ANTIBIOTIC   Parenteral only (IV)   See listing for **penicillin p 249**
  Combination drug   **piperacillin sodium** & **tazobactam**

Zovirax

ANTIVIRAL (Herpes)   See **acyclovir p 23**

Z-Pak
  Zithromax

ANTIBIOTIC, Macrolide   See **azithromycin p 49**
  (pack of 6- 250 mg tabs)

Zyban

AID TO SMOKING CESSATION   See **bupropion p 65**

Zyloprim

ANTIGOUT   See **allopurinol p 27**

Zyprexa/Zyprexa IM

ANTIPSYCHOTIC, Second Generation   See **olanzapine p 233**

Zyprexa Zydis (ODT)	ANTIPSYCHOTIC, Second Generation	See **olanzapine p 233**
Zyrtec	ANTIHISTAMINE	See **cetirizine p 81**
Zyvox	ANTIBIOTIC, Oxazolidinone	See **linezolid p 195**

LABORATORY VALUES

<u>"Reference intervals" depend on the analytical method, specimen type and the specific laboratory performing the test. Always interpret test results relative to the laboratory's reference interval.</u>

Laboratory test results are influenced by many factors including medications. Always interpret results relative to the patient's condition and clinical situation. Values are for **blood/serum** unless otherwise stated.

*These tests indicate possible blood dyscrasia (any abnormal or pathological condition of the blood).

CONSTITUENT	REFERENCE RANGE	CAUSE/SIGNIFICANCE OF ABNORMAL VALUES
Activated Partial Thromboplastin Time (APTT)	26-37 seconds	See PTT, p 366.
Alanine Amino Transferase ALT	M: 4-40 U/L F: 4-31 U/L	↑ c̄ hepatitis, jaundice, cirrhosis, hepatic cancer, MI, severe burns, trauma, shock, mononucleosis, pancreatitis, obesity.
Albumin Alb <u>Depletion c̄ protein malnutrition:</u> <u>Mild</u> = 3-3.4 gm/dL <u>Moderate</u> = 2.1-3 gm/dL <u>Severe</u> < 2.1 gm/dL < 3 gm/dL ↓ binding of acidic drugs, resulting in ↑ free drug level = increased effects of drug.	3.5-5.0 gm/dL	↑ c̄ dehydration. ↓ c̄ edema, hepatic disease, malabsorption, diarrhea, burns, eclampsia, ESRD, malnutrition, low pro intake, stress, over-hydration, cancer. ↓ values normal in pregnancy. ↓ values normal c̄ aging, nephrotic syndrome.
Alkaline Phosphatase alk phos or ALP	Adult: 40-120 U/L Child: 60-530 U/L	<u>Marked</u> ↑ c̄ hepatic disease or metastasis, Paget's disease of bone, metastatic bone disease. <u>Moderate</u> ↑ c̄ hypercalcemia (indicates possible hyperparathyroidism), pancreatitis, hepatitis. <u>Also</u> ↑ c̄ bone growth (children/ pregnancy), Vit D def, rickets, osteomalacia, active AIDS infection. ↓ c̄ hypophosphatemia, malnutrition, cretinism, hypothyroidism, pernicious anemia, Vit C def/scurvy, milk-alkali syndrome, Zn def, Vit D excess.

Ammonia NH_3	Adult: 7-27 µmol/dL Child: 0-64 µmol/dL	↑ c̄ hepatic disease or coma (cirrhosis or severe hepatitis), severe heart failure, azotemia, pericarditis, pulmonary emphysema, acute bronchitis, Reye's syndrome, urea cycle defects. Also ↑ c̄ high protein diet, vigorous exercise, valproic acid therapy.
Amylase	30-110 U/L	↑ c̄ acute (or exacerbation of chronic) pancreatitis, mumps, perforated peptic ulcer, alcohol poisoning, renal insufficiency, acute cholecystitis, AIDS. ↓ c̄ hepatitis, cirrhosis, pancreatic insufficiency, toxemia of pregnancy, severe burns.
Anion gap $AG = [Na^+] - ([Cl^-] + [TCO_2])$	7-15 mmol/L	↑ in renal failure, ketoacidosis, lactic acidosis, poisoning c̄ ethylene glycol, methanol or salicylates. ↓ c̄ multiple myeloma, hypoalbuminemia, hyponatremia, bromide ingestion.
Anti-nuclear Antibodies ANA	<1:80	↑ c̄ systemic lupus erythematosus, Sjogren syndrome, scleroderma, rheumatiod arthritis, juvenile rheumatoid arthritis, systemic sclerosis, dermatomyositis/polymyositis, mixed connective tissue disease, hepatitis, leukemia, multiple sclerosis, primary biliary cirrhosis.
Aspartate Amino Transferase AST	M: 10-37 U/L F: 10-31 U/L	↑ c̄ cell injury/death: MI (4-10 X normal, ↓ to base by 4th day), acute cirrhosis, hepatitis, pancreatitis or renal disease, cancer, alcoholism, burns, trauma, crushing injury, muscular dystrophy, gangrene. ↓ c̄ uncontrolled DM (c̄ acidosis), beriberi (Thi def).
B-Type Natriuretic Peptide		↑ in congestive heart failure. Correlates with degree of left ventricular func. Elevated values ↓ with effective drug therapy for CHF.
BNP	< 100 pg/mL	
NT-proBNP 0-74 yrs ≥ 75 yrs	< 125 pg/mL < 450 pg/mL	

Bicarbonate HCO_3	22-29 mmol/L	↑ c̄ <u>metabolic alkalosis</u> (↓ acids/ ↑ HCO_3 in extracellular fluid), respiratory acidosis/suppression, emphysema, vomiting, aldosteronism, salicylate overdose (early). ↓ c̄ <u>metabolic acidosis</u>, renal failure, diabetic ketoacidosis, lactic acidosis, diarrhea, respiratory alkalosis/stimulation (hyperventilation, hysteria, lack of O_2, fever), primary hyperparathyroidism, salicylate overdose (late), starvation.
Bilirubin bil	Direct ≤ 0.3 mg/dL Total 1.0 mg/dL	↑ c̄ hepatitis, jaundice, cirrhosis, biliary obstruction, drug toxicity, hemolysis, prolonged fasting.
Blood Urea Nitrogen BUN	8-23 mg/dL	↑ (azotemia) c̄ renal failure (> 50 = serious impairment), shock, dehydration, infection, DM, chronic gout, excessive pro intake/catabolism, MI. ↓ c̄ hepatic failure, malnutrition, malabsorption, overhydration (excessive IV fluids), pregnancy, SIADH.
C-Reactive Protein CRP Risk factor for atherosclerotic event (MI, CVA or PVD)	regular CRP < 0.8 mg/dL high sensitivity CRP low risk: < 1mg/L average risk: 1-3 mg/L high risk: > 3 mg/L	↑ c̄ arterial inflammation, bacterial infections (appendicitis, otitis media, pyelonephritis, pelvic inflammatory disease), cancer, Crohn's disease, myocardial infarction, pancreatitis, rheumatic fever, rheumatoid arthritis, obesity.
Calcium (Total) Ca	8.4-10.2 mg/dL	↑ (hypercalcemia) c̄ cancer, hyperparathyroidism, adrenal insufficiency, hyperthyroidism, Paget's disease of bone, prolonged immobilization, excessive Vit D or Ca intake, LT use of thiazide diuretics, respiratory acidosis, milk-alkali syndrome. Chronic renal failure, granulomatous diseases. ↓ (hypocalcemia) c̄ hypoalbuminemia, elevated phosphorus, alkalosis, diarrhea, hypoparathyroidism, sprue, osteomalacia, malabsorption, diarrhea, acute pancreatitis, hypomagnesemia, starvation, steroid use, Vit D def.

Carbon Dioxide (CO₂)   22-29 mmol/L   See bicarbonate (HCO₃), p 356.
  Measure of blood alkalinity/acidity

Celiac Disease Panels
  IgA
  If IgA is ≥ 7 mg/dL then order
  Tissue transglutaminase Ab IgA   < 20 U/mL   ↑ with celiac disease in patients who are not IgA deficient.
                                                ↓ with celiac disease in patients who are IgA deficient.

  Deamidated gliadin peptide Ab IgA<20 U/mL   ↑ with celiac disease in patients who are not IgA deficient.
                                                ↓ with celiac disease in patients who are IgA deficient.

  If IgA is < 7 mg/dL then order
  Tissue transglutaminase Ab IgG   <20 U/mL   ↑ with celiac disease, useful when IgA deficient.
  Deamidated gliadin peptides Ab IgG<20 U/mL   ↑ with celiac disease, useful when IgA deficient.

Chloride   98-107 mEq/L   ↑ c̄ dehydration, eclampsia, anemia, hyperventilation,
  Cl   or mmol/L   cardiac decompensation, renal insufficiency,
                                                aspirin toxicity, diarrhea, diabetes insipidus,
                                                Cushing's syndrome, metabolic acidosis.
                                                ↓ c̄ diabetic acidosis, fever, acute infections, metabolic
                                                alkalosis, protracted vomiting, K deficiency.
                                                Chronic respiratory acidosis, SIADH.

*Cholesterol, total   desirable: 120-199 mg/dL   ↑ c̄ hyperlipidemia, obstructive jaundice, DM,
  chol   borderline: 200-239   hypothyroidism, obesity, high fat diet, tuberculosis.
   Strong risk factor   high risk: ≥ 240   Nephrotic syndrome, chronic renal failure,
   for CAD   child: 70-175   acute myocardial infarction, alcohol intake.
   In public screening   ↓ c̄ malabsorption, malnutrition, hepatic disease, stress,
   a patient c̄   anemia, sepsis, low fat diet, pregnancy, AIDS.
  CHOL ≥ 200 mg/dL should be further evaluated by a physician.

Cholesterol-High Density   low: < 40 mg/dL   ↑ c̄ regular, vigorous exercise, estrogen or insulin
Lipoprotein fraction   high: > 60 mg/dL   therapy, moderate alcohol intake.
   HDL   ↓ c̄ starvation, obesity, liver disease, diabetes mellitus,
                                                hyperthyroidism, smoking, AIDS.

Cholesterol-Low Density   optimal: <100 mg/dL   A **calculated value** (Friedwald formula)
Lipoprotein fraction above optimal: 100-129 mg/dL $\underline{LDL = total\ CHOL - HDL\ CHOL - (TG/5)}$
    LDL   borderline: 130-159 mg/dL   ↑ c̄ familial type II hyperlipidemia, high fat diet,
                 high :   160-189 mg/dL   hypothyroidism, hepatic disease, acute trauma, DM,
         very high: $\geq$ 190 mg/dL   pregnancy. ↓ in AIDS.

*Complete Blood Count (CBC) Consists of: WBC, RBC, Hb, HCT, MCV, MCH, MCHC,
*CBC Differential   Diff WBC = # of neutrophils, lymphocytes, monocytes,
  CBC c̄ diff   eosinophils, basophils as % of total WBC count.
  (see White Blood Cells)   (Many labs include platelets in CBC).

CK-MB mass   0-5 ng/mL   ↑ c̄ acute myocardial infarction, cardiac trauma,
  Cardiac specific CK isoform   renal failure, strenuous exercise.

Creatinine   adult: 0.4-1.2 mg/dL   ↑ c̄ acute & chronic renal disease, muscle damage,
  crea   hyperthyroidism, muscle mass, starvation, diabetic
                                       acidosis, high meat intake, gigantism, acromegaly.
                                       ↓ c̄ pregnancy.

Creatinine clearance   Male: 85-125 mL/min   ↑ in acromegaly and burns.
  GFR   Female: 75-115 mL/min   ↓ in CHF, glomerular (renal) disease, eclampsia, gout,
                                       multiple myeloma.

Creatine Phosphokinase   F: 20-180 U/L   ↑ c̄ MI or cardiac trauma, acute CVA, ALS, muscular
  CPK/CK   M: 20-200 U/L   dystrophy, hypothyroidism, vigorous exercise,
  Index of muscle/myocardium   electric burns/shock, chronic alcoholism,
   injury/disease.   hypokalemia, pulmonary edema.

Ferritin   F: 12-150 ng/mL   ↑ c̄ inflammatory diseases, chronic renal disease,
                     M: 30-320 ng/mL   malignancy, hepatitis, Fe overload, hemochromatosis.
                                       ↓ c̄ Fe def anemia.

Fibrinogen   150-430 mg/dL   ↑ c̄ inflammation, nephrotic syndrome, hepatitis,
                                   cirrhosis, pregnancy, estrogen therapy.
                                   ↓ c̄ liver disease, DIC, fibrinolytic therapy.

*Folic acid Folate Fol	2.8-40 ng/mL	↓ c̄ megaloblastic or hemolytic anemias, malnutrition, folate antagonist drug (eg anticonvulsant, methotrexate, oral contraceptives), malabsorption (eg sprue/celiac disease), alcoholic hepatic disease, hyperthyroidism, Vit C def, dialysis, febrile states, pregnancy, cancer.
gamma glutamyl transpeptidase GGT	M: 7-51 U/L F: 7-33 U/L	↑ c̄ hepatic disease, hepatotoxicity, biliary tract obstruction, pancreatitis, alcoholism.
Gastrin Upper limit of normal is very method dependent and may be as high as 300 pg/mL in some assays.	fasting level 0-100 pg/mL	↑ in Zollinger-Ellison syndrome, pyloric obstruction, following vagotomy, in some patients with peptic ulcer disease, drugs that inhibit stomach acid secretion, non-fasting state, following gastroscopy, in some insulin dependent diabetes, pheochromocytoma, some cancers of the colon, pancreas, breast or lung.
*Globulin	2.3-3.5 gm/dL	↑ c̄ infection, dehydration, Hodgkin's, Lupus, multiple myeloma, collagen disease, chronic alcoholism, shock, tuberculosis, leukemia. ↓ c̄ malnutrition.
Glucose, fasting Fasting blood sugar FBS	70-99 mg/dL	↑ c̄ DM, Cushing's syndrome, Thi def, acromegaly, gigantism, chronic hepatic dysfunction, severe infections, hyperthyroidism, pancreatitis, chronic hepatic disease, prolonged physical inactivity, chronic malnutrition, K def, drugs (eg corticosteroids, high dose antihypertensives, cyclosporine). ↓ c̄ insulin overdose, islet-cell carcinoma, bacterial sepsis, hypothyroidism, Addison's disease, extensive liver disease, glycogen storage disease, alcohol abuse, starvation, vigorous exercise, pancreatitis, oral hypoglycemic drugs.

Glucose-6-Phosphate Dehydrogenase G6PD (in RBC)	12.1 ± 2.09 IU/gm Hb[49] 4.6-13.5 IU/gm[62]	↑ c̄ pernicious anemia, chronic blood loss, other megaloblastic anemias. ↓ c̄ inherited G6PD def (X chromosome linked, ↑ in black males) = ↑ susceptibility to hemolytic anemia/hemolysis.
Glycated hemoglobin Hb A1$_C$ Index of LT glucose control (2-3 months)	4.0-6.0%	↑ c̄ poorly controlled/newly diagnosed DM, thalassemia, iron deficiency. Treatment goal: < 6.0%. The American Diabetes Association suggests additional action: > 8.0%. <u>Poor control:</u> > 12.0% ↓ c̄ sickle-cell anemia, other hemolytic anemias.
Growth hormone GH	Child: 0.1-8.8 ng/mL Adult male: 0.01-1.0 ng/mL Adult female: 0.03-10.0 ng/mL	↑ c̄ acromegaly, gigantism. ↓ c̄ hypothalmic, pituitary lesions, hypothyroidism.
H. pylori antibody, IgG	< 1.8 EV: Negative 1.8-2.2 EV: Equivocal >2.2 EV: Positive	↑ c̄ chronic superficial gastritis, gastric and duodenal ulcers, low grade B-cell gastric lymphomas.
Haptoglobin	30-200 mg/dL	↑ c̄ a variety of malignant neoplasms, infections, collagen vascular diseases, inflammation, obstructive jaundice. ↓ in hemolysis from any cause, megaloblastic anemia, ineffective erythropoiesis, congenital deficiency.
*Hematocrit HCT	F: 34-45% M: 41-51%	↑ c̄ dehydration, polycythemia, shock. ↓ c̄ anemia (< 30), blood loss, hemolysis, leukemia, hyperthyroidism, cirrhosis, over hydration.
*Hemoglobin Hb	F: 12.1-15.6 g/dL M: 14.6-17.5 g/dL	↑ c̄ severe burns, polycythemia, CHF, thalassemia, COPD, dehydration. ↓ c̄ anemia, hyperthyroidism, cirrhosis, many systemic diseases (eg leukemia, Lupus, Hodgkin's disease), HIV/AIDS.
Hb A1$_C$		See glycated hemoglobin above.

Homocysteine Homocystine Elevation indicates patient 　at ↑ risk for cardiovascular 　and thrombotic disease.	Fasting: 4-12 µmol/L	↑ c̄ homocystinuria (N-5, 10-methylene-tetra-hydrofolate def, aberrant Vit B_{12} metabolism, cystathionine-beta synthetase deficiency), folic acid def, drug therapy (phenobarbital, phenytoin). ↓ c̄ vitamin suppl (folic acid, Vit B_6, Vit B_{12}).
Insulin Fasting 4-27 µIU/mL 　30 min after 75g glucose: 20-112 µIU/mL 　60 min after 75g glucose: 29-88 µIU/mL 　90 min after 75g glucose: 26-84 µIU/mL 　120 min after 75g glucose: 22-79 µIU/mL		↑ c̄ acromegaly, cirrhosis, glucocoticoid excess, hyperparathyroidism, insulinoma, metabolic syndrome, polycystic ovary disease, Type 2 diabetes mellitus, (glucose measurements are the preferred method to detect insulin resistance). ↓ in growth hormone def, protein malnutrition, Type 1 diabetes mellitus.
International Normalized Ratio (INR) (for PT) Measures response to anticoagulant therapy (eg warfarin)	2-3 conventional 2.5-3.5 intensive anticoagulation (eg patients c̄ mechanical heart valves)	$INR = \left[\dfrac{Patient\ PT}{Mean\ Normal\ PT}\right]^{ISI}$ Where Patient and Mean Normal PT are in secs. Where ISI is the International Sensitivity Index for the thromboplastic product used.
Iron Fe	F: 30-160 µg/dL M: 50-170 µg/dL	↑ c̄ excessive Fe intake, hemolytic anemias, hepatic disease, estrogen use, hemochromatosis. ↓ c̄ Fe def anemia, chronic diseases (eg Lupus, rheumatoid arthritis), infections, hepatic disease, surgery, MI.
Ketones, URINE Acetone	0, negative	↑ c̄ diabetic ketoacidosis, fever, prolonged vomiting, diarrhea, ↑ fat-pro/ ↓ CHO diet, starvation, anorexia, drug therapy (eg levodopa, insulin).
Lactate	Plasma 0.5-2.2 mmol/dL	↑ c̄ lactic acidosis, strenuous exercise, sepsis, stress, toxins, NRTI (nucleoside reverse transcriptase inhibitor), metformin therapy.

Lactic Dehydrogenase LDH/LD	105-230 U/L	↑ c̄ MI, leukemia, megaloblastic or hemolytic anemias, pulmonary infarction, cancer, renal failure, shock c̄ anoxia, mononucleosis, muscular dystrophy. <u>Minor</u> ↑ c̄ cirrhosis, hepatitis, jaundice.
Lipoprotein (a) Lp (a)	< 30 mg/dL	↑ level associated c̄ increased risk for myocardial infarction, stroke, coronary artery disease, vein graft, re-stenosis and retinal artery occlusion.
Lipase	16-63 U/L	↑ c̄ acute (or exacerbation of chronic) pancreatitis, perforated peptic ulcer, renal insufficiency, acute cholecystitis, gallstones, AIDS. ↓ c̄ viral hepatitis, protein malnutrition, pancreatic insufficiency.
Lipoprotein-associated phospholiase A_2 (PLAC™)	< 235 ng/mL	↑ concentration associated c̄ ↑ increased risk for myocardial infarction & ischemic stroke.
Magnesium Mg	1.3-2.1 mEq/L	↑ c̄ renal failure, diabetic acidosis, hypothyroidism, Addison's, dehydration, overuse of Mg suppl or antacid. ↓ c̄ chronic diarrhea, alcoholism, pancreatitis, renal disease, hepatic cirrhosis, toxemia of pregnancy, hyperthyroidism, malabsorption, ulcerative colitis, K-depleting diuretics, malnutrition.
*Mean Corpuscular Hemoglobin (MCH)	26-33 pg/RBC	↑ See Mean Corpuscular Volume (MCV) below. ↓ See Mean Corpuscular Volume (MCV) below.
*Mean Corpuscular Hemoglobin Concentration MCHC	32-37 gm/dL (gm Hb/dL RBC)	↑ usually indicates hereditary spherocytosis. ↓ c̄ Fe def anemia, thalassemia minor, sideroblastic anemia, Pyr-responsive anemia, lead poisoning.

Mean Corpuscular Volume (MCV)	78-93 µm³/RBC (cubic microns/RBC)	↑ c̄ megaloblastic anemia due to Fol or Vit B_{12} def, liver disease, reticulocytosis, myelofibrosis. Spurious c̄ cold agglutinins. ↓ c̄ Fe def anemia, hereditary spherocytosis, thalassemia minor, sideroblastic anemia, Pyr-responsive anemia, lead poisoning.
Methemoglobin (ferrihemoglobin) Used to evaluate cyanosis	0-3%	↑ c̄ congenital methemoglobin reductase def, agents that cause oxidation of hemoglobin such as amyl nitrate, dapsone, nitroglycerin, aniline, naphthalene, nitrates, nitrites, nitrous oxide, others.
Methylmalonic acid	Serum: <0.4 µmol/L Urine: 0-3.6 mmol/mol creatinine	↑ c̄ Vit B_{12} def, methylmalonic acidemia.
Microalbumin, URINE	<30 mg/24 hour <30 mg/g creatinine	↑ c̄ diabetic nephropathy, congestive heart failure, various cancers, multiple myeloma, galactosemia, hypothyroidism, sickle cell disease, hypertension, glomerulonephritis, nephrotic syndrome, eclampsia, systemic lupus erythematosus.
Myoglobin	0-116 ng/mL	↑ c̄ skeletal or cardiac muscle damage, trauma, surgery, MI.
N-Telopeptide cross-links NTx	Serum: Premenopausal female: 6.2-19.0 nM BCE Adult male: 5.4-24.2 nM BCE Urine: Premenopausal female: 17-94 nM BCE Postmenopausal female: 26-124 nM BCE Adult male: 21-83 nM BCE	↑ c̄ osteoporosis, Paget's disease, metastatic bone disease, hyperparathyroidism, hyperthyroidism, immobilization. ↓ c̄ bisphosphonates, calcitonin, calcium, estrogen, Vit D.

Osmolality, serum	Child: 271-296 mOsm/kg Adult: 280-298 mOsm/kg	↑ c̄ hypernatremia, dehydration, hyperglycemia, diabetes insipidus, mannitol therapy, azotemia, ingestions (ethanol, ethylene glycol, methanol). ↓ c̄ overhydration, hyponatremia. SIADH.
Osmolality, urine	0-1 month: 50-645 mOsm/kg >1 month: 50-1200 mOsm/kg	↑ c̄ hypernatremia, dehydration, hyperglycemia, mannitol therapy, SIADH. ↓ c̄ overhydration, hyponatremia, diabetes insipidus.
pH Arterial Venous	7.35-7.45 7.31-7.41	↑ (alkalemia) c̄ respiratory or metabolic alkalosis, vomiting, ↓ K or Cl, high fever, hyperventilation, anoxia, cerebral hemorrhage. ↓ (acidemia) c̄ respiratory or metabolic acidosis, diabetic ketoacidosis, renal failure, diarrhea, respiratory depression, airway obstruction, shock, CHF.
Phosphorus, inorganic P (Phosphate PO_4)	2.3-4.3 mg/dL	↑ c̄ ESRD & severe nephritis, hypocalcemia, hypervitaminosis D, bone tumors, Addison's, hypoparathyroidism, acromegaly, sickle cell anemia. ↓ c̄ hyperparathyroidism (c̄ ↑ Ca), alcoholism, hypovitaminosis D, rickets or osteomalacia, hyperinsulinism, acute gout, overuse of P binders, Cushing's syndrome, salicylate poisoning, DM, alcoholism.
Platelets	177-406 x 1000/μL	↑ (thrombocytosis) c̄ malignancy (leukemia, lymphoma, solid tumor), polycythemia vera, post splenectomy rheumatoid arthritis, iron deficiency anemia. ↓ (thrombocytopenia) c̄ hemolytic or pernicious anemia, chemotherapy, infection, leukemia, inherited thrombocytopenia disorder, hypersplenism, hemorrhage, Lupus, disseminated intravascular coagulation.

| Potassium | 3.5-5.0 mEq/L | ↑ (hyperkalemia) c̄ renal failure, tissue damage, acidosis, Addison's, uncontrolled DM, internal hemorrhage, overuse of K suppl, acute AIDS. |
| K | | ↓ (hypokalemia) c̄ GI loss, IV fluid s̄ K suppl, alcohol abuse, malabsorption, malnutrition, diarrhea, vomiting, chronic stress or fever, K depleting diuretic, steroid, estrogen use, hepatic disease c̄ ascites, excessive licorice intake, renal disease. |

| Prealbumin (Transthyretin) | 18-38 mg/dL | ↑ c̄ renal failure, Hodgkin's disease. |
| Prealbumin is a better indicator of dietary change than albumin. Half-life is 2-3 days. Value not affected by Fe def. | < 10 mg/dL indicates significant malnutrition | ↓ c̄ acute catabolic states, hepatic disease, stress, infection, surgery, malnutrition, low protein intake. |

| Procalcitonin | <0.5 ng/mL | ↑ c̄ severe sepsis or septic shock |
| | > 2.0 ng/mL indicates severe sepsis/septic shock | |

| Protein electrophoresis | No paraprotein detected | Paraproteins can be detected in multiple myeloma, primary amyloidosis, lymphoma, macroglobulinemia of Waldenstrom, monoclonal gammopathy of unknown significance. |

| Protein, Total | 6.3-8.2 gm/dL | ↑ c̄ dehydration, diseases that ↑ globulin. |
| TP | | ↓ c̄ protein def, severe hepatic disease, malabsorption, diarrhea, severe burns or infection, edema, nephrotic syndrome. |

PSA	0-4 ng/mL	↑ c̄ benign prostatic hypertrophy, prostatic cancer, prostatitis, urinary retention. Digital rectal exam may falsely ↑.
Prostate specific antigen		4-10 ng/mL - increased risk of prostate cancer.
		> 10 ng/mL - highest risk of prostate cancer.

| PT | 12.0-15.5 seconds | ↑ c̄ prothrombin def, Vit K def, liver disease, decreased fibrinogen, anticoagulant therapy, biliary obstruction, salicylate intoxication, hypervitaminosis A, DIC disease, AIDS. |
| Prothrombin Time | | |

PTT   26-36 seconds
   Partial Thromboplastin time
   Screen for coagulation/clotting
   disorders & to monitor
   heparin therapy.

↑ c̄ Vit K def, hemophilia, hepatic disease, DIC disease, antibiotic therapy, clotting factor defect or deficiencies, AIDS.
↓ c̄ extensive cancer (except c̄ hepatic involvement), acute hemorrhage, early DIC.

*RBC   F: 3.9-5.5
   Red Blood Cell Count   million/mm^3
   erythrocytes   M: 4.7-6.1

↑ c̄ polycythemia, dehydration, severe diarrhea.
↓ c̄ anemia, hemorrhage, Fe def, systemic disease (eg Hodgkin's, leukemia, Lupus).

Reticulocyte Count   Percent of Total
                      Erythrocytes
       Adults: 0.4%-2.3%
    Children: 0.8%-2.8%

↑ c̄ hemolytic anemias, 3-4 days post hemorrhage, sickle cell disease.
↓ c̄ Fe def anemias, aplastic anemia, untreated pernicious anemia, chronic infection, radiation therapy, endocrine problems, tumor in bone marrow, myelodysplastic syndromes.

Serum Glutamic Oxaloacetic Transaminase (SGOT)   See Aspartate Amino Transferase (AST), p 355.

Serum Glutamic Pyruvic Transaminase (SGPT)   See Alanine Amino Transferase (ALT), p 354.

Sodium   136-144 mEq/L
   Na

↑ (hypernatremia) c̄ dehydration & low fluid intake, diabetes insipidus, Cushing's syndrome, coma, primary aldosteronism.
↓ (hyponatremia) c̄ edema, severe burns, severe diarrhea/vomiting, diuretics, SIADH, water intoxication, Addison's disease, severe nephritis, starvation, hyperglycemia, malabsorption, AIDS.

Specific Gravity   1.016-1.022
   URINE   (c̄ normal fluid
   SG   intake)

↑ SG (concentrated urine) c̄ DM, nephrosis, fever, dehydration, vomiting, diarrhea, low fluid intake.
↓ SG (dilute urine) c̄ diabetes insipidus, chronic pyelo- or glomerulo-nephritis, severe renal damage, water intoxication.

Testosterone			
	Male		↑ c̄ polycystic ovary syndrome, congenital adrenal hyperplasia, androgen resistance, in women c̄ Cushing's syndrome, hirsutism, adrenal or ovarian androgen secreting tumors.
	Tanner Stage I	< 30 ng/dL	
	Tanner Stage II	<150 ng/dL	
	Tanner Stage III	100 -320 ng/dL	
	Tanner Stage IV, V	200-970 ng/dL	
	20-39 years	400-1080 ng/dL	↓ c̄ male hypogonadism, in men c̄ Cushing's syndrome or those receiving corticosteroid therapy, AIDS wasting.
	40-59 years	350-890 ng/dL	
	60 & over	350-720 ng/dL	
	Female		
	Tanner Stage I	< 10 ng/dL	
	Tanner Stage II	< 30 ng/dL	
	Tanner Stage III	< 35 ng/dL	
	Tanner Stage IV, V	15-40 ng/dL	

20-39 years- 15-70 ng/dL, 40-59 years- 4-70 ng/dL, 60 & over- 4-60 ng/dL

Thyroxine T_4 Free	0.8-1.5 ng/dL	↑ c̄ hyperthyroidism, toxic goiter, anorexia nervosa, hyperemesis gravidarum.
		↓ c̄ hypothyroidism, pre-eclampsia, chronic renal failure.

Total triiodothyronine T_3	70-180 ng/dL	↑ c̄ hyperthyroidism, thyroid hormone therapy.
		↓ c̄ chronic renal failure, hyperparathyroidism, hypothyroidism, nephrotic syndrome, nonthyroidal illness, protein calorie malnutrition.

Thyroid-stimulating hormone TSH	0.4-5.0 µU/mL	↑ c̄ primary hypothyroidism.
		↓ c̄ hyperthyroidism, secondary hypothyroidism, thyroid hormone therapy.

Tissue Transglutaminase Antibody		↑ c̄ celiac disease, dermatitis herpetiformis, Crohn's disease.
IgA	<7.0 AU	
IgG	<30 EU	

Total Iron-Binding Capacity TIBC	240-450 µg/dL	↑ c̄ Fe def, pregnancy, Fe def anemia.
		↓ c̄ chronic inflammatory states, Fe overload, hemochromatosis.

Transferrin	212-360 mg/dL	↑ c̄ inadequate Fe stores, Fe def anemia, acute hepatitis, polycythemia, oral contraceptive use, pregnancy. ↓ c̄ pernicious & sickle-cell anemia, infection, cancer, hepatic disease, malnutrition, nephrotic syndrome, thalassemia. <u>Mild</u> ↓ = 150-200. <u>Moderate</u> ↓ = 100-150. <u>Severe</u> ↓ = < 100.
Triglycerides TG	(fasting range) desirable: < 150 mg/dL borderline: 150-199 mg/dL high: 200-499 mg/dL very high: ≥ 500 mg/dL	↑ c̄ hyperlipidemias, hepatic disease, pancreatitis, poorly controlled DM, hypothyroidism, MI, alcoholism, high sugar &/or fat intake, AIDS. ↓ c̄ malnutrition, malabsorption syndrome, hyperthyroidism, COPD.
Troponin Either Troponin I or Troponin T Cardiac specific markers	Troponin I ≤ 2.0 ng/mL Troponin T ≤ 0.1ng/mL	↑ 4-10 hr after MI onset. Also ↑ in unstable angina, chronic renal failure (T more frequently than I). Not ↑ in skeletal muscle disease or injury.
Uric Acid	F: 2.5-6.1 mg/dL M: 3.7-7.8 mg/dL	↑ c̄ renal failure, gout, anorexia, leukemias, acute infectious disease, metastatic cancer, severe eclampsia, shock, diabetic ketosis, metabolic acidosis, lead poisoning, stress, alcoholism, rigorous exercise, polycythemia, psoriasis, asymptomatic hyperuricemia. ↓ c̄ antigout drugs (eg allopurinol, probenecid), Wilson's disease, cancer. Healthy adults are often below references.
Vitamin B_{12} Vit B_{12}	210-911 pg/mL	↑ (> 1100 pg/mL) c̄ hepatic disease, some leukemias, cancer (especially c̄ hepatic metastasis), pregnancy, oral contraceptives. ↓ (< 100 pg/mL) c̄ pernicious anemia, malabsorption syndromes, primary hypothyroidism, ↓ gastric mucosa (eg gastrectomy or stomach cancer), vegetarian diet, achlorhydria.

Vitamin D, 25 Hydroxy	20-80 ng/mL Optimal > 30 ng/mL Toxic >150 ng/mL		↑ c̄ statin use, vitamin D dependent rickets, vitamin D, 25OH intoxication. ↓ dietary deficiency, liver disease, nephrotic syndrome, primary sclerosing cholangitis.
Vitamin D, 1, 25-Dihydroxy	15-75 pg/mL		↑ granulomatous disease, hyperparathyroidism, idiopathic hypercalciuria, lymphoma, vitamin D $1,25(OH)_2$ intoxication. ↓ dietary deficiency, hyperphosphotemia, hypomagnesemia, hypoparathyroidism, liver disease, malabsorption, renal failure, vitamin D dependent rickets.
White Blood Cells WBC Leukocyte Count	3200-10,600/µL		↑ (leukocytosis) c̄ leukemia, bacterial infection, hemorrhage, trauma or tissue injury, cancer. ↓ (leukopenia) c̄ some viral infections, chemotherapy, radiation, bone-marrow depression, HIV, AIDS.

		Absolute	
	Relative %	Value #/µL	
*WBC diff	Neutrophils 44-76%	1300-7000	The relative percentage or number of each type of
Differential	Eosinophils 0-6%	0-400	leukocyte (white blood cell) in the blood.[49]
Leukocyte	Basophils 0-2%	0-100	Formula:
Count	Lymphocytes 15-43%	800-3100	
	Monocytes 2-8%	100-500	

Absolute value = Relative percent X total WBC ct
WBC/mm^3 = (%) X (cells mm^3)

Zinc Zn	M: 50-291 µg/dL F: 65-256 µg/dL	↑ c̄ CHD, arteriosclerosis, osteosarcoma. ↓ c̄ malnutrition, dialysis, protein-losing enteropathy, inflammatory bowel disease, nephrotic syndrome, burns or trauma, prolonged TPN, alcoholism, alcoholic cirrhosis or pancreatitis, anorexia, pernicious or sickle cell anemia, cancer c̄ hepatic metastasis, tuberculosis, thalassemia, hypoalbuminemia.

Edited by William L. Roberts MD, PhD, Dir Clinical Chemistry, ARUP Laboratories; Professor of Pathology, University of Utah, Salt Lake City, UT. References: 7, 52, 58, 63, 67, 92.

COMPARISON OF HEIGHT-WEIGHT TABLES

Height	Metropolitan 1983 Weights for Ages 25-59 Men	Women	Gerontology Research Center Weight Range for Men and Women by Age (Years) 20-29	30-39	40-49	50-59	60-69
ft-In	lb		lb				
4-10		100-131	84-111	92-119	99-127	107-135	115-142
4-11		101-134	87-115	95-123	103-131	111-139	119-147
5-0		103-137	90-119	98-127	106-135	114-143	123-152
5-1	123-145	105-140	93-123	101-131	110-140	118-148	127-157
5-2	125-148	108-144	96-127	105-136	113-144	122-153	131-163
5-3	127-151	111-148	99-131	108-140	117-149	126-158	135-168
5-4	129-155	114-152	102-135	112-145	121-154	130-163	140-173
5-5	131-159	117-156	106-140	115-149	125-159	134-168	144-179
5-6	133-163	120-160	109-144	119-154	129-164	138-174	148-184
5-7	135-167	123-164	112-148	122-159	133-169	143-179	153-190
5-8	137-171	126-167	116-153	126-163	137-174	147-184	158-196
5-9	139-175	129-170	119-157	130-168	141-179	151-190	162-201
5-10	141-179	132-173	122-162	134-173	145-184	156-195	167-207
5-11	144-183	135-176	126-167	137-178	149-190	160-210	172-213
6-0	147-187		129-171	141-183	153-195	165-207	177-219
6-1	150-192		133-176	145-188	157-200	169-213	182-225
6-2	153-197		137-181	149-194	162-206	174-219	187-232
6-3	157-202		141-186	153-199	166-212	179-225	192-238
6-4			144-191	157-205	171-218	184-231	197-244

From: Environmental Nutrition, Vol II, #3, March 1988.

Values in these tables are for height without shoes and weight without clothes.

Weight ranges are the weight for small frame at the lower limit and large frame at the upper limit.

Segmental Weights for Limbs
Use to estimate body weight for amputees

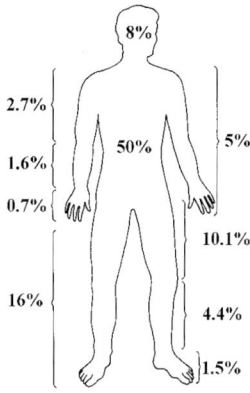

$$Wt_E = Wt_O/1-P$$

Wt_E = estimate of total body weight
Wt_O = observed body weight
P = percentage of total body weight represented by missing limb
References upon request

IDEAL BODY WEIGHT CALCULATION

Build	Height	Calculation
F: Medium Frame	1st 5 ft	Allow 100 lbs & add 5 lbs/inch
Large Frame		Add 10%
Small Frame		Subtract 10%
M: Medium Frame	1st 5 ft	Allow 106 lbs & add 6 lbs/inch
Large Frame		Add 10%
Small Frame		Subtract 10%

Paraplegic: subtract 5-10% from ideal body weight

BODY MASS INDEX (BMI)
Corrects body weight for height, correlated $\bar{c}$ body fat.

$$BMI = \frac{weight\ (kilograms)}{height^2\ (meters)}$$

$$BMI = \left[\frac{weight\ (lb.)}{height\ (in.)^2}\right] \times 703$$

NUTRITIONAL ASSESSMENT STANDARDS FOR ADULT FEMALES

Height ft+in	Ideal Body Weight[a] lbs (- or + 10%)	kg	Calories[b] 25-35/kg	Fluid Minimum[b,c] 30 mL/kg/day	Cups[d]	Protein Minimum[b] 0.8-1.0 g/kg/day
4'9"	85 (77-94)	38.6	970-1350	1160	4.75	31-39
4'10"	90 (81-99)	40.9	1020-1430	1230	5.0	33-41
4'11"	95 (86-105)	43.2	1080-1540	1300	5.5	35-43
5'0"	100 (90-110)	45.5	1140-1590	1360	5.75	36-45
5'1"	105 (95-116)	47.7	1190-1670	1430	6.0	38-48
5'2"	110 (99-121)	50.0	1250-1750	1500	6.25	40-50
5'3"	115 (104-127)	52.3	1310-1830	1570	6.5	49-52
5'4"	120 (108-132)	54.5	1360-1910	1640	6.75	44-55
5'5"	125 (113-138)	56.8	1420-1990	1710	7.0	45-57
5'6"	130 (117-143)	59.1	1480-2070	1770	7.5	47-59
5'7"	135 (122-149)	61.4	1540-2150	1840	7.75	49-61
5'8"	140 (126-154)	63.6	1590-2230	1910	8.0	52-64
5'9"	145 (131-160)	65.9	1650-2310	1980	8.25	53-66
5'10"	150 (135-165)	68.1	1700-2380	2050	8.5	54-68
5'11"	155 (140-171)	70.5	1760-2470	2110	8.75	56-71
6'0"	160 (144-176)	72.7	1820-2540	2180	9.0	58-73

a- Lower weight for small frame, higher weight for large frame.
b- Calories, fluid and protein amounts are for medium frame. Subtract 10% for small frame, add 10% for large frame.
c- Fluid minimum reflects minimum fluid standard for median calorie intake.
d- To convert from cups to ounces, multiply by 8. eg: 5 cups equal 40 ounces.

NUTRITIONAL ASSESSMENT STANDARDS FOR ADULT MALES

Height ft+in	Ideal Body Weight[a] lbs (- or + 10%)	kg	Calories[b] 25-35/kg	Fluid Minimum[b,c] 30 mL/kg/day	Cups[d]	Protein Minimum[b] 0.8-1.0 g/kg/day
5'2"	118 (106-130)	53.6	1340-1880	1610	6.75	43-54
5'3"	124 (112-136)	56.4	1410-1970	1690	7.0	45-56
5'4"	130 (117-143)	59.1	1480-2070	1770	7.5	47-59
5'5"	136 (122-150)	61.8	1550-2160	1860	7.75	49-62
5'6"	142 (128-156)	64.5	1610-2260	1940	8.0	52-65
5'7"	148 (133-163)	67.3	1680-2360	2020	8.5	54-67
5'8"	154 (139-169)	70.0	1750-2450	2100	8.75	56-70
5'9"	160 (144-176)	72.7	1820-2540	2180	9.0	58-73
5'10"	166 (149-183)	75.5	1890-2640	2260	9.5	60-75
5'11"	172 (155-189)	78.1	1950-2730	2350	9.75	62-78
6'0"	178 (160-196)	80.9	2020-2830	2430	10.0	65-81
6'1"	184 (166-202)	83.6	2090-2930	2510	10.5	67-84
6'2"	190 (171-209)	86.4	2160-3020	2590	10.75	69-86
6'3"	196 (176-216)	89.1	2230-3120	2670	11.0	71-89
6'4"	202 (182-222)	91.8	2300-3200	2760	11.5	73-92
6'5"	208 (186-228)	94.5	2370-3270	2890	12.0	75-94

a- Lower weight for small frame, higher weight for large frame.
b- Calories, fluid and protein are for medium frame. Subtract 10% for small frame, add 10% for large frame.
c- Fluid minimum reflects minimum fluid standard for median calorie intake.
d- To convert from cups to ounces, multiply by 8. eg: 5 cups equal 40 ounces.

Table created by: Linda Kautz Osterkamp, PhD, RD, FADA, Christine H. Smith, PhD, RD & Zaneta M. Pronsky, MS, RD, LDN, FADA

POTENTIAL INTERACTIVE INGREDIENTS

Food may contain ingredients which interact with drugs. Drugs may contain excipients. These are ingredients that are added to give form, consistency or to act as a diluent. Excipients may cause reactions as noted in this table.

Albumin (egg or human): In some medications. May cause allergic reaction. Human albumin is a blood product.

Alcohol (ethanol): CNS depressant used as a solvent in medications. All alcohol and alcohol containing products and drugs must be avoided with medications such as disulfiram (Antabuse) or limited with other drugs to prevent additive CNS or hepatic toxicity. See individual drug listings and the chart on p 376.

Aspartame: Artificial sweetener composed of the amino acids aspartic acid and phenylalanine. PKU (phenylketonuria) patients lack the enzyme phenylalanine hydroxylase. If aspartame is ingested in significant quantities by PKU patients, accumulation of phenylalanine causes toxicity to brain tissue.

Benzyl Alcohol: Bacteriostatic agent used in parenteral solution. It causes allergic reactions in some people. Benzyl alcohol has been associated with a fatal "Gasping Syndrome" in premature infants.

Caffeine: Caffeine belongs to the methylxanthine family of drugs. Methylxanthines are CNS and heart muscle stimulants, cerebral vasoconstrictors and diuretics. Coffee, green and black teas, guarana, maté and cola nut are sources of caffeine and may affect medication action. See caffeine p 67 and Caffeine Content table p 379.

Lactose: Lactose is used as a filler in some medications. The natural sweetener in milk, lactose is hydrolyzed in the small intestine by the enzyme lactase to glucose and galactose. Lactose intolerance (due to lactase deficiency) results in GI distress when lactose is ingested. Lactose in medication(s) may cause this reaction.

Licorice -- Glycyrrhiza glabra: Natural extract of glycyrrhiza root used in "natural" licorice candies. Two or more twists per day (approximately 100 g) of natural licorice (usually imported), can ↑ cortisol concentration resulting in pseudohyperaldosteronism and ↑ sodium reabsorption, water retention, K excretion and ↑ BP. This antagonizes the action of diuretics and antihypertensives. Resultant hypokalemia may alter the action of some drugs.

Maltodextrin: In the United States it is considered to be gluten free since it can only be manufactured from corn or rice.

Mannitol: The alcohol form of the sugar mannose. Mannitol is absorbed more slowly, yielding 1.6 calories/gram. Due to slow absorption, mannitol can cause soft stools and diarrhea.[52]

Oxalate: A salt or ester of oxalic acid. Oxalate-containing foods must be avoided with some minerals due to formation of nonabsorbable complexes or oxalate kidney stones. See High Oxalate Foods table p 381.

Phytate (phytic acid): Phosphorus-containing compound found in the outer husks of cereal grains. The amount of phytate increases with the maturity of the seed. Phytate containing foods need to be avoided with some minerals (Ca, Fe, Mg, Zn) due to formation of non-absorbable complexes. See High Phytate Foods table p 382.

Saccharin: Artificial sweetener. Extensive human research has found no evidence of carcinogenicity.

Sorbitol: The alcohol form of glucose. Absorbed more slowly than sucrose, yields 2.6 cal/g. Sorbitol's low glycemic response inhibits the rise in blood glucose. Due to slow absorption, sorbitol can cause soft stools/ diarrhea.[52]

Starch: Starch, from wheat, corn or potato, is added to medication as a filler, binder or diluent. Celiac disease patients have a lifelong intolerance to gluten, a protein component of wheat, barley, rye or oat flour. In celiac disease, gluten ingestion leads to damage of the lining of the small intestine. See Gluten table p 380.

Sulfites: Sulfiting agents are used in foods, beverages and pharmaceuticals as preservatives. Sulfites may cause severe hypersensitivity reactions in some people, particularly asthmatics. Sulfites include sulfur dioxide, sodium sulfite, sodium and potassium metabisulfite. FDA regulations ban the use of sulfites on fresh fruits and vegetables served raw. The FDA requires the listing of sulfites when present in foods or drugs.

Tartrazine: Tartrazine is FD&C Yellow No. 5, an artificial color additive, which causes severe allergic reactions in some people (1 in 10,000). The FDA requires the listing of tartrazine on labels when present in foods or drugs.

Tyramine and other pressor agents (dopamine, phenylethylamine, histamine): Tyramine is the decarboxylated product of the amino acid tyrosine. It is a vasoconstrictor which, in combination with some drugs [eg monoamine oxidase inhibitors (MAOI)], may cause a hypertensive crisis: dangerous increases in blood pressure , increased heart rate, flushing, headache, stroke and death. Highest in aged, fermented or spoiled foods. See Pressor Agents table p 383.

Vegetable Oil: Soy, sesame, cottonseed, corn or peanut oil is used in some drugs as solvents or vehicles. Hydrogenated vegetable oil is a tablet/capsule lubricant. May cause allergic reactions in sensitive people.

Drug-Alcohol (Ethanol) Interactions

Interactions between alcohol and medication may range from mild to potentially life threatening. Particularly worrisome is the combination of alcohol and medications that affect the central nervous system since alcohol alone may have a profound effect on coordination, alertness and thinking. Drug-alcohol interactions may produce intensification of a drug effect or lead to therapeutic failure. Medication interactions with alcohol are not necessarily predictable from individual to individual. The amount of alcohol consumed and the frequency of consumption often play a role in the severity of the adverse effects produced by the combination of medication and alcohol. The following table is not all inclusive, but offers examples of commons types of drug-alcohol interactions.

Additive CNS depression (enhanced sedation, confusion, respiratory depression, impaired coordination)
antiemetics eg metoclopramide (**Reglan**); prochlorperazine (**Compazine**)
antihistamines eg diphenhydramine (**Benadryl**)
anticonvulsants eg carbamazepine (**Tegretol),** lamotrigine, (**Lamictal**)
antidepressants (MAO inhibitor) eg phenelzine (**Nardil**)
antidepressants (Tricyclic) eg amitriptyline (**Elavil**), nortriptyline (**Pamelor**)
Antiparkinson Agents eg benztropine (**Cogentin**)
antipsychotic agents eg halperidol (**Haldol**), olanzapine (**Zyprexa**)
barbituates eg phenobarbital, butalbital (**Fiorinal, Fioricet**)
benzodiazepine (antianxiety) eg alprazolam (**Xanax**), diazepam (**Valium**)
benzodiazepine (hypnotics) eg flurazepam (**Dalmane**), temazepam (**Restoril**)
cannabinoids eg dronabinol (**Marinol**)
central a-2 adrenergic receptor agonist eg clonidine (**Catapres**)
narcotic analgesics eg oxycodone (**Oxycontin, Oxy IR, Percocet**); morphine (**MS Contin, Roxanol, Avinza**)
phenothiazines eg chlorpromazine (**Thorazine**)
sedative/hypnotic agents eg zolpidem (**Ambien**), eszopiclone (**Lunesta**)
skeletal muscle relaxants eg cyclobenazeprine (**Flexaril**), metaxalone (**Skelaxin**)

Increased risk of Hepatotoxicity

acetaminophen (**Tylenol**)
antifungal (azole) agents eg ketaconazole (**Nizoral**)
carbamazepine (**Tegretol**)
etretinate (**Tegison**)
HMG CoA reductase inhibitors eg lovastatin (**Mevacor**)

isoniazid
methotrexate (**Rheumatrex**)
rifampin (**Rifadin**)
sulfonamide antibiotics
valproic acid (**Depakene**), divalproex (**Depakote**)

Increased risk of GI irritation, bleeding

aspirin
corticosteroids eg methylprednisilone (**Medrol**)

NSAIDS eg ibuprofen (**Motrin**), naproxen (**Naprosyn**)
methotrexate (**Rheumatrex**)

Disulfiram-alcohol type reactions (flushing, headache, tachycardia, increased respiration and cardiac output)

cephalosporins eg cefotetan (**Cefotan**), cefamandole (**Mandol**)
chlorpropamide (**Diabinese**)
isoniazid
procarbazine (**Matulane**)[6]

furazolidone (**Furoxone**)
ketaconazole (**Nizoral**)
trimethoprim (**Bactrim**, **Trimpex**)

chloral hydrate
griseofulvin eg (**Grisactin**)
metronidazole (**Flagyl**)

Decreased drug effect with chronic alcohol ingestion

anesthesia agents eg propofol (**Diprivan**)
barbiturates eg phenobarbital
isoniazid (INH)

anticonvulsants (hydantoin) eg phenytoin (**Dilantin**)
doxycycline (**Vibramycin**)
warfarin (**Coumadin**)

Increased drug effect with acute alcohol ingestion

Alpha1-Adrenergic blockers eg doxazosin (**Cardura**, **Cardura XL**)
heparin
lithium (eg **Lithobid**, **Eskalith**)
oral hypoglycemic agents eg glyburide (**Diabeta**)
  glipizide (**Glucotrol**, **Glucotrol XL**)
tamulosin (**Flomax**)   tetracycline

barbiturates eg phenobarbital
insulin eg **Humulin**
nitrates eg isosorbide mononitrate (**Imdur**)
phenytoin (**Dilantin**)
propoxyphene (**Darvocet**)
warfarin (**Coumadin**)

TABLE CONTINUED ON NEXT PAGE

Drugs that intensify the CNS effects of alcohol (sedation, confusion, respiratory depression, etc)

antiulcer agents (H2 antagonists) eg cimetadine (**Tagamet**)
cisapride (**Propulsid**)
metoclopropamide (**Reglan**)
tricyclic antidepressants eg amitriptyline (**Elavil**)

bupropion (**Wellbutrin**)
erythromycin
oral contraceptives
verapamil (**Calan**, **Isoptin**, **Verelan**)

Miscellaneous interactions with alcohol

acitretin (**Soriatane**): Ethanol & acitretin form etretinate which has a longer half life & increases risk of teratogenicity

amantadine (**Symmetrel**): Increased CNS depression and orthostatic hypotension.

antihypertensive agents: Enhanced antihypertensive effects with possible hypotension.

bromocriptine (**Parlodel**): Increased risk of nausea & abdominal pain possibly due to enhanced dopamine receptor sensitivity.

etretinate (**Tegison**) & isotretinoin (**Accutane**): Increased risk of hypertriglyceridemia.

glipizide (**Glucotrol**): Ethanol may prolong, but not augment, hypoglycemic reaction.

loop diuretics eg furosemide (**Lasix**): Increased diuretic & hypotensive effects.

medication in solution with alcohol: Increased alcohol effects eg cyclosporine oral solution (**Neoral**, **Sandimmune**) 9.5-12.5% alcohol.

metformin (**Glucophage**): Increased risk of lactic acidosis.

nitrates eg isosorbide mononitrate (**Imdur**): Enhanced antihypertensive effects with possible hypotension.

phenothiazines: Increased risk of dystonic reactions.

phenytoin (**Dilantin**): Increased risk of folate deficiency.

Table is not all inclusive, also see references such as 3, 6, 9b, 10, 13, 93.
Compiled by Sr. Jeanne P. Crowe, PharmD, RPh

CAFFEINE CONTENT OF FOODS AND BEVERAGES

Item	mg Caffeine Range
Coffee (5 oz cup)	
Brewed: drip	70-130
Instant:	50-70
Decaffeinated	2-3
Starbucks Coffee Frappuccino (8 oz)	82
Tea/Tea products	
Iced tea	65-75
Instant (5 oz cup)	25-35
Leaf or Bag	30-50
SoBe Power/Energy/Adrenaline Rush (16 oz)	86-115
Coffee or chocolate enteral products 8 oz or 1 bar	2-10
Energy Drinks (8.0-8.4 oz)	
SoBe Power, KMX, Red Devil,	
Glaceau Vitamin Water	32-48
Red Bull, E Maxx, Amp, SoBe No Fear,	
SoBe Adrenaline Rush Red Celeste, Monster Energy	64-80
Rip It	100
Spike Shooter	300

Soft Drinks (12 oz diet and regular)

Item	mg Caffeine Range
Jolt	72
Diet Pepsi Max	69
Mountain Dew Live Wire	48.2
Mello Yello, Mountain Dew, Coca Cola, Dr. Pepper, Mr. Pibb, Pibb Xtra, Nitro Water, RC Cola, Shasta Cola, Pepsi One, Slice (orange), Water Joe	33-48
Big Red, Pepsi Cola,	27
Barq's Root Beer and Diet Barq's Root Beer	23
Celeste Cola,	18-19.4
Caffeine free Diet coke, club soda, Gatorade, Sierra Mist, Sprite, Fanta (all flavors), Pepsi Vanilla, Fresca (orange/grape/strawberry), PowerAde, ginger ale, root beer, 7-Up, tonic water, seltzer, sparkling water	0

Item	mg Caffeine Range
Chocolate or Coffee Products	
cocoa hot (5 oz)	2-15
dry (1 oz)	6
chocolate milk (8 oz)	8
milk chocolate (1 oz)	1-15
dark chocolate, semi-sweet (1 oz)	5-35
baking chocolate (1 oz)	57
chocolate flavored syrup (2 Tbsp)	5
chocolate malted-milk powder (3 hp Tbsp)	8
chocolate chips, semi-sweet (2 oz)	12-15
chocolate pudding (5 oz can)	7
chocolate ice cream (1 C)	4-8
chocolate cold cereal (100 g)	1-11
coffee ice cream (1 C)	30-60
Dannon coffee yogurt (8 oz)	45

See also caffeine medication entry, p 67 and caffeine section, p 374.
References: 28, 55a, 56, 57, 61, 73, 102, 132, 133 & manufacturer's information

POTENTIAL GLUTEN CONTAINING INGREDIENTS OF MEDICATION

It is IMPERATIVE that persons with gluten sensitivity such as CELIAC DISEASE/SPRUE/DH avoid **WHEAT, RYE, OATS, BARLEY** and all derivatives of these gluten grains if intestinal damage is to be prevented. *Inactive pharmaceutical ingredients* produced from these grains may contain a small but significant amount of gluten. The source of each ingredient, if not specified, must be checked with the manufacturer. Ingredients derived from corn, rice, potato and tapioca are permitted. *A parenteral formulation may be an alternative in an emergency until a safe gluten-free formulation can be determined.*

Potential sources of gluten which may be contained in medication are listed below.

<u>Inactive ingredients **MORE LIKELY** to be a source of gluten</u>

Dextri-Maltose- May contain barley malt.	**Flour**	**Pregelatinized Starch**
Dusting Powder	**Gluten**	**Starch**

<u>Inactive ingredients **LESS LIKELY** to be a source of gluten</u>

Caramel Coloring- Usually from corn. May rarely contain barley malt or starch hydrolysates.

Dextrin- Usually from corn; can be made from wheat.

Sodium Starch Glycolate- Usually from potato; can be made from any starch.

<u>Inactive ingredients **LEAST LIKELY** to be a source of gluten</u>

Alcohol- Theoretically, the distillation process separates alcohol from gluten, but alcohol may cause problems in some celiacs.

Maltodextrin- Usually made from corn or rice, rarely wheat (outside the United States). If made in the United States is certified gluten free.

Compiled by: Crowe, Sr. Jeanne Patricia, PharmD, RPh & Falini, Nancy Patin, MA, RD

HIGH OXALATE (OXALIC ACID) FOOD SOURCES

Fruits

Blackberries, blueberries, cranberries, *green gooseberries, dewberries, raw or canned strawberries, red and black raspberries, red currants, canned fruit cocktail, Concord grapes, *lemon peel, *lime/orange peel, damson plums, unspecified plums, canned or stewed *rhubarb, tangerines.

Vegetables

*Amaranth; beans in tomato sauce, **Beans:** boiled/raw green, wax, dried. *Beets, *beetroot; *cassava root, celery, *Swiss chard, chicory, *collards, dandelion greens, eggplant, escarole, kale, *leek, *okra, *parsley, parsnips, sweet green pepper and chilies, pokeweed, sweet potato, *purslane, rutabagas, *spinach boiled/frozen, summer squash, watercress.

Beverages (5 - 10 oz)

Beer: Guiness Stout, draft- Lager, Pilsner, Tuborg. Juices (that contain high oxalate berries eg cranberry), Ovaltine and other mixes, tea (oxalate content ↑ c̄ ↑ brewing time), coffee powder (Nescafe), colas.

Miscellaneous

Nuts: *almonds, *peanuts, *pecans. *Wheat germ, *poppy seeds, *peanut butter, *chocolate, *dry cocoa, *fig newton, fruit cake, graham crackers, pop corn, *soybean crackers, *sunflower seeds, *pepper (> 1 tsp/day), grits (white corn), whole wheat flour.

40-50 mg/day = low-oxalate intake. * = > 70 mg/100 gm.

Adapted from Brzezinski E, et al, **Oxalate Content of Selected Foods 3rd Ed,** UCSD Medical Center, San Diego, CA.

FOOD ITEM	PHYTIC ACID (mg)
Grain/Grain Products	
wheat bran, crude - 1 oz (28 gm)	843
wheat germ - 1 T (6 gm)	244
barley, whole grain - 3.5 oz (100 gm)	970
barley, pearl, raw - 3.5 oz (100 gm)	491
oats, raw - 3.5 oz (100 gm)	943
corn chips - 1 oz (28 gm)	178
Cereals- 1 oz All Bran	679
Shredded Wheat	415
wheat flakes	411
oatmeal (cooked) .5 cup	113
Bread, rye 1 slice	235
Nuts, Nut products and Seeds	
nuts: 3.5 oz (100 gm)	
almonds	1280
brazil nuts	1799
coconut, raw	270
hazelnuts	604
peanuts	748
walnuts	760
peanut butter - 1T (16 gm)	200
sesame seeds, raw - 1 oz (28 gm)	1319

FOOD ITEM	PHYTIC ACID (mg)
Vegetables 3.5 oz (100 gm)	
rice, wild, raw	2200
rice, brown, raw	890
rice, white, long-grain, raw	340
rice, white, short-grain, raw	140
kidney beans, raw	1200-2060
garbanzo beans, raw	280
navy beans, raw	280
peas, dried, raw	851
pinto beans, raw	620-1950
white beans, raw	1030
Miscellaneous 3.5 oz (100 gm)	
cocoa, dry pwd 1 T (5 gm)	94
soybean meal	1400-1600
soybean protein concentrate	1240-2170
soybean protein isolate	430-1170

The phytic acid content varies according to plant part and state of maturity at harvest.[55] References: 13, 52, 55 (14th edition).

PRESSOR AGENTS IN FOODS AND BEVERAGES
(Tyramine, Dopamine, Histamine, Phenylethylamine)

FOODS THAT MUST BE AVOIDED

aged cheeses: eg Cheddar, Bleu, Gorgonzola, Stilton
aged meats: eg dry sausage such as salami, mortadella. Chinese dried duck
soy sauce
fermented soya bean, soya bean paste
tofu/fermented bean curd
Miso Soup
fava beans, snowpea or broad bean pods (contain dopamine)
sauerkraut, kim chee
tap beer, Korean beer
concentrated yeast extracts (Marmite, Vegemite)
banana peel
all casseroles made with aged cheese

FOODS THAT MAY BE USED WITH CAUTION

red or white wine, 2-4 oz per day
coffee, cola*
pizza (homemade or gourmet pizzas may have higher content)
bottled beer, 2- 12 oz bottles max
alcohol-free beer, 2- 12 oz bottles max

FOODS NOT LIMITED (Based on current analyses)

unfermented cheeses (cream, cottage, ricotta, processed)
smoked white fish, salmon, carp, smoked anchovies
pickled herring
fresh meat, poultry or fish
canned figs, raisins
fresh pineapple
beetroot, cucumber
sweet corn, mushrooms
salad dressings, tomato sauce
Worcestershire sauce
baked raised products, English cookies
boiled egg, yogurt, junket, ice cream
avocado, figs, banana, raspberries
Brewer's yeast (vitamin supplements)
curry powder
peanuts, chocolate

All packaged or processed meats eg hot dogs, bologna, liverwurst (Store in refrigerator immediately & eat as soon as possible).

HISTAMINE: Content is highest in improperly stored or spoiled fish, tuna.

*Caffeine, a weak pressor agent, in quantities > 500 mg per day may exacerbate reactions.
See also Tyramine p 351. References: 9, 10, 21, 52, 59, 97, 98, 99 and
Rapaport M, "Dietary restrictions and drug interactions with monamine oxidase inhibitors: the state of the art"
2007 J Clin Psychiatry 68 Suppl 8:42-6.

OSMOLALITIES OF SELECTED BEVERAGES AND FOODS

Osmolality refers to the number and size of particles per kilogram of water. Expressed in osmoles or milliosmoles per kg water. Extracellular fluid is 280 to 300 mOsms/kg water. Normal serum is 275 to 325.

Patients with limited gastrointestinal tolerance should receive hyposmolar or mildly hyperosmolar liquids (< 400 mOsm). Because of high osmolality some food/liquids may need to be diluted initially.

Beverage	Dilution	mOsm/kg
Juices		
prune	1:3	1,076
cranberry	1:3	836
pineapple	-	772
apple	-	705
tomato, grapefruit	-	619
orange	-	601
V-8	-	578
low-calorie cranberry	-	287
Coffee/Tea (1 cup)		
coffee with 1 tsp sugar	-	128
tea with 1 tsp sugar	-	106
coffee	-	83
tea	-	8
Enteral Formulas		
isotonic (Choice DM, Isocal, Jevity, Osmolite, Ultracal)	-	270-310
1.0 cal/mL (Boost, Ensure, Resource)	-	430-670
1.5 (Boost Plus, Ensure Plus, Resource Plus)	-	600-690
2.0 (Nepro, Nutren, Novasource)	-	665-790

References: 16, 32, 52, 61 & manufacturer's information

Beverage	Dilution	mOsm/kg
Broth		
↑ Na, low-fat chicken	-	452
regular chicken	-	389
Jello		
cherry, (≥ sugar)	1:4	735
sugar-free	-	57
Milk/Milk Products		
human milk	-	277-303
ice cream	-	1,150
Carnation Instant Breakfast		
made c̄ nonfat milk	-	617
made c̄ whole milk	-	653
eggnog	-	695
nonfat milk Lactaid	-	375
whole milk Lactaid	-	413
nonfat milk	-	280
whole milk	-	277
Soft Drinks		
cola	-	714
Gatorade	-	280-360
ginger ale	-	565
diet ginger ale/cola	-	43-50
Water ice, cherry	1:3	1,064

pH and ACID CONTENT OF BEVERAGES

Active peptic ulcer or GERD: Some juices and most carbonated beverages have a pH low enough (< 3.5) to activate pepsin. Acid content is comparable to or exceeds the basal gastric secretion. Avoidance of extrinsic sources of acid may decrease patient discomfort.

Fruit or vegetable products	pH	mEq acid/cc	Carbonated beverages	pH	mEq acid/cc
vinegar (cider)	3.1-3.2	0.60-.64	orange soda	2.8	0.056-.058
grapefruit, pineapple, orange	3.4-3.8		cola (average)	2.4	0.037-.057
0.12-.17			diet cola (can)	2.9	0.042
cranberry	2.6-2.8	0.080-.081	(soda open 1 hour)	2.9-3.1	0.057-.082
grape, apple, apricot nectar	3.3-3.8	0.055-.096	7-Up	3.0-3.1	0.048-.055
orange drink	2.6	0.055	ginger ale (can)	2.7-2.9	0.041-0.054
tomato	4.3	0.049-.059	club soda	3.7	0.046
peach nectar	3.6	0.038-.039	**Other beverages**		
prune	4.1-4.2	0.031-.036	coffee (whole)	4.9-5.1	0.004-.006
pear nectar	3.7	0.021-.022	Sanka (instant)	5.1-5.4	0.004-.006
Milk			cocoa (instant)	6.7-6.9	0.001-.002
skim	6.5-6.7	0.007-.009	tea (instant)	6.8-6.9	0.001-.002
half & half cream	6.6-6.7	0.005-.007	tap water	7.6-8.2	————
whole	6.6-6.7	0.005-.006			

References: Manufacturer's information; New England Journal of Medicine; 11/21/85, p. 1351

MAGNESIUM (Mg) SIGNIFICANT DIETARY SOURCES*

Fruits and Vegetables

Avocado, banana, adzuki beans, beet greens, blackeye peas (cowpeas), cassava (raw), chickpeas (garbanzo beans), figs (dried), great northern beans, kidney beans, lentils, lima beans, lupins, mung beans, navy beans, okra, pigeonpeas, pink beans, pinto beans, potato with skin (baked or microwaved), potato flour, raisins, seaweed, soybeans, spinach, Swiss chard, white beans, yellow beans.

Grains and Grain Products

(More than 80% of the Mg is lost by removal of the germ and outer layers of cereal grains).[47]

Amaranth, barley, buckwheat, buckwheat flour, bulgar, granola, millet, oats (whole grain), oat bran, rice (brown), rice (wild), rice bran, rye flour, triticale flour, wheat bran, wheat germ, whole wheat flour.
Whole wheat pasta.
High bran cereals (eg All Bran, 100% Bran, Bran Buds, Bran Chex, bran flakes, raisin bran).

Nuts and Seeds

Pumpkin seeds, peas, lentils, sunflower seeds, sesame seeds, almonds, cashews, flax seeds, hazel nuts, brazil nuts, peanuts, black walnuts, pistachios, soybeans, English walnuts, macadamia nuts, pecans.

Other

Molasses, malt syrup, hummus, peanut butter, soybean products: sauce, flour, natto, miso, tempeh, raw tofu. Oysters, shrimp, halibut, yeast, dry milk.

* 30 mg or more magnesium/100 g   See also **magnesium p 202.**

References: 16, 47b, 52, 55a, 55b, Nutritionist V data base and website http://fnic.nal.usda.gov

POTASSIUM (K) SIGNIFICANT DIETARY SOURCES

Vegetables and Fruits
Standard servings provide approximately 150-300 mg potassium

apple, raw, with skin	celery, Pascal type raw 2 stalks	seaweed
asparagus	kale	spinach, turnip greens
artichoke	mushrooms, raw boiled	squash, winter
bamboo shoots, raw	okra pods, cooked	sweet potato canned
beets, cooked drained	tomato, tomato juice	tomato paste
broccoli	potato chips	vegetable juice 6 oz
cauliflower	pumpkin, cooked	

Standard servings provide approximately 300-500 mg potassium

apricots, raw	cantaloupe	kiwifruit	potato
avocado 1/3 whole	carrots, carrot juice	orange juice	prune juice 5 oz
banana 1 small	grapefruit juice	orange, 1	strawberries
Brussels sprouts, raw, cooked	honeydew	pineapple juice	sweet potato
dried fruit: apple, apricots, dates, pear, peach, prune, raisins			(fresh baked)
beans: adzuki, black, kidney, lentil, lima, pinto, red, soy, white			tangerine juice

Cereal and Breads
Serving sizes average approximately 200-300 mg K

All Bran	Bran Flakes	Mueslix	Raisin Bran
Bread pumpernickel, 2 slices	Cheerios	Quaker 100% natural cereal with raisins	
	Fiber One with Raisin Bran Clusters		

Dairy foods
Serving sizes average approximately 200-400 mg K

Milk, plain 1%, whole or fat free, 1 cup		Yogurt, plain, 1 cup
Milk, evaporated, 1/2 cup	Cottage cheese, low fat, 1 cup	Ricotta, whole milk or part skim, 1 cup

Miscellaneous   100-200 mg K

almonds, 12-15	coffee, 10 oz	pecans	pumpkin seeds
Brazil nuts, 5 medium	filberts, hazelnuts	peanuts	tea, 14 oz
cashews	fruitcake	peanut butter	tofu
chestnuts, 4 large	molasses, 1/2 T	potato, mashed	sunflower seeds
		from granules	walnuts

Reference: website http://fnic.nal.usda.gov
Table prepared by Zaneta Pronsky, MS, RD, FADA & Keith-Thomas Ayoob, EdD, RD, FADA

See also **KCl p 260**

VITAMIN K SIGNIFICANT DIETARY SOURCES*

Fats and Oils

(Exposure to fluorescent and sunlight rapidly destroys vitamin K in oils).

Canola (rapeseed) oil, soybean oil

Vegetables

(Higher concentrations of Vitamin K are found in the outer leaves and peels of vegetables).

Highest sources: cooked spinach, collards, kale, turnip greens, beet greens, mustard greens.

Raw forms of these vegetables are lower in Vitamin K, per equal measure.

Other sources: Asparagus, bran, broccoli, Brussels sprouts, cabbage (green raw), chayote leaf, chickpeas (garbanzo beans), chive (raw), coriander leaf, cucumber peel, endive, green tomato, lettuce, lentils, mint, mung beans, nettle leaves, oats, purslane, romaine lettuce, scallions (green onions), seaweed (extremely high levels), soybeans, Swiss chard, watercress.

Other

Beef liver, chicken liver, pork liver, egg yolk, green tea leaves, algae (purple laver and hijiki), apples with green peel.

* 50 μg or more Vit K/100 g   See also **Vitamin K p 342**

References: 3a, 47, 52, 55, 78, 81a, 81b, 93 and website http://fnic.nal.usda.gov

NOTES

Grapefruit - Drug Interactions

Many drugs interact with grapefruit (juice, segments, extract and certain related citrus fruits, eg Seville oranges, tangelos, minneolas, pummelos and certain exotic oranges). Components in grapefruit called furanocoumarins (two of which are bergamottin and 6'7'-dihydroxybergamottin) irreversibly inhibit cytochrome p450 (CYP) 3A4 isoenzymes (3A4) in the intestinal wall, decreasing the pre-systemic metabolism of affected drugs taken up to 72 hours after grapefruit consumption. Intestinal 3A4 activity remains inhibited during this time as the body produces enzymes. For drugs that are normally poorly absorbed due to significant pre-systemic 3A4 metabolism, grapefruit intake can lead to significantly higher blood levels, potentially resulting in increased therapeutic effects, adverse effects and/or toxicity. In experimental studies, use of furanocoumarin-free grapefruit juice (produced by heat treatment or UV irradiation) with drugs proven to interact with normal grapefruit juice did not lead to increased blood levels, providing further confirmatory evidence for their role in enzyme inhibition. Limited evidence indicates that following intake of very large amounts of grapefruit, hepatic 3A4 may also be inhibited. If a drug is known to be metabolozed by 3A4 and has low oral bioavailability, it may be possible to predict an interaction with grapefruit. Grapefruit weakly inhibits intestinal cell wall p-glycoprotein (p-GP), an efflux pump in enterocytes that actively secretes some absorbed drugs back into the gut lumen. Not all 3A4-metabolized drugs are p-GP substrates. Organic anion transporting polypeptide (OATP) is a drug transporter system inhibited by grapefruit. Drugs handled by OATP1A2 and OATP2B1 may have *decreased* absorption when taken with grapefruit, potentially leading to loss of efficacy. Emerging information indicates bergamottin also inactivates CYP 2C9, 2D6 and 3A5 isoenzymes, and may potentially cause drug interactions with substrates of these isoenzymes.

1- Manufacturer recommends avoidance.

2- Avoid with grapefruit/related citrus unless instructed to do so by a physician.

3- Serum plasma level monitoring required/recommended.

4- Minor interaction, clinically significant unclear.

5- Interaction suspected, but no formal studies.

6- No formal studies, but lacks a cardiotoxic metabolite.

7- Not metabolized by CYP 3A4, no interaction suspected.

8- No interaction documented/suspected when administered parenterally.

9- Withdrawn from market.

10- Blood levels/bioavailability <u>decreased</u>.

11- Risk higher in CYP 2D6 poor metabolizers.

Avoid grapefruit with the following

amiodarone (Cordarone)[8]
astemizole (Hismanal)[5, 9]
budesonide (Entocort)[8]
buspirone (BuSpar)
cerivastatin (Baycol)[5, 9]
cilostazol (Pletal)[5]
cisapride (Propulsid, Prepulsid)[9]
colchicine[5]
dronedarone (Multaq)
eletriptan (Relpax)[5]

etoposide (Vepesid)[8, 10]
everolimus (Afinitor, Zortress)[5]
halofantrine (Halfan)
ixabepilone (Ixempra)[1]
lapatinib (Tykerb)[1,5]
lovastatin (Mevacor)
mifepristone (Mifeprex)[5]
nifedipine (Procardia)[1]
nilotnib (Tasigna)
pazopanib (Votrient)[5]
pimozide (Orap)[5]

primaquine
quinidine (Quinaglute, Quinidex)[8, 10]
ranolazine (Ranexa)[1]
simvastatin (Zocor)[8]
sirolimus (Rapamune)[1,5]
sunitinib (Sutent)
temsirolimus (Torisel)[5]
terfenadine (Seldane)[9]
tolvaptan (Samsca)[5]
ziprasidone (Geodon)[5]

Use grapefruit with caution

albendazole (Albenza)
alfentanil (Alfenta)[8]
alfuzosin (Uroxatral)[5]
almotriptan (Axert)[5]
aprepitant (Emend)[5]
aripiprazole (Abilify)[5]
atorvastatin (Lipitor)
buproprion (Wellbutrin, Zyban)[5]
carbamazepine (Tegretol)[3]
cinacalcet (Sensipar)[5]
clobazam (Onfi)[5]
clomipramine (Anafranil)[8]
cyclosporine (Neoral)[2, 3, 8]
darifenacin (Enablex)[5]
dasatinib (Sprycel)[5]
delavirdine (Rescriptor)
dextromethorphan
diazepam (Valium)[8]
docetaxel (Taxotere)
dofetilide (Tikosyn)[5]

eszopiclone (Lunesta)[5]
ethinyl estradiol[4,8]
etravirine (Intelence)[5]
felodipine (Renedil, Plendil)
fexofenadine (Allegra)[10]
fluvoxamine (Luvox)
gefitinib (Iressa)
guanfacine (Intuniv, Tenex)[5]
indinavir (Crixivan)[10]
itraconazole (Sporanox)[10]
levothyroxine (Eltoxin,
  Levoxyl, Synthoid)[4,8]
losartan (Cozaar)
manidipine
maraviroc (Selzentry)
methadone (Dolophine)[5]
methylprednisolone (Medrol)[8]
midazolam (Versed)[9]
nicardipine (Cardene)[8]
nimodipine (Nimotop)

propafenone (Rythmol)[5,11]
quetiapine (Seroquel)[5]
quinine
ramelteon (Rozerem)[5]
rilpivirine (Edurant)[5]
rivaroxaban (Xarelto)[5]
rolflumilast (Daliresp)[5]
saquinavir (Invirase)[2]
sertraline (Zoloft)
sildenafil (Viagra, Revatio)
solifenacin (Vesicare)[5]
tacrolimus (Prograf)[2, 3, 8]
tadalafil (Adcirca, Cialis)
tamoxifen (Nolvadex)[5]
tamsulosin (Flomax)[5]
telaprevir (Incivek)[5]
ticagrelor (Brilinta)[5]
tolterodine (Detrol)[5]
trazodone (Desyrel)
triazolam (Halcion)

TABLE CONTINUED ON NEXT PAGE (TURN PAGE)

efavirenz (Sustiva)[5]
erlotinib (Tarceva)[5]
erythromycin (E-mycin)[8]

nisoldipine (Sular)
oxybutynin (Ditropan)[5]
oxycodone (OxyContin)

vardenafil (Levitra)
verapamil (Calan, Isoptin, Verelan)[8]
vilazodone (Viibryd)[5]

Medications with no significant interaction with grapefruit

Drugs in this section have all been studied with GJ, and found to have minimal/negligible interaction.

acebutolol (Monitan, Sectral)[4]
aliskiren (Tekturna)
alprazolam (Xanax)[4]
amlodipine (Norvasc)[4]
amprenavir (Agenerase)[4, 10]
caffeine[4,8]
carvedilol (Coreg)[4]
clarithromycin (Biaxin)
clozapine (Clozaril)[4]
digoxin (Lanoxin)[8]
diltiazem (Cardizem)[4,8]
eplerenone (Inspra)[4]

fentanyl (Actiq)[4,8]
glyburide (Diabeta)
haloperidol (Haldol)[8]
imatinib (Gleevec/Glivec)
lansoprazole (Prevacid)[4,8]
montelukast (Singulair)[5]
nicotine (*via oral route*)
omeprazole (Losec, Prilosec)[4]
phenytoin (Dilantin)[8]
pitavastatin (Livalo)[4]
pravastatin (Pravachol)

prednisone (Deltasone)
quazam (Doral)[4]
repaglinide (Prandin, Gluconorm)[4]
scopolamine (Hyoscine)[4,8]
17-β estradiol[4,8]
telithromycin (Ketek)[4]
theophylline (Theo-Dur, Uniphyl)
tretinoin (Vesanoid)
warfarin (Coumadin)[8]

Medications considered safe for use with grapefruit

cetirizine (Zyrtec, Reactine)[6]
desloratadine (Aerius, Clarinex)[7]

fosaprepitant (Emend for injection)
fluvastatin (Lescol)[7]
loratadine (Claritin)[6]

praziquantel (Biltricide)
rosuvastatin (Crestor)[7]

Tables compiled by Dean Elbe BSc (Pharm), PharmD, BCPP, Clinical Pharmacist, Vancouver, BC, Canada

References: 1, 3, 3a, 7, 9b, 10, 43, 46, 49, 50, 73, 76, 78, 80, 93, 109

DRUGS NOT COMPATIBLE WITH TUBE FEEDING

The following drugs, combined with enteral products*, cause thickening or clumping by visual inspection. This may clog the feeding tube, most frequently with highly acidic syrups (pH < 4.0) & bulk-forming agents. Delivery method, tube diameter, formula composition, tube placement and flushing protocol also influence compatibilty.

aluminum hydroxide (Amphogel)
al-mg hydroxide (Mylanta Double Strength)
   (regular strength- compatible)
calcium glubionate (Neo-Calglucon Syrup)
chlorpromazine (Thorazine Conc)
ciprofloxacin (Cipro) susp
dicyclomine (Bentyl Liquid)
Dimetane/Dimetapp Elixir
ferrous sulfate (Feosol Elixir)
Fleet Phospho-soda (Na biphosphate + Na phosphate)
guaifenesin (Robitussin Syrup)

lansoprazole (Prevacid)- cap contents or granule packet
lithium carbonate (Cibalith-S syrup)
magaldrate (Riopan)**
mandelamine suspension (see below)
metoclopramide syrup (Reglan Syrup)
Paregoric Elixir (opium, 45% alcohol)
potassium chloride (some liquid forms)
   (KCl Liquid 10 & 20%, Klorvess Syrup)
pseudoephedrine (Sudafed Syrup)
sevelamer (Renagel)
thioridazine (Mellaril Soln)[70] (conc- compatible)[71]
zinc sulfate (capsules)

<u>Administer separately from tube feedings due to possible reduced bioavailability</u>: methyldopa,[69] phenytoin susp (Dilantin), tetracycline, theophylline, warfarin (Coumadin), diazepam solution, omeprazole (Prilosec), pantoprazole (Protonix), penicillin V. All fluoroquinolones: ciprofloxacin (Cipro), gatifloxacin (Tequin), levofloxacin (Levaquin), lomafloxacin (Maxaquin).[39]

<u>Possible bezoar formation</u>: sucralfate susp

* Ensure, Ensure HN, Ensure Plus, Ensure Plus HN, Enrich, Osmolite, Osmolite HN, Two-Cal HN.

Elemental products, Vital and Vivonex TEN were also tested. No incompatibility was found with these products, except c̄ mandelamine susp (incompatible c̄ Vital).
** Compatible c̄ Osmolite HN, but not Osmolite.   References: 7, 8, 10, 25, 32, 39, 69, 70, 71, 138

The following products, Ensure HN, Ensure plus HN, Osmolite HN, which were used in the original research are no longer available. Other products have taken their place and their formulas may have changed.

REFERENCES 17th EDITION

1. *Pharmacist's Letter* Stockton, Ca thru Vol 28 (11), March, 2012
2. **Handbook of Nonprescription Drugs**, 13th Ed (Washington, DC, Am Pharm Assoc, 2002)
3. **Drug Interaction Facts**, Tatro DS, Editor (St Louis, MO, Facts and Comparisons, thru December, 2009)
3a. **Drug Interaction Facts Herbal Supplements and Food** (thru December 2007)
4. Herr SM, **Herb-Drug Interaction Handbook**, 3rd Ed (Nassau, NY, Church Street Books, 2005)
5. Gilbert DN, et al, **The Sanford Guide to HIV/AIDS Therapy** 18th Ed (Sperryville, VA, Antimicrobial Therapy, Inc 2010)
6. **AHFS Drug Information 2012** McEvoy GK, Editor (Bethesda, MD, Am Soc of Health Pharmacists, 2012)
7. **Facts and Comparisons** (St Louis, MO, Facts & Comparisons, thru February, 2012)
8. **Nutrition and Drug Therapy: Clinical Pharmacology, Drug Compatibility and Stability** (Silver Spring, MD, ASPEN, 1992)
9 a. *The Medical Letter on Drugs and Therapeutics* New Rochelle, NY thru Vol 54 (1386), March, 2012
   b. **The Medical Letter Handbook of Adverse Drug Interactions**, Kim RB, Editor, 2008
10 a. **Physicians' Desk Reference**, 66th Ed (Montvale, NJ, Physicians' Desk Reference, Inc, 2012)
   b. **PDR for Nutritional Supplements** Second Ed, 2001
11. Pelton R, LaValle J, Hawkins EB, Krinsky DL, **Drug-Induced Nutrient Depletion Handbook** 2nd Ed (Hudson, OH, Lexi-Comp, 2001)
12. Isada CM et al, **Infectious Diseases Handbook** 5th Ed (Hudson, OH, Lexi-Comp, 2001)
13. **USPDI, Drug Information for the Health Care Professional** Vol I 27th Ed (Rockville, MD, 2007)
14. Smith CH "Drug-Food/Food-Drug Interactions" Chapter 30, **Geriatric Nutrition** (NYC, NY, Raven Press, 1995)
15. Fraunfelder FW, "Twice-yearly exams unnecessary for patients taking quetiapine" 2004 Am J Ophthalmol 138(5):870-1
16. **Manual of Clinical Dietetics**, 6th Ed (Chicago, IL, Am Diet Assoc, 2000)
17. Keltner NL, Folks DG, **Psychotropic Drugs** 4th Ed (St Louis, MO, Elsevier Mosby, 2005)
18. Pandit MK, Burke J, Gustafson AB, et al, "Drug-induced disorders of glucose tolerance" 1993 Ann Int Med 118:529-539
19. Bezchlidnyk KZ, "Should psychiatric patients drink coffee?" 1981 CMAJ 124:4 Feb 15, 1981
20. Nakhjavani M et al, "Short term effects of spironolactone on blood lipid profile: a 3-month study on a cohort of young women with hirsutism" Br J Clin Pharmacol 2009 Oct;68(4):634-7
21. Gelenberg AJ, *Biological Therapies in Psychiatry Newsletter* (St Louis, MO, Mosby) thru Vol 32 (12) December, 2009
22. Srinivasan K, et al "Effect of imipramine on linear and nonlinear measures of heart rate variability

in children" Pediatr Cardiol. 2004 Jan-Feb;25(1):20-5

23. Fuller MA, Sajatovic M, **Drug Information for Mental Health** (Hudson, OH Lexi-Comp, Inc 2001)
24. Strain EC, Mumford GK, Silverman K, et al, "Caffeine dependence syndrome" 1994 JAMA 272:1043-8
25. Lourenco R, "Enteral feeding: drug/nutrient interaction" 2001 Clin Nutr 20(2):187-193
26. Gahart BL, Nazareno AR, **Intravenous Medications**, 25th Ed (St Louis, MO, Mosby, 2009)
27. Murray JJ, Healy MD, "Drug-mineral interactions: a new responsibility for the hospital dietitian" 1991 J Am Diet Assoc 91(1):66-73
28. Leclercq I, Desager JP, Horsmans Y, "Inhibition of chlorzoxazone metabolism, a clinical probe for CPY2E1, by a single ingestion of watercress" 1998 Clin Pharmacol Ther 64(2):144-9
29. Brunser O et al,"Effect of a milk formula with prebiotics on the intestinal microbiota of infants after an antibiotic treatment" 2006 Pediatr Res 59(3):451-6
30. Raitt MH, et al, "Fish oil supplementation and risk of ventricular tachycardia and ventricular fibrillation in patients with implantable defibrillators: a randomized contolled trial" 2005 JAMA 292(23):2884-91
31. Stone KA, "Lithium-Induced Nephrogenic Diabetes Insipidus" 1999 J Am Board Fam Pract 12(1):43-47
32. **Nutrition Support Handbook**, Teasley-Strausburg KM, Editor (Cincinnati, OH, Harvey-Whitney, 1992)
33. Richter WO, Jacob BG, Schwandt P, "Interaction between fibre and lovastatin" 1994 The Lancet 338:706
34. Henkin Y, Como JA, Oberman A, "Secondary dyslipidemia inadvertent effects of drugs in clinical practice" 1992 JAMA 267(7):961-968
35. Holden K, **Parkinson's Disease, Guidelines for Medical Nutrition Therapy** (Ft Collins, CO, Five Star Living, 2000)
36. Rabey JM, Vered Y, Shabtai H, et al, "Broad Bean (Vicia faba) consumption and Parkinson's Disease" 1993 in **Advances in Neurology** 681-684 (NY, Raven Press)
37. Fava M, Judge R, Hoog SL, et al "Fluoxetine versus sertraline and paroxetine in major depressive disorder: changes in weight with long-term treatment" 2000 J Clin Psychiatry 61(11):863-7
38. Bartel PR, Ubbink JB, Delport R, et al, "Vitamin B-6 supplementation and theophylline-related effects in humans" 1994 Am J Clin Nutr 60(1):93-99
39. Wright DH, Pietz SL, Konstantinides FN, Rotschafer JC, "Decreased in vitro fluoroquinolone concentrations after admixture with an enteral feeding formulation" 2000 JPEN 24(1):42-48
40. Roth MS, Martin AB, Katz JA, "Nutritional implications of prolonged propofol use" 1997 Am J Health-Syst Pharm 54:694-5
41. Pinto JT, Rivlin RS, "Drugs that promote renal excretion of riboflavin" 1987 Drug Nutr Inter 5:143-151
42. Writing Group for the Women's Health Initiative Investigators. "Risks and benefits of estrogen plus

progestin in healthy postmenopausal women" 2002 JAMA 288:321-333

43. Penzak SR, Gubbins PO, Gurley BJ, et al, "Grapefruit Juice decreases the systemic availability of itraconazole capsules in healthy volunteers" 1999 Ther Drug Monit 21:304-9

44. Laheij RJ, et al, "Risk of community-acquired pneumonia and use of gastric acid-suppressive drugs" 2004 JAMA 292(16):1955-60

45. Bennett WM, "Drug interactions and consequences of sodium restriction" 1997 Am J Clin Nutr 65(suppl):678S-681S

46. Harris RZ, Jang GR, Tsunoda S "Dietary Effects on Drug Metabolism and Transport" Clinical Pharm 42(130) 1071-1088, 2003

47a. National Academy of Sciences, **1989 Recommended Dietary Allowances**, 10th Ed (Washington, DC, 1989)
   b. - e. Institute of Medicine, **Dietary Reference Intakes** (Washington, DC, National Academy Press)
   b. 1997 **for Calcium, Phosphorus, Magnesium, Vitamin D and Fluoride**
   c. 1998 **for Thiamin, Riboflavin, Niacin, Vitamin B$_6$, Folate, Vitamin B$_{12}$, Pantothenic Acid, Biotin and Choline**
   d. 2000 **for Vitamin C, Vitamin E, Selenium and Carotenoids**
   e. 2001 **for Vitamin A, Vitamin K, Arsenic, Boron, Copper, Iodine, Iron, Manganese, Molybdenum, Nickel, Silicon, Vanadium and Zinc**

48. Jick SS, Kremer HM, Vasilakis-Scaramozza C, "Isotretinoin use and risk of depression, psychotic symptoms, suicide and attempted suicide" 2000 Arch Dermatol 136(10):1231-6

49. Garg SK, Kumar N, Bhargava VK, Prabhakar SK, "Effect of grapefruit juice on carbamazepine bioavailability in patients with epilepsy" 1998 Clin Pharmacol Ther 64(3):286-8

50. Bailey DG, Arnold MO, Spence JD, "Grapefruit juice and drugs: how significant is the interaction?" 1994 Clin Pharm 26(2):91-98

51. Menon IS, Kendal RY, Dewar HA, Newell DJ, "Effect of onions on blood fibrinolytic activity" 1968 BMJ 3:351

52. Mahan LK, Escott-Stump S, **Krause's Food, Nutrition, & Diet Therapy**, 12th Ed (Phila, PA, Elsevier, 2008)

53. Johnson BF, Rodin SM, Hoch K, Shekar V, "The effect of dietary fiber on the bioavailability of digoxin in capsules" 1987 J Clin Pharmacol 27(7):487-90

54. Ghirlanda G, Oradei A, Manto A, et al, "Evidence of plasma CoQ10-lowering effect by HMG-CoA Reductase Inhibitors: a double blind, placebo controlled study" 1993 J Clin Pharmacol 33:226-9

55. Pennington JAT, **Bowes & Church's Food Values of Portions Commonly Used**, 14th Ed (NYC, NY, Harper & Row, 1989)

56. "Caffeine Content of Foods and Drugs" Sept, 2007 CSPI at **http://www.cspinet.org/new/cafchart.htm**

57. Consumer Information, Coca-Cola Co, Consumer Info. Center, PO Box 1734, Atlanta, GA 30301, 2001

58. Aronof GR, **Drug Prescribing in Renal Failure** 5th Ed (Phila, PA, Amer College of Physicians, 2007)

59a. McCabe BJ, "The MAOI Diet" 1987 Biol Ther Psych 10(2)

b. "Dietary tyramine and other pressor amines in MAOI regimes: a review" 1986 J Am Diet Assoc 86:1059

c. & Tsuang MT, "Dietary considerations in MAO inhibitor regimens" 1982 J Clin Psych 43:5

60. Apeland T, Mansoor MA, Strandjord RE, "Antiepileptic drugs as independent predictors of plasma homocysteine levels" 2001 Epilepsy Res 47(1-2):27-35

61. Pepsi Cola, "What's in our soft drinks?" pamphlet, 1998

62. Hagg S, Spigset O, Dahlqvist MT, et al, "Effect of caffeine on clozapine pharmacokinetics in healthy volunteers" 2000 Br J Clin Pharmacol 49(1):59-63

63. **ARUP Laboratories/User Guide** 2009 (Salt Lake City, UT, ARUP Labs, 2009)

64. Morii M, Ueno K, Ogawa A, et al, "Impairment of mycophenolate mofetil absorption by iron ion" 2000 Clin Pharmacol Ther 68(6):613-6

65. Pan SH, Lopez RR, Sher LS, et al, "Enhanced oral cyclosporine absorption with water-soluble vitamin E early after liver transplantation" 1996 Pharmacotherapy 16(1):59-65

66. Lingtak-Neander C, "Drug-Nutrient Interactions in Transplant Recipients" 2001 JPEN 25(3):132-142

67. Henry JB, **Clinical Diagnosis and Management by Laboratory Methods** 21th Ed (Phila, PA, W.B. Saunders, 2006)

68. De Abajo FJ, Garcia-Rodriguez LA, Montero D, "Association between selective serotonin reuptake inhibitors and upper gastrointestinal bleeding: population based case-control study" 1999 BMJ 319:1106-9

68a. Dalton SO et al, "Use of selective serotonin reuptake inhibitors and risk of upper gastrointestinal bleeding" 2003 Arch Intern Med 163:59-64

69. Holtz L, Milton J, Sturek JK, et al, "Compatibility of medications with enteral feedings" 1987 JPEN 11(2):183-6

70. Cutie AJ, Altman E, Lenkel L, et al, "Compatibility of enteral products with commonly employed drug additives" 1983 JPEN 7(2):186-191

71. Burns PE, McCall L, Wirsching R, et al, "Physical compatibility of enteral formulas with various common medications" 1988 J Am Diet Assoc 88(9):1094-6

72. Friedman RD, Young DS, **Effects of Disease on Clinical Laboratory Tests**, 4th Edition (Washington, DC, AACC Press, 2001)

73. *Environmental Nutrition,* NYC, NY, Environmental Nutrition, Inc thru Vol 32 (11):2009

74. Force RW, et al, "Increased Vitamin B_{12} requirement associated with chronic acid suppression therapy" 2003 Ann Pharmacother 37:490-493

75. Consumer Laboratories product testing at: http://www.consumerlab.com/results/index.asp

76. Bailey DG, Dresser GK, Munoz C, et al, "Reduction of fexofenadine bioavailability by fruit juices" 2000 Clin Pharmacol Ther 68(5):468-477

77. Urdaneta E, Idoate I, Larralde J, "Drug-nutrient interactions: inhibition of amino acid intestinal absorption by fluoxetine" 1998 Br J Nutr 79(5):439-46

78. Bailey DG, Dresser GK, "Interactions between grapefruit juice and cardiac drugs" 2004 Am J Cardiovasc Drugs 4(5):281-297

79. Scranton RE, Young M, Lawler E, et al, "Statin use and fracture risk: study of a US veterans population" 2005 Arch Intern Med 165(17):2007-12

79a. Majima T, Shimatsu A, Komatsu Y, et al "Short-term effect of pitavastatin on biochemical markers of bone turnover in patients with hypercholesteremia" Intern Med 2007 46(24):1967-1973

80. Malhotra S, Bailey DG, Paine MF, Watkins PB, "Seville orange juice-felodipine interactions: comparison with dilute grapefruit juice and involvement of furocoumarins" 2001 Clin Pharm & Ther 89(1):14-22

81a. Booth SL, Sadowski JA, Weihrach JL, "Vitamin K1 (Phylloquinone) content of foods: a provisional table" 1993 J Food Comp Anal 6:109-120

81b. Booth SL, Charnley JM, Sadowski JA, "Dietary Vitamin K1 and stability of oral anticoagulation: proposal of a diet with constant Vitamin K1 content" 1997 Thromb Haemost 77(3):504-9

82. Ortiz Z, Shea B, Suarez-Almazor ME, et al, "The efficacy of folic acid and folinic acid in reducing methotrexate gastrointestinal toxicity in rheumatoid arthritis" 1998 J Rheumatol 25(1):36-43

83. Johnston KL, Clifford MN, Morgan LM, "Coffee acutely modifies gastrointestinal hormone secretion and glucose tolerance in humans: glycemic effect of cholorogenic acid and caffeine" 2003 Am J Clin Nutr 78:728-733

84. Fick DM, et al, "Updating the Beers Criteria for potentially inappropriate medication use in older adults: results of a US consensus panel of experts." 2003 Arch Intern Med 163(3):2716-2724

85. Moon CH, Jung YS, Kim MH, et al, "Mechanism for antiplatelet effect of onion: AA release inhibition, thromboxane A(2)synthase inhibition and TXA(2)/PGH(2) receptor blockade" 2000 Prostaglandins Leukot Essent Fatty Acids 62(5):277-83

86. Seelig MS, "Interrelationship of magnesium and estrogen in cardiovascular and bone disorders, eclampsia, migraine and premenstrual syndrome" 1993 J Am College Nutr 12(4):442-58

87. Sherman SI, Malecha SE, "Absorption and malabsorption of levothyroxine sodium" 1995 Am J Thera 2:814-818

88. Addolorato G, Caputo F, Capristo E, et al, "Baclofen efficacy in reducing alcohol craving and intake: a preliminary double-blind randomized controlled study" 2002 Alcohol Alcohol 37(5):504-8

89. Chan LN, "Drug-nutrient interaction in clinical nutrition" 2002 Current Opinion in Clin Nutr and Metabolic Care 5:327-332

90. Haagsma CJ, Blom HJ, Van Riel PL, et al, "Influence of sulphasalazine, methotrexate, and the

combination of both on plasma homocysteine concentrations in patients with rheumatoid arthritis"
1999 Ann Rheum Dis 58:79-84

91. Cheymol G, "Clinical pharmacokinetics of drugs in obesity. An update"
1993 Clin Pharmacokinet Aug;25(2):103-14

92. Singh N, Singh PN, Hershman JM, "Effect of calcium carbonate on the absorption of levothyroxine"
2000 JAMA 283(21):2822-2825

93. Jellin JM, Gregory P, Batz F, Hitchens K, et al, **Natural Medicines Comprehensive Database** 9th Ed
(Stockton, Ca, Therapeutic Research Faculty 2007)

94. Bard RL, Bleske BE, Nicklas JM, "Food: an unrecognized source of loop diuretic resistance"
2004 Pharmacotherapy 24(5):630-7

95. Weerma RK, et al, "Increased incidence of azathioprine-induced pancreatitis in Crohn's diseae
compared with other diseases" 2004 Aliment Pharmacol Ther 20:843-50

96. Crowe JP, Falini NP, "Gluten in pharmaceutical products" 2001 Am J Health Syst Pharm 58(5):396-401

97. Da Prada M, Zurcher G, "Tyramine content of preserved and fermented foods or condiments of
Far Eastern cuisine" 1992 Psychopharmacology 106:S32-4

98. Gardner DM, et al, "The making of a user friendly MAOI diet" 1996 J Clin Psych 57(3):99-104

99. Shulman KI, Walker SE, "Refining the MAOI diet: tyramine content of pizzas and soy products"
1999 J Clin Psychiatry 60(3):191-3

100. Maki KC, et al, "Effects of oral albuterol on serum lipids and carbohydrate metabolism in healthy men"
1996 Metabolism 45(6):712-7

101. O'Connell MB, Madden DM, Murray AM, et al, "Effects of proton pump inhibitors on calcium
carbonate absorption in women: a randomized crossover trial" 2005 Am J Med 118(7):778-81

102. Caudle AG, Bell LN, "Caffeine and theobromine contents of ready-to-eat chocolate cereals"
2000 J Am Diet Assoc 100(6):690-692

103. Dharmarajan TS, Adiga K, Norkus EP, "Vitamin B12 deficiency" 2003 Geriatrics 58(3):30-38

104. Darbar D, Dell'Orto S, Morike K, et al, "Dietary salt increases first-pass elimination of oral quinidine"
1997 Clin Pharm Ther 61(3):292-300

105. Exner DV et al, "Lesser response to angiotensin converting enzyme inhibitor therapy in Black as
compared to White patients with left ventricular dysfunction" 2001 N Eng J Med 344(18):1351-1357

106. Kall MA, Vang O, Clausen J, "Effects of dietary broccoli on human in vivo drug metabolizing enzymes:
evaluation of caffeine, oestrone and chlorzoxanone metabolism" 1996 Carcinogenesis 17(4):793-9

107. Heaney RP, "Effects of caffeine on bone and the calcium economy" 2002 Food Chem Toxicol 40(9):1263-70

108. Renner B et al, "Caffeine accelerates absorption and ebhances the analgesic effect of acetaminophen"
2007 J Clin Pharmacol 47(6):715-26

109. Hori H, et al, "Grapefruit juice-fluvoxamine interaction" 2003 J Clin Psychopharmacol 23:422

110. Pace A, Savarese A, Picardo M, et al, "Neuroprotective effect of vitamin E supplementation in patients treated with cisplatin chemotherapy" 2003 J Clin Oncol 21(5):927-31

111. Lilja JJ, Raaska K, Neuvonen PJ, "Effects of orange juice on the pharmacokinetics of atenolol" 2005 Eur J Clin Pharmacol 61(5-6): 337-340

112. Hidaka M, Okumura M, Fujita K, et al, "Effects of pomegranate juice on human cytochrome p450 3A (CYP3A) and carbamazepine pharmacokinetics in rats" 2005 Drug Metab Dispos 33(5):644-8,

113. Kotake T et al, "Serum amiodarone and desethylamiodarone concentrations following nasogastric versus oral administration" 2006 J Clin Pharm & Ther 31: 237-243

114. Wallace AW, Victory JM, Amsden GW, "Lack of bioequivalence when levofloxacin and calcium-fortified orange juice are co-administered to healthy volunteers" 2003 J Clin Pharmacol 43(5):539-544

115. Hansson O, Sillanpaa M, "Pyridoxine and serum concentration of phenytoin and phenobarbitone" 1976 Lancet 1:256

116. Wilder BJ, Leppick I, Hietpas TJ, et al, "Effect of food on absorption of Dilantin Kapseals and Mylan extended phenytoin sodium capsules" 2001 Neurology 57:582-589

117. Nirogi RV et al, Effect of food on bioavailability of a single dose of clopidogrel in healthy male subjects" 2006 Arzneimittelforschung 56(11):735-9

118. Jeppsen RB, "Toxicology and safety of Ferrochel and other amino acid chelates" 2001 Arch Latinoam Nutr Mar:51(1 Suppl 1):26-34

119. Slain D, Amsden JR, Khakoo RA, et al, "Effect of high-dose vitamin C on the steady-state pharmacokinetics of the protease inhibitor indinavir in healthy volunteers" 2005 Pharmacotherapy 25(2):165-70

120. Nielsen FH, Milne DB, "A moderately high intake compared with a low intake of zinc depresses magnesium balance and alters indices of bone turnover in postmenopausal women." 2004 Eur J Clin Nutr 58(5):703-10

121. Benito-Garcia E, Heller JE, Chibnik LB et al, "Dietary caffeine intake does not affect methotrexate efficacy in patients with rheumatoid arthritis" 2006 J Rheumatol 33(7):1275-81

122. Marchioli R, Barzi F, Bomba E et al, "Early protection against sudden death by n-3 polyunsaturated fatty acids after myocardial infarction: time-course analysis of the results of the Gruppo Italiano per lo Studio della Sopravvivenza nell'Infarto Miocardico (GISSI)-Prevenzione 2002 Circulation. Apr 23; 105(16):1897-903

123. Fukatsu S, Fukudo M, Masuda S et al, "Delayed effect of grapefruit juice on pharmacokinetics and pharmacodynamics of tacrolimus in a living-donor liver transplant recipient." 2006 Drug Metab Pharmacokinet Apr;21(2):122-5

124. Flowers CM et al, "Seizure activity and off-label use of tiagabine" 2006 N Engl J Med 354:773-774

125. Tannergren C, Engman H, Knutson L et al, "St John's wort decreases the bioavailability of R- and S-verapamil through induction of the first-pass metabolism" 2004 Clin Pharmacol Ther 75(4):298-309

126. Eussen SJ, De Groot LC, Clarke R et al, "Oral cyanocobalamin supplementation in older people with vitamin B12 deficiency: a dose-finding trial" 2005 Arch Intern Med 165(10):1167-72

127. Holick MF, Biancuzzo RM, Chen TC, et al, "Vitamin D2 is as effective as vitamin D3 in maintaining circulating concentrations of 25-hydroxyvitamin D" 2007 J Clin Endocrinol Metab

127a. Holick MF "Vitamin D Deficiency" 2007 N Engl J Med(357):266-81

128. Zhaoping Li, et al, "Cranberry does not affect prothrombin time in male subjects on warfarin" 2006 J Am Diet Assoc 106:2057-61

128a. Ansell J, McDonough M, Zhao Y, et al. "The absence of interaction between warfarin and cranberry juice: a randomized trial" J Clin Pharmacol. 2009 Jul;49(7):824-30

129. Seki N, Hamano H, Iiyama Y, et al, "Effect of lactulose on calcium and magnesium absorption: a study using stable isotopes in adult men" 2007 J Nutr Sci Vitaminol Feb;53(1):5-12

130. Fay MA, Sheth RD, Gidal BE, "Oral absorption kinetics of levetiracetam: the effect of mixing with food or enternal nutrition formulas" 2005 Clin Ther 27(5):594-8

131. Gardyn J, Mittelman M, Zlotnik J, et al, "Oral contraceptives can cause falsely low vitamin B(12) levels" 2000 Acta Haematol 104(1):22-4.

132. McCusker RR, Goldberger BA, Cone EJ, "Caffeine content of energy drinks, carbonated sodas, and other beverages" 2006 J Anal Toxicol Mar;30(2):112-4

133. McCusker RR, Fuehrlein B, Goldberger BA, et al, " Caffeine content of decaffeinated coffee" 2006 J Anal Toxicol Oct;30(8):611-13

134. http://www.nlm.nih.gov/medlineplus/druginformation.html

135. Bailey DG, Dresser GK, Bend JR "Bergamottin, lime juice and red wine as inhibitors of cytochrome P4503A4 activity: comparison with grapefruit juice" 2003 Clin Pharmacol Ther 73(6):529-37

136. Grande LA et al "Attention- grapefruit!" The Lancet 373 p 1222 April 4, 2009

137. Hubulashvili D and Marzella N. "Romisplastim (NPlate), a treatment option for immune (idiopathic) thrombocytopenia pupura" P&t (Pharmacy and Therapeutics) Vol. 34, No. 9 September 2009, 482-485

138. Wohlt PD, et al, "Recommendations for use of medications with continuous enteral nutrition" 2009 Am J Health-Syst Pharm 66 1458-1467

139. Hypponen E et al "Intake of Vitamin D and risk of Type 1 diabtes: a birth-cohort study" 2001 Lancet; 358:1500-1503

ABBREVIATIONS and SYMBOLS 16th edition

abs	absorption	crea	creatinine
ADHD	attention deficit hyperactivity disorder	CrCl	creatinine clearance
AI	adequate intake	CRP	C-reactive protein
AIDS	acquired immunodeficiency syndrome	Cu	copper
Al	aluminum	CVA	cerebrovascular accident (stroke)
alb	albumin	CVD	cardiovascular disease
alk phos	alkaline phosphatase	CYP	cytochrome P-450
ALT	alanine aminotransferase	↓	decreased (low)
amt	amount	DC	discontinue/discontinuation
ANA	antinuclear antibody	def	deficiency
ANC	absolute neutrophil count	diff	differential
aPTT	active partial thromboplstin time	dL	deciliter
AST	aspartate aminotransferase	DM	Diabetes Mellitus
BCE	bone collagen equivalents	DR	delayed release form
bil	bilirubin	DRI	dietary reference intakes
BMI	body mass index	DVT	deep vein thrombosis
BP	blood pressure	EAR	estimated average requirement
BUN	blood urea nitrogen	EC	enteric coated
BW	body weight	ECG	electrocardiogram
$\bar{c}$	with	eg	for example
Ca	calcium	EIB	exercise induced bronchospasm
CAD	coronary artery disease	ENL	erythema nodosum leprosum
cal	calorie	ENT	ear, nose & throat
cap	capsule	EPS	extra pyramidal symptoms
CBC	complete blood count	ESRD	end stage renal disease
CHD	coronary heart disease	ECT	euglobulin clot test
Chem	chemistry	EV	ELISA value
CHF	congestive heart failure	F	female
CHO	carbohydrate	FBS	fasting blood sugar
chol	cholesterol	FDA	Food & Drug Administration
Cl	chloride	Fe	iron
CMV	cytomegalovirus	Fol	folic acid/folate
CNS	central nervous system	FSH	follicle stimulating hormone
CO_2	carbon dioxide	func	function
conc	concentrate or concentration	g	gram
CPK	creatinine phosphokinase	GERD	gastroesophageal reflux disease
Cr	chromium	GFR	glomerular filtration rate

GI	gastrointestinal		mM/mmol	millimole
GnRH	gonadotropin releasing hormone		Mn	manganese
G6PD	glucose-6-phosphate dehydrogenase		MNT	Medical Nutrition Therapy
Hb	hemoglobin		mol	mole
HCT	hematocrit		mOsm	milliosmole
HDL	high density lipoprotein		MRSA	Methcillin-resistant Staphyloccous aureus
HIV	Human Immunodeficiency Virus		MS	multiple sclerosis
HLA	Human Leucocyte Antigen		MVI	multi-vitamin
hr	hour		N	nitrogen
HR	heart rate		Na	sodium
HS	bedtime (hour of sleep)		ng	nanogram
HTN	hypertension		NG	nasogastric
Hx	history		NH_3	ammonia
IBD	inflammatory bowel disease		Nia	niacin
IBW	ideal body weight		NIDDM	non insulin dependent diabetes mellitus
IM	intramuscular		nM	nanometer
↑	increased (high)		NMS	neuroleptic malignant syndrome
INR	international normalized ratio (for PT)		NRTI	nucleoside reverse transcriptase inhibitor
IR	immediate release		NSAID	non-steroidal anti-inflammatory drug
IU	international units		N/V	nausea & vomiting
IV	intravenous		ODT	orally disintegrating tablet
K	potassium		p	page
kg	kilogram		P	phosphorus/phosphate
L	liter		PBI	protein-bound iodine
LDH	lactic dehydrogenase		PCP	Pneumocystis carinii pneumonia
LDL	low density lipoprotein		PEG	percutaneous endoscopic gastrostomy
LH	luteinizing hormone		pg	picogram
LT	long term		PHE	phenylalanine
LVEF	left ventricular ejection fraction		PI	package insert (manufacturer information)
M	male		PMDD	premenstrual dysphoric mood disorder
Mab	monoclonal antibody		pro	protein
MAOI	monoamine oxidase inhibitor		PSA	prostate specific antigen
MCH	mean corpuscular hemoglobin		pt	patient
MCV	mean corpuscular volume		PT	prothrombin time
mEq	milliequivalent		PTH	parathyroid hormone
mg	milligram		PTSD	posttraumatic stress disorder
Mg	magnesium		PTT	partial thromboplastin time
MI	myocardial infarction		PUFA	polyunsaturated fatty acid
min	minute		pwd	powder
mL	milliliter (cc)			

Pyr	pyridoxine (Vit B_6)
q	every
RBC	red blood cells or count
RDA	recommended dietary allowance
Rib	riboflavin (Vit B_6)
s̄	without
Sat	saturated
SC	subcutaneous
Se	selenium
SERM	selective estrogen receptor modulator
SIADH	syndrome of inappropriate secretion of antidiuretic hormone
SJS	Stevens-Johnson Syndrome
SJW	St. John's wort
SL	sublingual
SLE	systemic lupus erythematosus
SNRI	serotonin-norepinephrine reuptake inhibitor
soln	solution
SR	sustained release form
S/S	signs and symptoms
SSRI	selective serotonin reuptake inhibitor
ST	short term
suppl	supplement
susp	suspension
T_3	total triiodothyronine
T_4	total thyroxine
tab	tablet/caplet
TB	tuberculosis
TBW	total body weight
TD	tardive dyskinesia
TEN	toxic epidermal necrolysis
TF	tube feeding
TG	triglyceride
Thi	thiamine/thiamin
TIBC	total iron binding capacity
TMJD	temporomandibular joint dysfunction
TNF	tumor necrosis factor
TP	total protein
TPN	total parenteral nutrition
TSH	thyroid stimulating hormone
TT	thrombin time
U	Unit/Units
UA	urinalysis
ug	microgram
uL	microliter
UL	tolerable upper limit
um^3	cubic micrometer
umol	micromole
URTI	upper respiratory tract infection
UTI	urinary tract infection
uU	micro International Unit
Vit	vitamin
VLDL	very low density lipoprotein
VMA	vanillylmandelic acid
WBC	white blood cells
wt	weight
XR	extended release
yr/yrs	year/years
Zn	zinc

NOTES

NOTES